Clinical Psychiatry: Recent Advances and Future Directions

Editors

DAVID A. BARON
LAWRENCE S. GROSS

PSYCHIATRIC CLINICS OF NORTH AMERICA

www.psych.theclinics.com

September 2015 • Volume 38 • Number 3

ELSEVIER

1600 John F. Kennedy Boulevard • Suite 1800 • Philadelphia, Pennsylvania, 19103-2899

http://www.theclinics.com

PSYCHIATRIC CLINICS OF NORTH AMERICA Volume 38, Number 3
September 2015 ISSN 0193-953X, ISBN-13: 978-0-323-39581-6

Editor: Lauren Boyle
Developmental Editor: Kristen Helm

Psychiatric Clinics of North America (ISSN 0193-953X) is published quarterly by Elsevier Inc., 360 Park Avenue South, New York, NY 10010-1710. Months of issue are March, June, September, and December. Business and Editorial Offices: 1600 John F. Kennedy Blvd., Suite 1800, Philadelphia, PA 19103-2899. Periodicals postage paid at New York, NY and additional mailing offices. Subscription prices are $300.00 per year (US individuals), $546.00 per year (US institutions), $150.00 per year (US students/residents), $365.00 per year (Canadian individuals), $455.00 per year (international individuals), $687.00 per year (Canadian & international institutions), and $220.00 per year (Canadian & international students/residents). Foreign air speed delivery is included in all *Clinics'* subscription prices. All prices are subject to change without notice. **POSTMASTER:** Send address changes to *Psychiatric Clinics of North America*, Elsevier Health Sciences Division, Subscription Customer Service, 3251 Riverport Lane, Maryland Heights, MO 63043. **Customer Service: 1-800-654-2452 (US). From outside the United States, call 1-314-447-8871. Fax: 1-314-447-8029. E-mail: journalscustomerservice-usa@elsevier.com (for print support) and journalsonline support-usa@elsevier.com (for online support).**

Reprints. For copies of 100 or more, of articles in this publication, please contact the Commercial Reprints Department, Elsevier Inc., 360 Park Avenue South, New York, New York 10010-1710. Tel.: 212-633-3874, Fax: 212-633-3820, E-mail: reprints@elsevier.com.

Psychiatric Clinics of North America is covered in *MEDLINE/PubMed (Index Medicus), Current Contents/Social and Behavioral Sciences, Social Science Citation Index, Embase/Excerpta Medica,* and PsycINFO.

Contributors

EDITORS

DAVID A. BARON, MSEd, DO
Professor and Interim Chair, Department of Psychiatry and Behavioral Sciences, Keck School of Medicine, University of Southern California, Los Angeles, California

LAWRENCE S. GROSS, MD
Professor of Clinical Psychiatry, Department of Psychiatry and Behavioral Sciences, Keck School of Medicine, University of Southern California, Los Angeles, California

AUTHORS

LUJAIN ALHAJJI, MD
Resident, Department of Psychiatry and Behavioral Sciences, University of Miami Miller School of Medicine, Miami, Florida

RAJENDRA D. BADGAIYAN, MD
Professor and Director, Laboratory of Advanced Radiochemistry and Molecular and Functioning Imaging; Neurmodulation Scholar, Department of Psychiatry, University of Minnesota, Minneapolis, Minnesota

BERNHARD BAUNE, MD, PhD
Discipline of Psychiatry, University of Adelaide, Adelaide, South Australia, Australia

KENNETH BLUM, PhD
Volunteer Professor, Department of Psychiatry, McKnight Brain Institute, University of Florida College of Medicine, Gainesville, Florida; Adjunct Professor, Department of Psychiatry, Center for Clinical and Translational Science, Community Mental Health Institute, University of Vermont College of Medicine, University of Vermont, Burlington, Vermont; Chief Scientific Advisor, Division of Applied Clinical Research, Dominion Diagnostics, LLC, North Kingstown, Rhode Island; Member, Rivermend Health Scientific Advisory Board, Atlanta, Georgia

JOEL BRASLOW, MD, PhD
Professor, Department of Psychiatry and Biobehavioral Sciences; Department of History, Wilshire Center, University of California, Los Angeles, Los Angeles, California

JOHN BRIERE, PhD
Associate Professor, Department of Psychiatry and Behavioral Sciences, Keck School of Medicine, University of Southern California, Los Angeles, California

PETER F. BUCKLEY, MD
Dean, Medical College of Georgia, Georgia Regents University, Augusta, Georgia

STEVEN CHAN, MD, MBA
Resident, Department of Psychiatry and Behavioral Sciences, University of California, Davis School of Medicine and Health System, Sacramento, California

HARRIS EYRE, MBBS
Discipline of Psychiatry, University of Adelaide, Adelaide, South Australia, Australia; Semel Institute for Neuroscience, University of California, Los Angeles, Los Angeles, California

MARK S. GOLD, MD, FASAM
Adjunct Professor, Department of Psychiatry and Behavioral Sciences, Keck School of Medicine, University of Southern California, Los Angeles, California; Adjunct Professor, Department of Psychiatry, Washington University School of Medicine, St Louis, Missouri; Chairman, Rivermend Health Scientific Advisory Board, Atlanta, Georgia; Director of Research, Drug Enforcement Administration (DEA) Educational Foundation, Washington, DC

DONALD HILTY, MD
Professor and Vice-Chair of Education, Psychiatry and Behavioral Sciences; Director of Telepsychiatry and Distance Education, Telehealth, USC Care Health System, Keck School of Medicine, University of Southern California, Los Angeles, California

HANNA KIENZLER, PhD
Department of Social Science, Health and Medicine, King's College London, Strand, London, United Kingdom

HELEN LAVRETSKY, MD, MS
Director, Late Life Mood Stress and Wellness Research Program, Semel Institute for Neuroscience; Professor of Psychiatry, University of California, Los Angeles, Los Angeles, California

ROBERT M. McCARRON, DO
Associate Professor, Director, Integrated Medicine and Psychiatry Education Director, Pain Psychiatry, Division of Pain Medicine, Department of Anesthesiology; Department of Psychiatry and Behavioral Sciences; Department of Internal Medicine, University of California, Davis School of Medicine, Sacramento, California

BRIAN J. MILLER, MD, PhD, MPH
Associate Professor, Department of Psychiatry, Georgia Regents University, Augusta, Georgia

CHARLES B. NEMEROFF, MD, PhD
Leonard M. Miller Professor and Chairman, Department of Psychiatry and Behavioral Sciences, University of Miami Miller School of Medicine, Miami, Florida

TARA A. NIENDAM, PhD
Assistant Professor, Department of Psychiatry, UC Davis Imaging Research Center, University of California, Davis, Sacramento, California

JOSEPH JOHN PARKS III, MD
Director, Missouri Institute of Mental Health; Distinguished Professor of Science, University of Missouri–St. Louis, St Louis, Missouri

MICHELLE B. PARRISH, MA
Research Manager, Telepsychiatry and Health Informatics, University of California, Davis School of Medicine and Health System, Sacramento, California

BRADLEY S. PETERSON, MD
Professor of Pediatrics and Psychiatry, Institute for the Developing Mind, Children's Hospital Los Angeles, University of Southern California, Los Angeles, California

ERIC M. PLAKUN, MD
Leader, APA Psychotherapy Caucus; Associate Medical Director, Austen Riggs Center, Stockbridge, Massachusetts

MARK RAGINS, MD
Medical Director, MHA Village Integrated Service Agency, Long Beach, California

ALAN F. SCHATZBERG, MD
Kenneth T. Norris, Jr Professor, Department of Psychiatry and Behavioral Sciences, Stanford University School of Medicine, Stanford, California

CATHERINE SCOTT, MD
Assistant Professor of Clinical Psychiatry, Department of Psychiatry and Behavioral Sciences, Keck School of Medicine, University of Southern California, Los Angeles, California

RODERICK SHANER, MD
Medical Director, Los Angeles County Department of Mental Health; Clinical Professor of Psychiatry, Keck School of Medicine, University of Southern California, Los Angeles, California

ERICA Z. SHOEMAKER, MD, MPH
Assistant Professor of Clinical Psychiatry, Department of Psychiatry and Behavioral Sciences, University of Southern California, Los Angeles, California

KENNETH S. THOMPSON, MD
Pennsylvania Psychiatric Leadership Council, Pittsburgh, Pennsylvania

LAURA M. TULLY, PhD
Post Doctoral Scholar, Department of Psychiatry, UC Davis Imaging Research Center, University of California, Davis, Sacramento, California

JEROME V. VACCARO, MD
President, Right Path HC, Ingenuity Health, Mounts Kisco, New York

THOMAS WENZEL, Dr med
Professor, Division of Social Psychiatry, Department of Psychiatry and Psychotherapy, Medical University of Vienna, Vienna, Austria

ANDREAS WOLLMANN, Mag
Sigmund Freud University, Vienna, Austria

PETER M. YELLOWLEES, MBBS, MD
Professor of Clinical Psychiatry and Behavioral Sciences; Vice-Chair of Faculty Development; Former Director, Health Informatics Graduate Program, University of California, Davis School of Medicine and Health System, Sacramento, California

Contents

This overview highlights the current hot topics in schizophrenia research. One major drawback to progress is the ability to define and focus on the right patient group. Schizophrenia is a biased and heterogeneous (group of) condition(s), the boundaries of which remain uncertain. An initiative that will focus attention away from (mere) symptoms of the illness and toward its underlying neurobiological construct(s) is the Research Domain Criteria. A preliminary analysis from a large neurobiological study suggests that 3 distinct biological phenotypes underlie the clinical expression of 1 major psychosis. A firmer neurobiologically based foundation is needed to advance this field.

Antidepressant and anxiolytic drug development has largely stalled. This article reviews novel current programs for developing depressants and anxiolytics. Biological bases are discussed for these, as are recent results. Problems encountered are reviewed. Recently announced failed programs for other antidepressants are then discussed with an eye toward uncovering possible common elements that may explain their failures. Lastly, possible solutions for improving the likelihood of the success of antidepressant/anxiolytic agents are discussed.

Some of the latest advances in personalized psychiatry with future research directions are discussed in this article. Many factors contribute to the phenotypic psychiatric profile in individual patients. These overlapping factors include but are not limited to genetics, epigenetics, central nervous system circuit alterations, family history, past personal history, environmental influences including early life stress, and more recent life stressors. The authors discuss the role of pharmacogenomics, particularly in the cytochrome P450 enzyme system in relation to treatment response. Despite some promising advances in personalized medicine in psychiatry, it is still in its early phases of development.

> Psychotherapy and psychosocial treatment have been shown to be effective forms of treatment of a range of individual and complex comorbid disorders. The future role of psychotherapy and psychosocial treatment depends on several factors, including full implementation of mental health parity, correction of underlying false assumptions that shape treatment, payment priorities and research, identification and teaching of common factors or elements shared by effective psychosocial therapies, and adequate teaching of psychotherapy and psychosocial treatment.

> This article focuses on the shared molecular and neurogenetics of food and drug addiction tied to the understanding of reward deficiency syndrome. Reward deficiency syndrome describes a hypodopaminergic trait/state that provides a rationale for commonality in approaches for treating long-term reduced dopamine function across the reward brain regions. The identification of the role of DNA polymorphic associations with reward circuitry has resulted in new understanding of all addictive behaviors.

> Patients with mental illness, particularly serious mental illness, are more likely to suffer from common disorders without optimal treatment. Changes in preventive practice patterns cannot be fully realized on a large scale until clinicians are trained how to routinely provide this care. Psychiatrists may consider using preventive care strategies in the area of cardiovascular health, as cardiovascular disease is the most common cause of death and disproportionately affects patients with mental illness. At minimum, psychiatrists are well positioned to work collaboratively with primary care providers to address psychopathology that may interfere with adherence to the treatment plan.

> The last two decades have marked tremendous progress in our ability to prevent and intervene early in psychiatric illnesses. The interventions described in this article range from established, empirically-supported treatments to creative interventions early in their development and deployment. Some of these interventions are low-technology programs delivered in social settings (such as schools), and some rely on sophisticated emerging technologies such as neuroimaging. This article reviews

4 preventative interventions: 1) The use of structural brain imaging to identify children at risk for familial depression who are most likely to benefit from preventative cognitive behavioral therapy, 2) The Good Behavior Game, a school based program that, when implemented in 1st grade classrooms, cut the incidence of substance use disorders in students in half when those students were 19 years old, 3) The SPARX video game, which has the potential to be an accessible, appealing, and cost-effective treatment for the thousands of teens affected by mild to moderate depressive disorders, and 4) Intensive psychosocial treatments which can reduce the progression from the ultra high risk state to the first episode psychosis by 50% over 12 months. All of these interventions have tremendous potential to reduce the suffering and disability caused by psychiatric illness to both children and adults.

The world population is aging at a rate unprecedented in human history, placing substantial pressure on health systems across the world along with concurrent rises in chronic diseases. In particular, rates of cognitive disorders and late-life affective disorders are expected to increase. In tandem with aging, there are robust predictions suggesting that rates of age-related cognitive decline and dementia, and geriatric depression, will increase, with serious consequences. Clearly innovative prevention and treatment strategies are needed. This article reviews the latest promising clinical advances that hold promise for assisting the prevention and treatment of depression, cognitive decline, and dementia.

Complex trauma involves multiple exposures to adverse events over the lifespan. Such experiences are associated with a variety of psychological outcomes, including a decreased threshold for the development of posttraumatic stress disorder as well as self-capacity problems and dysfunctional behaviors. Psychological interventions that increase affect regulation, support titrated processing of memories and cognitions, and emphasize the therapeutic relationship seem to be most helpful for complex trauma effects. Pharmacologic treatments have some efficacy in the treatment of the posttraumatic stress components of complex posttraumatic outcomes, but are generally less successful in reducing self-related problems and symptoms.

Violence has been shown to be a global challenge resulting in long-lasting social, medical, and mental health sequelae. In this article, we focus on massive social violence, such as war and civil war. Social suffering and mental health problems related to violence as a global public health problem can be tackled only with a holistic approach that addresses the specific region, culture and group and the limited resources available in most countries. Research that can give a reliable assessment of complex long-term outcomes is still largely missing, and can be seen as a major and complex challenge for future study.

This article reviews the fiscal, programmatic, clinical, and cultural forces of health care reform that are transforming the work of public psychiatrists. Areas of rapid change and issues of concern are discussed. A proposed health care reform agenda for public psychiatric leadership emphasizes (1) access to quality mental health care, (2) promotion of recovery practices in primary care, (3) promotion of public psychiatry values within general psychiatry, (4) engagement in national policy formulation and implementation, and (5) further development of psychiatric leadership focused on public and community mental health.

Patient-centered health care questions how to deliver quality, affordable, and timely care in a variety of settings. Telemedicine empowers patients, increases administrative efficiency, and ensures expertise gets to the place it is most needed—the patient. Telepsychiatry or telemental health is effective, well accepted, and comparable to in-person care. E-models of care offer variety, flexibility, and positive outcomes in most settings, and clinicians are increasingly interested in using technology for care, so much so that telepsychiatry is now being widely introduced around the world.

PSYCHIATRIC CLINICS OF NORTH AMERICA

RELATED INTEREST

Child and Adolescent Psychiatric Clinics
January 2015 (Vol. 24, No. 1)
Top Topics in Child and Adolescent Psychiatry
Harsh K. Trivedi, *Editor*

THE CLINICS ARE AVAILABLE ONLINE!
Access your subscription at:
www.theclinics.com

Preface

Where Are We, and Where Are We Going? An Insider's View...

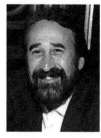 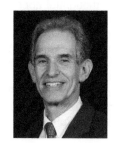

David A. Baron, MSEd, DO   Lawrence S. Gross, MD
Editors

We are excited to welcome you to this issue of *Psychiatric Clinics of North America*, highlighting recent advances and future directions in the field of psychiatry. We were very fortunate to have key thought leaders from around the world contribute their expertise on a wide range of topics. Each article is written as a stand-alone contribution and does not require reading in any particular order, although we are confident you will find them all informative and at times a bit provocative. Despite this intended non-homogenized approach, the reader will quickly identify common themes that emerge in virtually every article.

We start off with discussions on recent advances in schizophrenia and psychopharmacology. Drs Buckley and Miller present a progress report on key research discoveries in schizophrenia that have added to our understanding of this complex and challenging disorder. Dr Schatzberg uses his extensive expertise to offer insights into the development of new psychopharmacologic agents for depression and anxiety.

Drs Alhajji and Nemeroff address genetics, epigenetics, pharmacogenomics, and environmental influences as part of their discussion on personalized, or precision, medicine in the diagnosis and treatment of mood disorders. Interestingly, some of these same topics are cited by Dr Plakun in his thought-provoking commentary about biological reductionism as a potential barrier to patients receiving psychotherapy and psychosocial interventions.

Why does obesity continue to be one of the greatest preventable health risks worldwide, despite robust public health education efforts? Drs Gold, Badgaiyan, and Blum offer a compelling explanation of the biology of food addiction and the role of dopamine. Dr McCarron's contribution expands on important health risks in our patients, addressing an integrated care approach to the recognition and prevention of medical illness in the psychiatric setting.

Psychiatr Clin N Am 38 (2015) xiii–xiv
http://dx.doi.org/10.1016/j.psc.2015.06.001
0193-953X/15/$ – see front matter © 2015 Published by Elsevier Inc.

psych.theclinics.com

As our knowledge base increases, the theme of prevention has become part of the discussion in psychiatry—from childhood to geriatrics. The capacity to intervene at the genesis of psychopathology and possibly prevent future suffering is highlighted by Drs Shoemaker, Tully, Niendam, and Peterson. As advances in medical science have extended life expectancy, outliving your brain is a key factor in adding life to years, not merely years to life. In discussing clinical advances in geriatric psychiatry, Drs Eyre, Baune, and Lavretsky present a thoughtful approach focusing on prevention of cognitive and mood disorders in the elderly.

Violence and trauma continue to grow worldwide. Drs Briere and Scott share their insights in dealing with complex trauma, while Professor Wenzel and colleagues offer a global perspective on the psychiatric sequellae of social violence.

Few things will affect the provision of psychiatric care more than public policy and health care reform. Drs Shaner, Thompson, Braslow, Ragins, Parks, and Vaccaro share their insights on how health reform is reshaping public psychiatry. They review the history and recent changes, and they offer future directions for this highly complex, politically driven process.

The use of telecommunication to provide psychiatric care to patients with limited access to mental health services is a new solution to an old problem. Drs Hilty, Chan, Parrish, and Yellowlees present a comprehensive review of advances in telepsychiatry, expanding the discussion to include Internet and Web-based care along with emerging models of digital and social media communication.

We want to thank all of the authors for their outstanding work. We hope you, the readers, enjoy this issue as much as we enjoyed editing it.

David A. Baron, MSEd, DO
Department of Psychiatry and
Behavioral Sciences
Keck School of Medicine
University of Southern California
2250 Alcazar Street, Suite 2202
Los Angeles, CA 90033, USA

Lawrence S. Gross, MD
Department of Psychiatry and
Behavioral Sciences
Keck School of Medicine
University of Southern California
2250 Alcazar Street, Suite 2200
Los Angeles, CA 90033, USA

E-mail addresses:
dave.baron@usc.edu (D.A. Baron)
Lawrence.Gross@med.usc.edu (L.S. Gross)

Schizophrenia Research
A Progress Report

Peter F. Buckley, MD[a],*, Brian J. Miller, MD, PhD, MPH[b]

KEYWORDS

- Schizophrenia • Research discoveries • Treatment approaches
- Autoimmune diseases • Regenerative medicine • Head trauma • Early intervention
- Antipsychotics

KEY POINTS

- The collection and use of large collaborative databases has facilitated more detailed genetic inspections in schizophrenia.
- Recent studies highlight the immune hypothesis of schizophrenia, building on prior epidemiologic and postmortem research.
- Regenerative medicine is now coming into schizophrenia research.
- Emotional trauma in childhood is associated with a higher rate of schizophrenia in adulthood.
- One conspicuous change in recent years has been the refocusing of the field on the earliest stages of schizophrenia in the hopes of early intervention or even primary prevention in an effort to reduce long-term morbidity.

In keeping with the year-end synopsis focus of this special issue of *Psychiatric Clinics of North America*, this brief review focusses on key research discoveries and recent reports. Some discoveries advance our understanding of schizophrenia's causation and others advance treatment approaches. Collectively, this synthesis should also convey to the discerning reader an overall sense of the state of play of translational research and clinical practice for schizophrenia.

Although the neurobiology of mental illnesses in general—and in this instance schizophrenia—remains elusive, several recent studies point to some convergence in the genetics of schizophrenia. The collection and use of large collaborative databases have facilitated more detailed genetic inspections in schizophrenia. Two studies are illustrative. The Psychiatric Genomics Consortium conducted a large genomewide association study that found substantial overlap in risk loci between schizophrenia,

[a] Medical College of Georgia, Georgia Regents University, 1120 15th Street, AA-1006, Augusta, GA 30912, USA; [b] Department of Psychiatry, Georgia Regents University, 1120 15th Street, AA-1006, Augusta, GA 30912, USA
* Corresponding author.
E-mail address: pbuckley@gru.edu

Psychiatr Clin N Am 38 (2015) 373–377
http://dx.doi.org/10.1016/j.psc.2015.05.001
0193-953X/15/$ – see front matter © 2015 Elsevier Inc. All rights reserved.

mood disorders, autism, and attention deficit disorders.[1] In another large study involving 37,000 patients and 114,000 normal subjects, the Schizophrenia Working Group of the Psychiatric Genomics Consortium[2] found 108 gene loci that were associated with schizophrenia.[3] The loci implicated were in genes that involve dopamine synthesis, calcium channel regulation, and glutamate neuroreceptors. Additionally, there was substantial overlap with immunomodulatory genes, thus, adding to the growing literature on immune dysfunction in schizophrenia.

Other recent studies also highlight the immune hypothesis of schizophrenia, building on prior epidemiologic and postmortem research. Benrós and colleagues[4] examined a Danish registry of autoimmune diseases involving some 142,000 patients with known autoimmune diseases and some 39,000 patients with schizophrenia. They found strong relationships, including that 3.1% of patients with autoimmune diseases also had a positive family history of schizophrenia. Moreover, autoimmune diseases were observed in 3.6% of patients with schizophrenia. Another Danish registry study by Wium-Andersen and colleagues[5] found a substantial increase in C-reactive protein—a nonspecific marker of inflammation—in patients with schizophrenia. This immune hypothesis has gained traction in our field. In another broad overview, Steiner and colleagues[6] also highlight the overlap between immune dysfunction, schizophrenia, and glucose regulation. Kirkpatrick and Miller[7] provide a synthesis of findings to date, making the point of mind-body dualism in immune dysfunction in schizophrenia.

Although perhaps some skeptics might view recent immune findings as "old wine in a new bottle," it is different and encouraging to see that entirely new area of research—namely regenerative medicine—is now coming into schizophrenia research. This new area has considerable potential. To that end, Wright and colleagues[8] provide an exciting, yet scientifically terse, overview of emergent stem cell research in schizophrenia. Another, albeit small, study[9] of cultured fibroblasts from patients with first-episode schizophrenia replicated an earlier finding of elevation of plasma caspase-3 neurodegenerative enzyme in schizophrenia.[10]

Other known risk factors for schizophrenia have been studied recently. Orlovska and colleagues[11] found a 1.64-fold higher risk of schizophrenia in people who had suffered a head injury. Molloy and colleagues[12] also reported a similar effect in another large epidemiologic study. In addition, these authors[13] also found that emotional trauma in childhood is associated with a higher rate of schizophrenia in adulthood. This finding replicates earlier British work in this area and suggests that there is an inherent vulnerability to brain insults—infectious, traumatic, and psychological—that can predispose to later schizophrenia.

One conspicuous change in recent years has been the refocusing of our field on the earliest stages of schizophrenia in the hopes of early intervention or even primary prevention.[14] Although the field of prodromal research is burgeoning, it is still sobering (at least from a treatment perspective) that the conversion rates to psychosis remain too low—and too difficult to predict for any given patient—to espouse the use of antipsychotic medications in people who exhibit (merely) prodromal symptoms. To that point, Fusar-Poli and Yung[15] summarized the psychosis conversion rates over time among prodromal populations as follows: 18% conversion at 6 months, 21% at 1 year, 29% at 2 years, and 32% at 3 years. It seems that the conversion rate levels out after 3 years at an overall rate of 36%. This point is underscored by the 10-year conversion rate of almost 35% in the longitudinal PACE 400 Australian study.[16] It is debated that early cognitive decline might be a clinically detectable and core feature,[17,18] although this still seems too nonspecific to be of early diagnostic value.

Thus, the focus remains more on treating the first episode of schizophrenia—rather than beforehand—to reduce long-term morbidity.[19] Antipsychotic treatments options are now more varied, with an array of putative antipsychotic agents currently under development that have an ever-decreasing and more tenuous relationship to dopamine (D_2) receptor occupancy. Examples that are under development include brexpiprazole (a partial agonist), cariprazine (another partial agonist), bitopertin (a glycine reuptake inhibitor), ITI-007, TC5619, and OMS824 (a phosphodiesterase 10 inhibitor). Whether some or all of these putative drugs ever make it into clinical practice will become evident over the coming years. Nevertheless, the shift in focus away from singular reliance or D_2 receptor blockade as a "sine qua non" for drug development for schizophrenia is both interesting and opening up a broader array of potential therapeutic options.

In the meantime, there is no consensus as to which of the currently available antipsychotic drugs to use first. Leucht and colleagues[20] have conducted (yet another) meta-analysis of first- and second-generation antipsychotic (SGA) medications. They found that amisulpride, olanzapine, risperidone, and clozapine were superior in efficacy among the 16 antipsychotic drugs studied. In consideration of long-acting injectable (LAI) antipsychotic drugs, McEvoy and colleagues[21] found no difference in relapse rates over 2.5 years among patients receiving paliperidone palmitate or haloperidol decanoate. In another complementary study, Buckley and colleagues[22] also found no difference in relapse rates over 30 months in patients receiving either LAI risperidone or oral SGAs. In contrast, Meltzer and colleagues[23] found an improvement in clinical status among patients—who were a priori defined as treatment-refractory—receiving LAI risperidone. Overall, however, the role of long-acting injectable antipsychotic medications remains in debate.

Clozapine remains the treatment of choice for treatment-refractory patients. However, the high side-effect burden of clozapine and substantial small number of clozapine nonresponders have prompted efforts to determine better ways to introduce and manage clozapine therapy. Li and Meltzer[24] examined this from a pharmacogenetic perspective. They found that the single nucleotide polymorphism rs2237457 on chromosome 7 was associated with treatment resistance. Similarly, an earlier pharmacogenetic analysis of serotonin receptor genes predicted the development of weight gain on clozapine.[25] Taken together, these are provocative findings. The field, however, is still a far way off from personalized medicine.

Another strategy that is increasingly being used in clinical practice to reduce the side-effect burden of clozapine is to add another antipsychotic, thereby facilitating the reduction in dose of clozapine. Fleischhacker and colleagues[26] reported successful results in retention of clinical stability while reducing weight when aripiprazole was added to clozapine. Muscatello and colleagues[27] added ziprasidone to clozapine-treated patients, and they reported symptomatic benefits, although in this instance, there was no actual change in weight between the 2 groups. In a sample of patients with preexisting weight and metabolic abnormalities, the addition of metformin was helpful in managing these burdens.[28] However, this was a more general population of patients who were not on clozapine therapy. Additionally, switching to another antipsychotic drug over lower weight liability remains a trusted and effective strategy to mitigate the long-term weight burden of SGAs.[29]

CONCLUDING REMARKS

This brief overview hits the highlights of current hot topics in schizophrenia research. There is excitement in the field. However, progress is slow. One major drawback to progress is our ability to define and focus on the right patient group. All agree that schizophrenia is a biased and heterogeneous (group of) condition(s), the boundaries of which still remain uncertain. To that end, schizophrenia is challenging to research and, of course, to treat. A major initiative that will focus our attention away from (mere) symptoms of the illness and toward its underlying neurobiological construct(s) is the Research Domain Criteria.[30] A preliminary analysis from a large neurobiological study suggests that 3 distinct biological phenotypes underlie the clinical expression of one major psychosis.[31] This work is encouraging. A firmer neurobiologically based foundation is definitely needed to further advance our field.

REFERENCES

1. Cross-Disorder Group of the Psychiatric Genomics Consortium. Identification of risk loci with shared effects on five major psychiatric disorders: a genome-wide analysis. Lancet 2013;381(9875):1371–9.
2. Schizophrenia Working Group of the Psychiatric Genomics Consortium. Biological insights from 108 schizophrenia-associated genetic loci. Nature 2014; 511(7510):421–7.
3. Schizophrenia Working Group of the Psychiatric Genomics Consortium. Biological insights from 108 schizophrenia-associated genetic loci. Nature 2014; 511(7510):421–7.
4. Benrós ME, Pedersen MG, Rasmussen H, et al. A nationwide study on the risk of autoimmune diseases in individuals with a personal or a family history of schizophrenia and related psychosis. Am J Psychiatry 2014;171:218–26.
5. Wium-Andersen MK, Orsted DD, Nordestgaard BG. Elevated C-reactive protein associated with late- and very-late-onset schizophrenia in the general population: a prospective study. Schizophr Bull 2014;40(5):1117–27.
6. Steiner J, Bernstein HG, Schiltz K, et al. Immune system and glucose metabolism interaction in schizophrenia: a chicken-egg dilemma. Prog Neuropsychopharmacol Biol Psychiatry 2014;48:287–94.
7. Kirkpatrick B, Miller BJ. Inflammation and schizophrenia. Schizophr Bull 2013; 39(6):1174–9.
8. Wright R, Réthelyi JM, Gage FH. Enhancing induced pluripotent stem cell models of schizophrenia. JAMA Psychiatry 2014;71(3):334–5.
9. Gasso P, Mas S, Molina O, et al. Increased susceptibility to apoptosis in cultured fibroblasts from antipsychotic-naive first-episode schizophrenia patients. J Psychiatr Res 2014;48(1):94–101.
10. Jarskog LF, Selinger ES, Lieberman JA, et al. Apoptotic proteins in the temporal cortex in schizophrenia: high Bax/Bcl-2 ratio without caspase-3 activation. Am J Psychiatry 2004;161:109–15.
11. Orlovska S, Pedersen MS, Benros ME, et al. Head injury as risk factor for psychiatric disorders: a nationwide register-based follow-up study of 113,906 persons with head injury. Am J Psychiatry 2014;171(4):463–9.
12. Molloy C, Conroy RM, Cotter DR, et al. Is traumatic brain injury a risk factor for schizophrenia? A meta-analysis of case-controlled population-based studies. Schizophr Bull 2011;37:1104–10.
13. Kelleher I, Keeley H, Corcoran P, et al. Childhood trauma and psychosis in a prospective cohort study: cause, effect, and directionality. Am J Psychiatry 2013; 170(7):734–41.
14. McGorry PD. The next stage for diagnosis: validity through utility. World Psychiatry 2013;12(3):213–4.

15. Fusar-Poli P, Yung AR. Should attenuated psychosis syndrome be included in the DSM-5? Lancet 2012;379(9816):591–2.
16. Nelson B, Yuen HP, Wood SJ, et al. Long-term follow-up of a group at ultra high risk ("prodromal") for psychosis: the Pace 400 study. JAMA Psychiatry 2013; 70(8):793–802.
17. Heckers S. What is the core of schizophrenia? JAMA Psychiatry 2013;70(10): 1009–10.
18. Meier MH, Caspi A, Reichenberg A, et al. Neuropsychological decline in schizophrenia from the premorbid to the postmorbid period: evidence from a population-representative longitudinal study. Am J Psychiatry 2014;171(11):91–101.
19. Miller BJ, Buckley PF. First episode schizophrenia: considerations on the timing, selection, and duration of antipsychotic therapies. In: Kasper, Papadimitriou, editors. Schizophrenia. 2nd Edition. London: Informa Healthcare; 2009. p. 201–17.
20. Leucht S, Cipriani A, Spineli L, et al. Comparative efficacy and tolerability of 15 antipsychotic drugs in schizophrenia: a multiple-treatments meta-analysis. Lancet 2013;382(9896):951–62.
21. McEvoy JP, Byerly M, Hamer RM, et al. Effectiveness of paliperidone palmitate vs haloperidol decanoate for maintenance treatment of schizophrenia: a randomized clinical trial. JAMA 2014;311(19):1978–87.
22. Buckley PF, Schooler NR, Goff DC, et al. A Comparison of SGA Oral Medications and a Long-Acting Injectable SGA: the PROACTIVE Study. Schizophr Bull 2014; 41(2):449–59.
23. Meltzer HY, Lindenmayer JP, Kwentus J, et al. A six month randomized controlled trial of long acting injectable risperidone 50 and 100 mg in treatment resistant schizophrenia. Schizophr Res 2014;154(1–3):14–22.
24. Li J, Meltzer HY. A genetic locus in 7p12.2 associated with treatment resistant schizophrenia. Schizophr Res 2014;159(2–3):333–9.
25. Miller DD, Ellingrod VL, Holman TL, et al. Weight gain associated with the -759 C/T polymorphism of the 5HT2C receptor and clozapine. Am J Med Genet Part B Neuropsychiatric Genetics 2005;133B(1):97–100.
26. Fleischhacker WW, Heikkinen ME, Olié JP, et al. Effects of adjunctive treatment with aripiprazole on body weight and clinical efficacy in schizophrenia patients treated with clozapine: a randomized, double-blind, placebo-controlled trial. Int J Neuropsychopharmacol 2010;13(8):1115–25.
27. Muscatello MR, Pandolfo G, Mico U, et al. Augmentation of clozapine with ziprasidone in refractory schizophrenia: a double-blind, placebo-controlled study. J Clin Psychopharmacol 2014;34(1):129–33.
28. Jarskog LF, Hamer RM, Catellier DJ, et al. Metformin for weight loss and metabolic control in overweight outpatients with schizophrenia and schizoaffective disorder. Am J Psychiatry 2013;170(9):1032–40.
29. Stroup TS, McEvoy JP, King KD, et al. Schizophrenia Trials Network (inclusive of Buckley PF). A randomized trial comparing the effectiveness of switching from olanzapine, quetiapine, or risperidone to aripiprazole to reduce metabolic risk: comparison of antipsychotics for metabolic problems (CAMP). Am J Psychiatry 2011;168:947–56.
30. Insel T, Cuthbert B, Garvey M, et al. Research domain criteria (RDoC): toward a new classification framework for research on mental disorders. Am J Psychiatry 2010;167(7):748–51.
31. Tamminga CA, Pearlson G, Keshavan M, et al. Bipolar and schizophrenia network for intermediate phenotypes: outcomes across the psychosis continuum. Schizophr Bull 2014;40(S2):S131–7.

Development of New Psychopharmacological Agents for Depression and Anxiety

Alan F. Schatzberg, MD

KEYWORDS

- Antidepressants • Anxiolytics • Ketamine • NMDA antagonists
- Glutamatergic agents • Glucocorticoid antagonists • Obotulinum toxin
- Mu-opioid agents

KEY POINTS

- Antidepressant and anxiolytic drug development has largely stalled.
- There are several so-called start-up companies and small to mid-sized pharmaceutical companies that are still developing novel agents, and these are offering promise for the field.
- Most of our currently available agents for depression and anxiety are based on neurotransmitter models (norepinephrine or serotonin) of the disorders.
- A great deal of effort has gone into developing new agents that have alternative mechanisms of action that may provide relief for patients' symptoms via alternative neurobiological circuits or systems.
- Several failures in antidepressant development have occurred over the past 10 years. These failures may provide clues for future development, and it is reasonable to review several of them.
- Efforts have been expended at developing pharmacogenetic and other biological markers that can not only improve matching available drugs to patients but can stimulate new drug development for specific subtypes of disorders. Another approach has been to improve imaging tools that can be used to better screen compounds for pharmacological effects.

Conflicts of Interest: Dr A.F. Schatzberg has served as a consultant to Clintara, Forum (EnVivo), Genentech, Lundbeck/Takeda, McKinsey, Merck, Naurex, Neuronetics, One Carbon, Pfizer, and Sunovion. He has had equity in Amnestix, Cervel, Corcept (cofounder), Delpor, Merck, Neurocrine, Pfizer, Titan, and Xhale. He is a named inventor on pharmacogenetic use patents on glucocorticoid antagonists and on prediction of antidepressant response.
Department of Psychiatry and Behavioral Sciences, Stanford University School of Medicine, 401 Quarry Road, Stanford, CA 94305-5797, USA
E-mail address: afschatz@stanford.edu

Psychiatr Clin N Am 38 (2015) 379–393
http://dx.doi.org/10.1016/j.psc.2015.05.009
psych.theclinics.com

There has been much written in recent years regarding the somewhat sorry state of affairs in the development of new psychotropic agents.[1,2] In the past decade, we have seen fewer new clinical entities in development, in part because of the relatively high failure rates in separating drugs from placebo. Various reasons for these failures have been provided, including the poor validity of diagnostic categories, inflation of baseline measures to ensure patients will meet entry criteria, and poor consistency or reliability of ratings both within and across sites (see later discussion). Many large-scale pharmaceutical companies have become frustrated and have publicly announced their decision to stop active drug development in psychiatry. There are, however, several so-called start-up companies and small to mid-size pharmaceutical companies that are still developing novel agents, and these are offering promise for the field. Several of these have also resulted in partnerships between so-called Big Pharma and smaller companies. This review discusses several agents and strategies that are currently in development which highlight numerous issues commonly confronted in drug development in psychiatry.

Most of the currently available agents for depression and anxiety are based on neurotransmitter models (norepinephrine or serotonin) of the disorders. The original tricyclic antidepressants block the reuptake of norepinephrine and, to a lesser extent, serotonin, and often had anticholinergic and antihistaminic properties. The latter 2 accounted for much of the side effects seen with these agents, particularly the risk of death in overdose. Monoamine oxidase inhibitors also regulate the catabolism of the biogenic amines intracellularly, and provided another avenue to regulate these systems. Here, untoward interaction with various foods and other drugs could provoke hypertensive crises that were potentially lethal. The second-generation selective serotonin reuptake inhibitors (SSRIs) and serotonin norepinephrine reuptake inhibitors (SNRIs) have become the drugs of choice for depression and anxiety disorders, and these agents by and large block the reuptake of norepinephrine and serotonin while producing little in the way of anticholinergic or antihistaminic effects. Thus, they are much safer.

Unfortunately, large-scale clinical trials such as STAR*D and I-SPOT report relatively large percentages of subjects not responding to monotherapy with SSRIs and SNRIs, such that other methods to treat these nonresponding patients are required.[3,4] To this end, a great deal of effort has gone into developing new agents that have alternative mechanisms of action (MoAs) that may provide relief for patients' symptoms via alternative neurobiological circuits or systems. However, we are still at the point of not understanding which circuit or system is awry in an individual patient, and this lack of biological specificity makes difficult the development and practice of personalized medicine and even nonpersonalized medicine for the psychiatric patient. This article reviews 4 strategies that take different routes (**Box 1**). The first focuses on agents that affect the excitatory neurotransmitter glutamate and its circuits in the brain. The second explores glucocorticoid receptor antagonists in delusional depression. Glucocorticoids are steroid hormones that are found throughout the body. In the brain, they bind to both a high-affinity mineralocorticoid receptor and low-affinity glucocorticoid receptors and responsive elements on various neurotransmitter regulatory genes. The third examines botulinum toxin and its ability to modulate a potential brain circuit that involves outputs to facial muscles and includes the prefrontal cortex and the amygdala. The last approach involves the opioid system in the brain, and explores the use of partial μ agonists administered either alone or with an opioid antagonist. These 4 strategies represent varied approaches and offer some promise for future drug development. In addition several recent, failed development efforts with drugs that have a variety of alternative MoAs, and the lessons that can be gleaned from these efforts, are discussed.

Box 1
Conceptual approaches to drug development

- Synaptic-based neurotransmitter function (eg, monoamines [norepinephrine, serotonin, dopamine], glutamate)
  - Reuptake blockers (eg, for norepinephrine)
  - Mobilizers of release (eg, for dopamine)
  - Receptor agonists (eg, for dopamine)
  - Antagonists (eg, for serotonin and glutamate)
  - Receptor site cofactor site modulators (eg, for glutamate)
  - Receptor site transport modulators (eg, for glutamate)
  - Glial receptors to modulate release (eg, for glutamate)
- Neuroendocrine systems (eg, hypothalamic-pituitary-adrenal axis)
  - Receptor antagonists (eg, glucocorticoid receptor, CRH-R1)
  - Receptor agonists (mineralocorticoid receptor)
- Agents that may modulate brain circuits
  - Botulinum toxin
- Opioid system
  - Agonists or partial agonists
  - Antagonists
  - Agonist/antagonist combinations

KETAMINE AND GLUTAMATERGIC AGENTS

Glutamine is a key neurotransmitter that controls neuronal excitation. It is essential for normal functioning and has numerous receptors, presynaptic, postsynaptic, and glial, indicating how well it is preserved. These receptors include postsynaptic α-amino-3-hydroxy-5-methyl-4-isoxazolepropionic acid (AMPA) and N-methyl-D-aspartic acid (NMDA) receptors, and metabotropic receptors on glia. Glutamate has long been thought to play a role in schizophrenia, with numerous attempts being made to develop agents that modulate or downregulate the system. Although there have been some positive initial positive trials, many of these programs have failed with further study, generally because of a lack of separation from placebo. Several years ago Berman and colleagues[5] reported that intravenous administration of ketamine, an antagonist for the NMDA receptor, resulted in relatively rapid antidepressant effects. Ketamine is used generally as an anesthetic agent in both humans and animals. It is scheduled by the Drug Enforcement Agency as a class 3 substance, in part because it is abused on the street as "Special K."

This area of investigation remained relatively subdued until Zarate and colleagues[6] reported on a double-blind trial in unipolar refractory patients and followed these with others in bipolar depression.[7,8] In all of these trials, intravenous administration resulted in rapid improvement (in <120 minutes) in depressed mood in highly refractory cases. Responses lasted for several days, although they dissipated by 4 to 7 days (see **Table 1** for a summary of ketamine trials). Several positive predictors have been reported, 2 of which have been very strong augurs of response. For one, the development of dissociation during trials showed a predictive response,[9] indicating an

Table 1
Ketamine: published double-blind antidepressant studies

Study	N	Diagnosis	Design	Dose	Comparator	Results
Berman et al, 2000	9	Unipolar	Parallel; ratings for 3 d	0.5 mg/kg, given once IV	Placebo	Ketamine rapidly more effective and continued to day 3; high visual analog scale scores for intoxication on ketamine
Zarate et al, 2006	18	Unipolar	Crossover; ratings for 7 d	0.5 mg/kg, given once IV	Placebo	Rapid antidepressant effects by 110 min; waning over the week; 35% maintain response
Diazgranados et al, 2010	18	Bipolar I & II	Crossover; ratings for 7 d	0.5 mg/kg, given once IV	Placebo	Ketamine superior by 110 min; wanes by day 4
Zarate et al, 2012	15	Bipolar I & II	Crossover; ratings for 7 d	0.5 mg/kg, given once IV	Placebo	Separation by 40 min; wanes by day 4; dissociation most common side effect
Murrough et al, 2013	73	Unipolar	Parallel; ratings for 7 d	0.5 mg/kg, given once IV	Midazolam	Ketamine significantly greater antidepressant response; separation by 24 h; wanes somewhat by 1 wk
Sos, 2013	27	Hospitalized	Crossover; ratings for 7 d	0.5 mg/kg, given once IV	Placebo	Ketamine superior at days 1, 4, and 7; psychotomimetic effects related to antidepressant effects

Abbreviation: IV, intravenous.
Data from Refs.[5–8,13]

underlying biological effect, although which specific neurotransmitter system is involved is not entirely clear. Moreover, the drug's dissociative effects make blinding trials more difficult because placebo is not likely to produce similar effects. Another strong predictor has been a family history of alcohol abuse, as seen in several studies,[10] and this may reflect genetic variation in specific glutamate receptors. Other differential predictors include anxiety in unipolar (but not bipolar) subjects.[11] Anxiety on a dimensional basis has been reported in 2 major large-scale trials on typical antidepressants to be associated with poor response to antidepressant monotherapy and with various combinations.[4,12] Thus, ketamine may represent a novel approach to helping patients with anxious depression and others who have been nonresponsive to treatment.

The issue of the dissociative effects of the drug and the question of maintaining a blind was partially addressed in a study by Murrough and colleagues,[13] who compared midazolam with ketamine. Midazolam was associated with significantly less dissociation (30%) than ketamine (60%), but also produced significantly fewer antidepressant responders. Again a rapid antidepressant response for ketamine was observed, with waning by 1 week. Other side effects (eg, nausea) were somewhat more common with ketamine. These data confirm the efficacy of ketamine, although they may not fully have eliminated the issue of blinding.

Although the acute findings are exciting, they do not address long-term issues for patients who have responded. Several strategies have been considered, one of which involves repeated administration of ketamine past the first week. In one such trial, repeated administration of ketamine every other day for 2 weeks resulted in patients reexperiencing both dissociative and antidepressant effects.[14] Unfortunately, oral ketamine has not been particularly promising; however, an intranasal form (s-ketamine) is under investigation.

Of note is that other glutamatergic agents have not proved helpful for either acute treatment or follow-up to parenteral ketamine. For example, there are several failed trials with memantine, an NMDA antagonist approved for the treatment of Alzheimer disease. Riluzole, a glutamatergic agent approved for use in amyotrophic lateral sclerosis, was not effective after administration of ketamine, although there was some suggestion of response on the so-called survival analysis of relapse.[15] These data suggest that the effects of ketamine may be due to other pharmacological properties.

A recent perspectives paper debated on the possible mechanism of action of ketamine and its significance.[16] One hypothesis is that ketamine causes a surge in glutamate release that then results in binding to the AMPA receptor. This proposal could help explain the apparent quandary of why a glutamate antagonist that results in blockade of a stimulatory transmitter produces relief from depression. Another theory is that secondary messenger or other downstream effects (eg, m-TOR) explains why ketamine is effective while other NMDA antagonists are not.[17] These targets open up some potential avenues of novel drug development.

Perhaps more worrisome are other effects of ketamine that may carry a considerable risk of abuse. One is ketamine's binding to opioid receptors, particularly μ agonism. Recent rodent studies point to ketamine's analgesic effects as being blocked by μ-opioid antagonists.[18] This potential MoA for the antidepressant effect has not been explored in man. Although over 2 weeks tolerance to ketamine's antidepressant effects has not been seen,[14] it has not been studied prospectively beyond this time point. Moreover, medicine has witnessed many opiates that had been heralded as not being particularly addictive at the time of release onto the market but that proved to be problematic after release (eg, propoxyphene). Other opioid receptor effects (eg, κ) are not particularly problematic. Another MoA for the drug is sympathomimetic. Ketamine mobilizes midbrain dopamine release and acts as a stimulant in animal models,[19] which could connote a risk for abuse but could also lead to development of other potential stimulant antidepressants.

ALTERNATIVE GLUTAMATERGIC STRATEGIES

Following the ketamine lead, several large pharmaceutical and start-up companies have pursued other glutamatergic strategies, one of which has been to develop other

NMDA antagonists; however, as already mentioned this has not been effective to date. Another is the development of trapping agents that bind glutamate at the synapse and in a sense act as an antagonist. One such agent is AZD6765, which was first reported to have very short-term (<2 hours) antidepressant effects, but subsequent trials were not consistent in separating the effect from placebo, in part because of high placebo response rates.[20,21] A third approach is to develop agents that act on other glutamatergic receptors (eg, metabotropic glutamate receptors), which to date has yielded limited results. One intriguing approach involves agents that act as agonists or partial agonists at the glycine cofactor site at the NMDA receptor, one of which, GLYX-13, recently showed acute effects using intravenous administration at intermediate doses.[22] The manufacturer has since announced that a follow-on compound given orally appeared to exert similar efficacy. Another agent that inhibits the glycine transporter-I and acts as an agonist postsynaptically has been reported to have some efficacy.[23] These data suggest that alternative glutamatergic actions (particularly NMDA agonism rather than NMDA antagonism) may be important for antidepressant effects.

OBOTULINUM TOXIN

Obotulinum toxin has become commonly used for cosmetic reasons in the United States and abroad. Moreover, the agent has found several other interesting medical uses, such as treatment of migraine and bladder control. In the past few years, 2 double-blind comparison trials of Obotulinum toxin with placebo have been reported for the treatment of refractory depression, with encouraging results.[24,25] Although at face value this might be viewed as merely reflecting that improved appearance helps depressed mood by raising self-esteem, the effects are likely far more complex and tell us something about the relationship of facial expression to depression, an area that has been well recognized for centuries.

Charles Darwin wrote about this in his classic work, and noted the importance of emotional expression through the face for separating man from the lower animals. The so-called corrugator response involving the brow furrowing was described then and has been studied at times by investigators. For example, Greden and colleagues[26] noted some years ago in a cohort of depressed women that agitation was highly correlated with degree of brow furrowing, and that there were significant differences between patients and controls. The degree of furrowing could be measured objectively by electromyography. More recently, Davidson's group has reported that ability to downregulate the amygdalar response to negative faces on functional magnetic resonance imaging was highly correlated to the degree of furrowing, and that this relationship persisted over time.[27] These findings suggest not only that a biological process is involved in the corrugator muscle response but also that it may reflect a brain circuit that involves the prefrontal cortex, anterior cingulate, and the amygdala.

Dermatologists have noted antidepressant effects in some patients given obotulinum toxin in the brow for cosmetic reasons. There have now been 2 double-blind placebo-controlled trials that point to clinical effects. Both studies enrolled mainly women (80%–90%). In the first report from Germany, Wollmer and colleagues[24] noted the administration of obotulinum toxin resulted in improved mood by week 2 that persisted to the end point at 6 weeks (**Table 2**). Further statistical significance was observed to week 16. In the other study,[25] obotulinum toxin was significantly more effective than placebo at week 3 with separation in response noted to at least week 6. There were few untoward effects. The articles discuss possible violation of the blinding, but in both several methods were used to evaluate the findings, such as

Table 2
Botulinum toxin: randomized controlled double-blind trials

Study	N	Diagnosis	Design	Dose	Comparator	Results
Wollmer et al, 2012	30 (80% women)	Unipolar	Parallel; 6 wk end point; followed to 16 wk	29–39 units, given once	Saline	Significant separation by week 2 and continuing to week 16
Finzi and Rosenthal, 2014	69 (>90% women)	Unipolar	Parallel; 6 wk	29–40 units, given once	Saline	Significant separation by week 3 lasting to week 6

Data from Wollmer MA, de Boer C, Kalak N, et al. Facing depression with botulinum toxin: a randomized controlled trial. J Psychiatr Res 2012;46:574–81; and Finzi E, Rosenthal NE. Treatment of depression with onabotulinumtoxinA: a randomized, double-blind, placebo controlled trial. J Psychiatr Res 2014;52:1–6.

photographs of subjects rated independently by psychiatrists to assess changes in appearance. Reportedly the manufacturer is now conducting a trial in depressed women.

GLUCOCORTICOID ANTAGONISTS

Psychotic features are relatively common in depression, representing some 19% of subjects who meet criteria for major depression in community samples.[28] Current prevalence rates from 2 European surveys are 0.3% and 0.4%.[28,29] Some years ago, the author hypothesized that the development of delusions in major depression was due to excessive cortisol activity. Data in support of this hypothesis have been reviewed in detail elsewhere.[30] Based on these findings several groups have explored the use of mifepristone, a progesterone and glucocorticoid antagonist, to reverse the psychotic symptoms seen in the disorder. The drug is in phase III of development in an effort led by a biotechnology company that the author cofounded some 15 years ago. To date there have been 7 published reports of open-label[31–37] and double-blind trials. The results of the double-blind trials are summarized in **Table 3**.

Mifepristone in clinical trials is generally given for 7 days with outcomes assessed at 1, 4, and 8 weeks. In the initial pilot study of 5 subjects, a crossover design was used whereby the drug or placebo was given for 4 days.[31] The patients responded within 4 days and did not relapse on cessation. Subsequently, Flores and colleagues[32] reported positive results in a National Institute of Mental Health (NIMH)-funded trial; significantly greater improvement in psychosis was observed at week 1 on 600 mg/d of mifepristone in comparison with placebo. Increases in cortisol levels at week 1 were significantly correlated with continued improvement in psychosis at week 4.[30] The phase III trials of the company have been mixed. In the initial trial the drug was effective in improving psychosis at 1 week, extending to 4 and 8 weeks.[33] Subsequently, other studies have observed generally high placebo responses such that statistically significant separation was not observed. A priori application of data on therapeutic blood levels of mifepristone obtained in the first 2 studies to the third study that used 3 different doses (300 mg/d, 600 mg/d, and 1,200 mg/d) resulted in statistically significant separation from placebo in patients whose blood level at 1 week was above the so-called minimum therapeutic level of 1661 ng/mL. These data suggest that the

Table 3
Mifepristone treatment studies in PMD

Study	N	Design	Dose (mg/d)	Duration of Treatment and Outcome	Results
Belanoff et al, 2001	5	Crossover; mifepristone or placebo for 4 d; assessment at 4 and 8 d	600	4 d each Phase; outcome after each phase	4/5 patients on active drug showed improvement in total BPRS scores; little effect in initial placebo-treated subjects
Flores et al, 2006	30	Parallel; mifepristone or placebo for 2 d; assessed at baseline and day 8	600	8 d; outcome on day 8	Mifepristone significantly more effective than placebo in reducing BPRS PSS scores
DeBattista et al, 2006	221	Parallel; mifepristone or placebo for 7 d; assessed at days 7, 28, and 56; mifepristone blood levels explored	600	7 d; primary outcome at 1 and 4 wk; subset assessed at 1 and 8 wk	Mifepristone significantly more effective BPRS PSS at 7 and 28 d and at days 7 and 56
Blasey et al, 2009	258	Parallel; mifepristone or placebo for 7 d; assessed at days 7, 28, and 56; mifepristone blood levels explored	600	7 d; outcome at 1 and 8 wk	Mifepristone numerically but not statistically superior on BPRS PSS scores; therapeutic blood level observed; significant site by treatment effect
Blasey et al, 2011	433	Parallel; mifepristone vs placebo for 7 d; assessment at days 7, 28, and 56; mifepristone blood levels explored	300, 600, or 1200	7 d; outcome at 1 and 8 wk	Mifepristone numerically but not statistically significantly superior on BPRS PSS scores; applying a priori defined blood level, patients with levels above the cutoff separated statistically from placebo; suggests 1200 mg/d is optimal dose

Abbreviations: BPRS, Brief Psychiatric Rating Scale; PSS, Positive Symptom Subscale of BPRS.
Data from Refs.[31–35]

blood level is a mediator of response and suggests merit to the approach as long as patients are treated at adequate doses and blood levels. In that study, 1200 mg per day was needed to achieve sufficient numbers of patients attaining the therapeutic blood level. This approach is being assessed in one additional trial and across all phase III trials.[34] This initiative demonstrates some interesting issues in psychotropic drug development: the growing placebo response rates even in psychotic disorders[38]; the possible application of a drug blood level to assess response; and the potential use of a biological readout such as change in cortisol level to further assess the adequacy of treatment.

OPIOIDS: MIXED AGONIST/ANTAGONISTS

Before the advent of modern antidepressant therapy, opium was often used for the treatment of depression[39] but was quickly abandoned in favor of nonaddictive antidepressants such as the tricyclic antidepressants and second-generation SSRIs and SNRIs. Nevertheless, as already noted, many patients do not respond to available medications and require alternative strategies. Some years ago, Bodkin and colleagues[40] from McLean Hospital reported in a small series of patients that open-label buprenorphine, a μ partial agonist, was effective in about 70%. More recently, Reynolds' group reported that buprenorphine administered to refractory depressives aged 50 or older improved on buprenorphine.[41] The partial agonist properties have been thought to make the drug less abused, although concerns still abound regarding this strategy. Most recently, Alkermes, a biotechnology company interested in the treatment of drug abuse, has been exploring the combination of buprenorphine with a potent μ antagonist in refractory depression. The combination has been hypothesized to provide sufficient agonist effects to provide relief from depression, with the antagonist preventing the development of dependence. Preliminary data suggest the strategy may indeed be effective,[42] and a larger-scale trial has reportedly been completed.

Several years ago Larry Koran reported that oral morphine produced significantly greater relief of symptoms in obsessive-compulsive disorder (OCD), an effect that lasted for about 5 days. He noted that the NMDA antagonist effects of morphine might explain the clinical benefit.[43] More recently, Rodriguez and colleagues[44] observed that intravenous ketamine produced rapid relief from obsessive-compulsive symptoms in refractory OCD patients, consistent with a potential NMDA effect. However, the author has argued that ketamine may actually be acting as an opioid agonist and that an MoA might better explain its clinical effects.[16] He has also argued that this MoA for ketamine needs to be better studied for public health reasons. Moreover, the data on agents acting directly as opioid agonists or partial agonists (buprenorphine or morphine) coupled with the possible μ-opioid effects of ketamine indicate a trend toward an approach that may prove to be effective for the most severely ill or refractory patients, but which could prove to be problematic because of the risk for abuse and dependence. The practical pharmacological issues need to be studied, the risk versus benefit ratio needs to addressed, and the ethical and societal issues need to be discussed openly.

FAILED STRATEGIES AND FAILED DEVELOPMENT EFFORTS

Unfortunately, as indicated earlier, there have been several failures in antidepressant development over the past 10 years. These failures may provide clues for future development, and it is worthwhile reviewing some of them.

Corticotropin-Releasing Hormone Antagonists

Corticotropin-releasing hormone (CRH) is distributed widely in the brain with considerable concentration in the hypothalamus, hippocampus, prefrontal cortex, and amygdala. In the hypothalamic-pituitary-adrenal (HPA) axis, CRH in the hypothalamus stimulates the release of corticotropin from the pituitary, and corticotropin then stimulates the release of cortisol from the adrenal. Cortisol feeds back in a negative feedback loop at the level of the hypothalamus to control the release of CRH and at the level of the pituitary to control corticotropin release, and ultimately cortisol release, from the adrenal. By contrast, cortisol in the amygdala is under positive feedback control by cortisol, and this has been postulated to play a role in alcohol abuse.[45] Understandably there had been much anticipation and excitement about developing CRH-R1 antagonists for depression, anxiety, and alcohol abuse. However, these agents have not been effective in double-blind comparisons versus placebo in patients with depression or generalized anxiety disorder,[46,47] and several companies have canceled their development programs. It is possible that the systemic difficulties in separating drug from placebo that plague much of drug development may have played a part here, but there may be other reasons too. First, CRH-R1 is not the only receptor for CRH in brain. CRH-R2 binds with reasonable affinity, and may prove to be more important for mood and anxiety. Another concern has been whether these agents are entering the brain in sufficient concentrations. Moreover, the doses may not be sufficient to effect a blockade of CRH-R1 in key brain regions. Unfortunately, CRH-R1 ligands that can be used in PET have not been available to guide drug development. Using a marker such as a decrease in cortisol to judge efficacy may be insufficient or misleading for judging a dose if CRH-R1 outside the HPA axis is the putative target. Lastly, it is conceivable that these agents will be effective in patients who carry specific alleles for specific CRH-R1 single-nucleotide polymorphisms. Some recent data suggest that several CRH-R1 alleles may confer particular risk for developing either anxiety or depressive disorders.[48,49]

Taken together, developing CRH-R1 antagonists for depression or anxiety may require greater study of pharmacological properties and potential biological effects in man with better matching of patients to specific treatments.

AGOMELATINE

Agomelatine is a French melatonin R-1 and R-2 agonist and a serotonin (5-HT2) antagonist. The drug was approved in Europe at doses of 25 to 50 mg per day. In the United States, positive trials have been reported; however, 50 mg/d was associated with transient hepatotoxicity (elevated transaminases) that resulted in the drug being canceled. It remains on the market in Europe where the adverse effects on the liver apparently have not proved problematic. A recent meta-analysis of 9 studies (including 3 unpublished) concluded that the drug had a relatively small effect in reducing depressive symptoms.[50] Side effects can pose a great hurdle to companies in the United States, especially because of liability issues.

EDIVOXETINE AND LISDEXAMFETAMINE

Edivoxetine is a noradrenergic agent that was being developed as an adjunctive agent in patients who had failed to respond to monotherapy. It had positive results in phase II, partly as a monotherapy, but then failed to separate from placebo in 3 phase III adjunctive trials. Its failure was surprising in view of its being a potent noradrenergic drug and several other agents having been proved effective as adjuncts, for example, the atypical antipsychotics. Those trials had given the field some confidence that concentrating on refractory depressed subjects would decrease the placebo response in trials, but this was not the case for edivoxetine. Such failures are regrettably becoming more common and in part reflect issues in the conduct of clinical trials (**Box 2**). Its failure does raise the question, however, as to whether noradrenergic agents are weak antidepressants as monotherapy, and this has been suggested for reboxetine. Another catecholaminergic agent, lisdesamfetamine, recently failed as an augmentor in major depression. This drug, a dopaminergic agent with a unique oral absorption mechanism and profile, has in contrast been shown to be effective in binge-eating disorder[51] and was recently approved in the United States for that use.

These clinical development programs highlight the many difficulties in developing agents in psychiatry. Do we have the correct receptor target for improving the symptom set or syndrome? Do we have an agent that penetrates the blood-brain barrier and produces sufficiently high concentrations of drug in brain? Can we reliably measure symptom severity in patients? Is the conduct of the trial optimal? Are we overestimating symptomatology at baseline? Are we adding to nonspecific or placebo responses by having too much contact with patients? Is the risk-benefit ratio such that the drug will provide sufficient benefit and safety to be adopted? All of these are areas need to be addressed as we move forward in drug development if we are to have a new armamentarium.

Although some lament has been expressed about the state of affairs in psychiatric drug development, some innovative strategies have emerged that offer some hope for new agents. Efforts have been expended in developing pharmacogenetic and other biological markers that not only can improve matching available drugs to patients

---

Box 2
Failures in drug development

Reasons for Drug Development Failures

- Hypothesis of system involvement in disorder is misguided
- Agent has poor brain penetrance
- Limited data on pharmacologic effect in brain
- Optimal drug dose or blood/brain level is not established
- Poor tolerability/side effects

Diagnostic Issues

- Diagnosis is not valid or reliable
- Biological heterogeneity of specific diagnoses
- Comorbidity confuses optimal treatment
- Disorder subtyping not considered in trial design

Trial Conduct

- Symptom score inflation at baseline
- Poor interrater reliability
- Patients enrolled simultaneously in multiple studies
- Adherence to medication
- Blinding is compromised

but also can stimulate new drug development for specific subtypes of disorders. Another approach has been to improve imaging tools that can be used to better screen compounds for pharmacological effects in humans.

Ultimately, these approaches can lead to a truly personalized medicine in psychiatry. One general approach that has been advocated is to spend more time and effort early in the process on target validation of new agents or classes of agents (in part through application of imaging) to best understand the biology of the target system and the pharmacologic properties before embarking on large-scale phase III trials which have witnessed a great deal of failure in the past few years. Such an approach may conserve resources and optimize selection of drug candidates to advance into clinical trials, and is now being followed in NIMH-funded efforts in new treatment development that may prove more effective and cost-efficient. At any rate, only further study of the biology and genetics of specific disorders coupled with the development of new tools to assess both biological effect and clinical efficacy can help us negotiate difficult times in psychopharmacologic research.

REFERENCES

1. Schatzberg AF. Issues encountered in recent attempts to develop novel antidepressant agents. Ann N Y Acad Sci 2015;1345:67–73.
2. Nutt D, Goodwin G. ECNP Summit on the future of CNS drug research in Europe 2011: report prepared for ECNP by David Nutt and Guy Goodwin. Eur Neuropsychopharmacol 2011;21:495–9.
3. Rush AJ, Trivedi MH, Wisniewski SR, et al. Acute and longer-term outcomes in depressed outpatients requiring one or several steps: a STAR*D report. Am J Psychiatry 2006;163:1905–17.
4. Saveanu R, Etkin A, Duchemin AM, et al. The international study to predict optimized treatment in depression (i-SPOT-D): outcomes from the acute phase of antidepressant treatment. J Psychiatr Res 2015;61:1–12.
5. Berman RM, Cappiello A, Anand A, et al. Antidepressant effects of ketamine in depressed patients. Biol Psychiatry 2000;47:351–4.
6. Zarate CA Jr, Singh JB, Carlson PJ, et al. A randomized trial of an N-methyl-D-aspartate antagonist in treatment-resistant major depression. Arch Gen Psychiatry 2006;63(8):856–64.
7. Diazgranados N, Ibrahim L, Brutsche NE, et al. A randomized add-on trial of an N-methyl-D-aspartate antagonist in treatment-resistant bipolar depression. Arch Gen Psychiatry 2010;67:793–802.
8. Zarate CA Jr, Brutsche NE, Ibrahim L, et al. Replication of ketamine's antidepressant efficacy in bipolar depression: a randomized controlled add-on trial. Biol Psychiatry 2012;71:939–46.
9. Luckenbaugh DA, Niciu MJ, Ionescu DF, et al. Do the dissociative side effects of ketamine mediate its antidepressant effects? J Affect Disord 2014;159:56–61.
10. Luckenbaugh DA, Ibrahim L, Brutsche N, et al. Family history of alcohol dependence and antidepressant response to an N-methyl-D-aspartate antagonist in bipolar depression. Bipolar Disord 2012;14:880–7.
11. Ionescu DF, Luckenbaugh DA, Niciu MJ, et al. Effect of baseline anxious depression on initial and sustained antidepressant response to ketamine. J Clin Psychiatry 2014;75:932–8.
12. Fava M, Rush AJ, Alpert JE, et al. Difference in treatment outcome in outpatients with anxious versus nonanxious depression: a STAR*D Report. Am J Psychiatry 2008;165:342–51.

13. Murrough JW, Iosifescu DV, Chang LC, et al. Antidepressant efficacy of ketamine in treatment-resistant major depression: a two-site randomized controlled trial. Am J Psychiatry 2013;170:1134–42.
14. Murrough JW, Perez AM, Pillemer S, et al. Rapid and longer-term antidepressant effects of repeated ketamine infusions in treatment-resistant major depression. Biol Psychiatry 2013;74:250–6.
15. Mathew SJ, Murrough JW, aan het Rot M, et al. Riluzole for relapse prevention following intravenous ketamine in treatment-resistant depression: a pilot randomized, placebo-controlled continuation trial. Int J Neuropsychopharmacol 2010;13: 71–82.
16. Sanacora G, Schatzberg AF. Ketamine: promising path or false prophecy in the development of novel therapeutics for mood disorders? Neuropsychopharmacology 2015;40:259–67.
17. Li N, Lee B, Liu RJ, et al. mTOR-dependent synapse formation underlies the rapid antidepressant effects of NMDA antagonists. Science 2010;329:959–64.
18. Mehta AK, Halder S, Khanna N, et al. Antagonism of stimulation-produced analgesia by naloxone and N-methyl-D-aspartate: role of opioid and N-methyl-D-aspartate receptors. Hum Exp Toxicol 2012;31:51–6.
19. Tan S, Lam WP, Wai MS. Chronic ketamine administration modulates midbrain dopamine system in mice. PLoS One 2012;7(8):e43947.
20. Sanacora G, Smith MA, Pathak S, et al. Lanicemine: a low-trapping NMDA channel blocker produces sustained antidepressant efficacy with minimal psychotomimetic adverse effects. Mol Psychiatry 2013;19:978–85.
21. Sanacora G, Khan A, Atkinson S, et al. Adjunctive lanicemine (AZD6765) in patients with major depressive disorder and a history of inadequent response to antidepressants: primary results from a randomized, placebo controlled study (PURSUIT). Presented at American Society of Clinical Psychiatry. Hollywood (FL), June 2014.
22. Preskorn S, Macaluso M, Mehra DO, et al. Randomized proof of concept trial of GLYX-13, an N-methyl-D-aspartate receptor glycine site partial agonist, in major depressive disorder non responsive to a previous antidepressant agent. J Psychiatr Pract 2015;21:140–9.
23. Huang CC, Wei IH, Huang CL, et al. Inhibition of glycine transporter-I as a novel mechanism for the treatment of depression. Biol Psychiatry 2013;74(10):734–41.
24. Wollmer MA, de Boer C, Kalak N, et al. Facing depression with botulinum toxin: a randomized controlled trial. J Psychiatr Res 2012;46:574–81.
25. Finzi E, Rosenthal NE. Treatment of depression with onabotulinumtoxinA: a randomized, double-blind, placebo controlled trial. J Psychiatr Res 2014;52:1–6.
26. Greden JF, Genero N, Price HL. Agitation-increased electromyogram activity in the corrugator muscle region: a possible explanation of the "Omega sign"? Am J Psychiatry 1985;142:348–51.
27. Heller AS, Lapate RC, Mayer KE, et al. The face of negative affect: trial-by-trial corrugator responses to negative pictures are positively associated with amygdala and negatively associated with ventromedial prefrontal cortex activity. J Cogn Neurosci 2014;26:2102–10.
28. Ohayon M, Schatzberg AF. Prevalence of depressive episodes with psychotic features in the general population. Am J Psychiatry 2002;159:1855–61.
29. Perälä J, Suvisaari J, Saarni SI, et al. Lifetime prevalence of psychotic and bipolar I disorders in a general population. Arch Gen Psychiatry 2007;36:616–21.
30. Schatzberg AF. Anna-Monika Award Lecture, DGPPN Kongress, 2013: the role of the hypothalamic-pituitary-adrenal (HPA) axis in the pathogenesis of psychotic major depression. World J Biol Psychiatry 2015;16(1):1–10.

31. Belanoff JK, Flores BH, Kalezhan M, et al. Rapid reversal of psychotic depression using mifepristone. J Clin Psychopharmacolacol 2001;21:516–21.
32. Flores BH, Kenna H, Keller J, et al. Clinical and biological effects of mifepristone treatment for psychotic depression. Neuropsychopharmacology 2006;31: 628–36.
33. DeBattista C, Belanoff J, Glass S, et al. Mifepristone versus placebo in the treatment of psychosis in patients with psychotic major depression. Biol Psychiatry 2006;60:1343–9.
34. Blasey CM, Block TS, Belanoff JK, et al. Efficacy and safety of mifepristone for the treatment of psychotic depression. J Clin Psychopharmacolacol 2011;31: 436–40.
35. Blasey CM, DeBattista C, Roe R, et al. A multisite trial of mifepristone for the treatment of psychotic depression: a site-by-treatment interaction. Contemp Clin Trials 2009;30:284–8.
36. Belanoff JK, Rothschild AJ, Cassidy F, et al. An open label trail of C-1073 (mifepristone) for psychotic major depression. Biol Psychiatry 2002;52:386–92.
37. Simpson GM, El Sheshai A, Loza N, et al. An 8-week open-label trial of a 6-day course of mifepristone for the treatment of psychotic depression. J Clin Psychiatry 2005;66:598–602.
38. Rutherford BR, Pott E, Tandler JM, et al. Placebo response in antipsychotic clinical trials: a meta-analysis. JAMA Psychiatry 2014;71:1409–21.
39. Tenore PL. Psychotherapeutic benefits of opioid agonist therapy. J Addict Dis 2008;27:49–65.
40. Bodkin J, Zornberg GI, Lukas SE, et al. Buprenorphine treatment of refractory depression. J Clin Psychopharmacol 1995;15:49–57.
41. Karp JF, Butters MA, Begley AE, et al. Safety, tolerability, and clinical effect of low-dose buprenorphine for treatment-resistant depression in midlife and older adults. J Clin Psychiatry 2014;75:e785–93.
42. Ehrlich E, Turncliff R, Yangchun D, et al. Evaluation of opioid modulation in major depressive disorder. Neuropsychopharmacology 2015;40:1448–55.
43. Koran LM, Aboukaoude E, Bullock KM, et al. Double-blind treatment with oral morphine in treatment-resistant obsessive-compulsive disorder. J Clin Psychiatry 2005;66:353–9.
44. Rodriguez CI, Kegeles LS, Levinson A, et al. Randomized controlled crossover trial of ketamine in obsessive-compulsive disorder: proof-of-concept. Neuropsychopharmacology 2013;38:2475–83.
45. Vendruscolo LF, Barbier E, Schlosburg JE, et al. Corticosteroid-dependent plasticity mediates compulsive alcohol drinking in rats. J Neurosci 2012;32: 7563–71.
46. Binneman B, Feltner D, Kolluri S, et al. A 6-week randomized, placebo-controlled trial of CP-316,311 (a selective CRH1 antagonist) in the treatment of major depression. Am J Psychiatry 2008;165:617–20.
47. Coric V, Feldman HH, Oren DA, et al. Multicenter, randomized, double-blind, active comparator and placebo-controlled trial of a corticotropin-releasing factor receptor-1 antagonist in generalized anxiety disorder. Depress Anxiety 2010;27: 417–25.
48. Hsu D, Mickey BJ, Langenecker SA, et al. Variation in the corticotropin-releasing hormone receptor (CRHR1) gene influences fMRI signal responses during emotional stimulus processing. J Neurosci 2012;32:3253–60.
49. Schatzberg AF, Keller J, Tennakoon L, et al. HPA axis genetic variation, cortisol and psychosis in major depression. Mol Psychiatry 2014;19:220–7.

50. Koesters M, Guaiana G, Cipriani A, et al. Agomelatine efficacy and acceptability revisited: systematic review and meta-analysis of published and unpublished randomised trials. Br J Psychiatry 2013;203:179–87.
51. McElroy SL, Hudson JI, Mitchel JE, et al. Efficacy and safety of lisdexamfetamine for treatment of adults with moderate to severe binge-eating disorder: a randomized clinical trial. JAMA Psychiatry 2015;72:235–46.

Personalized Medicine and Mood Disorders

Lujain Alhajji, MD, Charles B. Nemeroff, MD, PhD*

KEYWORDS

- Major depressive disorder • Bipolar disorder • Personalized medicine
- Precision medicine • Pharmacogenomics • Epigenetics

KEY POINTS

- Personalized medicine integrates genetic information, epigenetic changes, identified biomarkers, environmental exposures, and clinical signs and symptoms to help predict disease vulnerability, make the correct diagnosis, and predict the response to specific treatments.
- Factors contributing to the diagnostic subtyping and treatment of major depressive and bipolar disorders include alterations in hypothalamic-pituitary-adrenal axis activity, serotonergic and other monoamine system markers, polymorphisms in the cytochrome P450 isoenzyme system, brain-derived neutrophic factor, and the circadian rhythm.
- Neuroimaging studies and certain cognitive-emotional domains are emerging as biomarkers for mood disorders that may predict disease subtypes and response to specific treatments.

INTRODUCTION

Personalized or precision medicine has several major aims: (1) To predict disease vulnerability, (2) to aid in accurate diagnosis of well-defined disease endophenotypes, and (3) to optimize treatment based on the individual patients biological characteristics. It has evolved more rapidly in some fields, such as oncology, than others; it involves integrating patients' genetic and epigenetic information, other biomarkers, environmental exposures, and clinical signs and symptoms (**Fig. 1**).

Genome-wide association studies (GWAS) have contributed to advances in personalized medicine in psychiatry by identifying genetic variants of disease that may contribute to disease vulnerability. The results have been promising in bipolar disorder and schizophrenia but considerably less so in major depression. Linkage studies preceded GWAS approaches and obtained information from family members with

Disclosure: See the last page of the article.
Department of Psychiatry and Behavioral Sciences, University of Miami Miller School of Medicine, 1120 Northwest 14th Street, Miami, FL 33136, USA
* Corresponding author. 1120 Northwest 14th Street, #1455, Miami, FL 33136.
E-mail address: cnemeroff@miami.edu

Psychiatr Clin N Am 38 (2015) 395–403
http://dx.doi.org/10.1016/j.psc.2015.05.003
0193-953X/15/$ – see front matter © 2015 Elsevier Inc. All rights reserved.

CLINICAL VIGNETTE: A MAN WITH MAJOR DEPRESSIVE DISORDER

JS is a 52-year-old married Caucasian man who presented to the outpatient clinic with a 1-year history of depressed mood, anhedonia, insomnia, fatigue, poor concentration, episodes of spontaneous crying, and excess feelings of guilt. JS identified his job loss as the main stressor precipitating this depressive episode. Since his job loss 1 year ago, he began spending most of his day isolating himself at home. He denied having any significant signs or symptoms of anxiety, mania, or psychosis. Furthermore, he adamantly denied having any suicidal thoughts, intent, or plans. He has had trials of multiple antidepressants, including sertraline, citalopram, and mirtazapine; but these were discontinued because of failure to improve his depression. He recalled that his father, who also suffered from depression, responded well to amitriptyline.

Amitriptyline was begun at 25 mg at bedtime and was titrated up to 75 mg at bedtime over the course of 3 weeks. During his next visit, JS reported some improvement in his symptoms, and the amitriptyline was increased to 100 mg at bedtime. Four days after the dose was increased to 100 mg, JS presented to the emergency department with a complaint of inability to urinate as well as dry mouth and constipation. His wife, who was present with him, confirmed that JS has been taking his medications as prescribed. The plasma concentration of amitriptyline was found to be 890 ng/mL in the toxic range. The emergency department physician discontinued amitriptyline, and JS was placed under electrocardiogram monitoring until his symptoms resolved 30 hours later.

After informed consent, JS underwent CYP2D6 genotype testing, which indicated that he was a poor metabolizer because of a polymorphism that rendered the CYP2D6 isoenzyme to have very low activity. JS was restarted on a reduced dose of amitriptyline 25 mg, with no reported side effects. The dose was gradually increased to 75 mg, which was associated with a gradual improvement in his depressive symptoms and therapeutic amitriptyline levels.

and without the specified disease. Thus far, these studies have been very useful for disorders with single-gene mendelian type of inheritance, for example, Huntington's disease, but much less so when analyzing psychiatric disorders because of the multifactorial nonmendelian-style disease inheritance and heterogeneity of disease

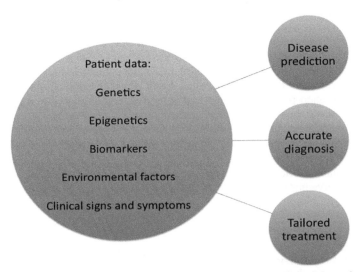

Fig. 1. Personalized medicine. The many different factors that contribute into each patient's clinical profile, including genetic variations, epigenetic alterations, biomarker changes, clinical signs and symptoms, and environmental influences. Once these factors are obtained from each patient, predisposition to disease can theoretically be predicted in order to reach an accurate diagnosis and in turn choose the most suitable therapy.

manifestations. Candidate gene association studies assess specific alleles or genetic markers, for example, single nucleotide polymorphisms (SNPs) and copy number variations, and measure whether these occur more frequently in family based studies or case-control trials. It is the authors' view that in spite of controversy in this area, this approach has been shown to be more informative in psychiatry research than the other approaches described earlier.

It is important to note that large-scale GWAS studies can successfully identify highly statistically significant differences in the frequency of certain genetic polymorphisms in the disease group compared with the control group. The absolute difference in the frequency is almost always quite small; individually, these variations constitute a very small percentage of disease heritability. There are many areas in medicine whereby personalized medicine has made remarkable advances and is clinically applicable. It is perhaps best demonstrated in oncology, whereby genetic mutations in BRCA1, BRCA2, and HER2 can predict breast cancer and its response to specific treatment.

MAJOR DEPRESSIVE DISORDER AND BIPOLAR DISORDER

The lifetime prevalence rate of major depressive disorder (MDD) is approximately 11% to 13% in men and almost twice that in women with the genetic component risk of 30% to 40%.[1] Approximately 10% of the population older than 12 years report taking antidepressants in the United States, although the rate of response is highly variable among patients.[2,3] Bipolar disorder affects approximately 1% to 3% of the population depending on the diagnostic criteria used. Numerous family studies have confirmed that bipolar disorder is highly familial, with the risk increasing to 10-fold in first-degree family members of patients with bipolar disorder. Bipolar disorder is known to have a strong genetic heritability, which contributes to approximately 60% to 85% of the risk.[4]

ALTERATIONS IN DRUG-METABOLIZING ENZYMES

One major focus of pharmacogenomics has been the hepatic cytochrome P450 enzyme (CYP450) system, particularly the polymorphic CYP450 2D6 isoenzyme, which is responsible for the metabolism of most antidepressants. This isoenzyme is responsible for metabolizing tricyclic antidepressants (TCAs), many selective serotonin reuptake inhibitors (SSRIs), serotonin-norepinephrine reuptake inhibitors, and antipsychotics. Multiple studies have scrutinized CYP450 2D6 polymorphisms as a predictor of tolerability and side effect burden of antidepressants. Patients with polymorphisms of this isoenzyme are classified into 4 categories: (1) poor (PM), (2) intermediate, (3) extensive, and (4) ultrarapid metabolizers (URM). CYP-2D6 PMs are at a higher risk of developing side effects because of slower metabolism, increased half-life, and increased bioavailability. In contrast, CYTP450 2D6 URMs are more likely to exhibit a poor response to therapy because of the shortened half-life and decreased bioavailability. These factors should be taken into consideration when patients show severe side effects at low doses or lack of efficacy at maximally approved doses. Despite these findings, evidence for routine screening for CYP450 genetic polymorphisms is still not compelling.[5]

CHANGES IN THE SEROTONERGIC SYSTEM

There is a vast literature implicating serotonergic circuit dysfunction in the pathophysiology of MDD and suicidal behavior. Alterations reported include

1. Reduced cerebrospinal fluid concentrations of the major serotonin metabolite 5-hydroxyindoleacetic acid
2. Reduced density of the serotonin transporter in the brain and platelets
3. Reduced plasma tryptophan concentrations, the rate-limiting step in serotonin biosynthesis
4. Alterations in the density of postsynaptic serotonin receptor subtypes
5. Increased activity of monoamine oxidase

Multiple studies have assessed polymorphisms in the serotonergic system and susceptibility to MDD, especially in the 5-hydroxytryptamine (serotonin) transporter (5-HTT) gene. For example, Hoefgen and colleagues[6] conducted a case-control trial in patients with German descent and found that, in patients with MDD, there was an increased frequency of polymorphism in the short allele of the 5' promoter region of the 5-HTT gene. In addition, in a landmark study, Caspi and colleagues[7] conducted a prospective longitudinal study to assess the relationship between 5-HTT gene polymorphism and the influence of child abuse and neglect on the development of MDD and related symptoms, including suicidality. They reported that those who with the short allele polymorphism of the 5-HTT promoter region, either homozygotes or heterozygotes, are more likely to develop depressive symptoms in combination with early life stress than those who were homozygous for the long allele. This finding has been widely reported by the authors' group and others[8,9]; but discordant reports have also appeared. This polymorphism does not predict treatment response.

THE HYPOTHALAMIC-PITUITARY-ADRENAL AXIS

Hyperactivity of the hypothalamic-pituitary-adrenal (HPA) axis has been repeatedly observed in depressed patients. Some of the most important components of this complex mammalian endocrine system are the FK506-binding protein (FKBP5), corticotropin-releasing hormone (CRH), its major receptor CRHR1, and the corticotropin-releasing hormone-binding protein (CRHBP).[10] FKBP5 is a cochaperone of the heat shock protein-90 in the mature glucocorticoid receptor complex and codes for a protein that causes glucocorticoid receptor subsensitivity.[11] Binder and colleagues[11] reported that depressed patients who were homozygous for the rs1360780 SNP of FKBP5 exhibited a more rapid response to SSRIs, TCAs, and mirtazapine compared with noncarriers. Furthermore, 2 FKBP5 SNPs, rs1360780TT and rs3800373GG, were found to be associated with a higher rate of suicide attempts in a sample of depressed, treatment-resistant adolescents.[12] FKBP5 SNPs also determine the likelihood of development of post-traumatic stress disorder (PTSD) in adult victims of child abuse.[13]

CRHR1 is a G-protein–coupled receptor, which mediates the main effect of CRH, thereby playing a major role in the regulation of the HPA axis as well as the behavioral, endocrine, and immune response to stress. Liu and colleagues[14] reported that 3 SNPs in the CRHR1 gene were considerably overrepresented in depressed Hans-Chinese patients compared with controls. The authors' group reported that polymorphisms in the CRHR1 gene predicted vulnerability to MDD in patients with a history of child abuse and neglect.[15] A small Swedish study scrutinized the association between CRHBP SNPs in 89 patients with major depression and matched controls. They found that 2 SNPs in the CRHBP gene were significantly associated with a diagnosis of major depression, with a frequency of 53% in patients compared with 35% in controls.[16] This finding was later replicated in a second study, but the results were not statistically significant.[17] The authors' group reported that CRHBP SNPs predicted treatment response to citalopram in the Sequenced Treatment Alternatives to Relieve Depression (STAR*D) Study.[18]

In addition to its contribution to the pathophysiology of MDD, the HPA axis has also been postulated to play a role in bipolar disorder. For example, adolescent offspring of parents who are bipolar exhibit higher baseline cortisol levels.[19] Furthermore, Willour and colleagues[20] conducted an association study in a family sample with bipolar disorder whereby there were 317 bipolar pedigrees and 554 bipolar offspring. Five SNPs of the FKBP5 gene were identified, which showed evidence for association with bipolar disorder. In addition, 4 other SNPs within FKBP5 were also identified to have an association with bipolar disorder; however, they varied depending on the number of depressive episodes in the past and history of suicide attempts.

CIRCADIAN RHYTHM GENES ALTERATIONS

Not surprisingly, there has also been much focus on changes in circadian rhythm genes in relation to bipolar disorder. Mansour and colleagues[21] carried out a small case-control association study, in which 234 patients with bipolar I disorder were sampled and compared with 180 controls. Forty-four SNPs of 8 circadian rhythm genes were assayed, and there were associations with SNPs for aryl hydrocarbon receptor nuclear translocator-like (ARNTL) and timeless circadian clock (TIMELESS). Another family study was conducted by Shi and colleagues,[22] and 3 SNPs within or near the circadian locomotor output cycles kaput (CLOCK) gene were found to be associated with bipolar disorder. However, these associations did not reach genome-wide significance after correction for multiple testing. Benedetti and colleagues[23] recorded the diurnal activity and nocturnal sleep in 39 patients diagnosed with bipolar disorder and studied the role of the SNP rs1801260 within the CLOCK gene. This specific SNP was associated with higher activity levels in the evening, delayed sleep onset, and reduced total amount of sleep per night.

EPIGENETIC MODIFICATIONS

Epigenetics is arguably the most rapidly evolving field in all of biology. It involves heritable genetic changes that are caused by factors other than changes in the DNA sequence, most notably involving DNA methylation and histone modification, which regulates gene transcription. Stress in general and childhood trauma in particular has been shown to be associated with epigenetic modifications, which may increase the risk of developing mood disorders. For example, histone remodeling of the brain-derived neurotrophic factor (BDNF) gene has been suggested to play a role in the development of depression.[24] In a 2006 study, social defeat stress in mice was followed by a 4-week treatment with the TCA imipramine. Defeat stress was associated with downregulation of BDNF gene transcription, which was reversed with imipramine treatment.[24] Other epigenetic studies examined changes in the neuron-specific glucocorticoid receptor (NR3C1) promoter region. McGowan and colleagues[25] obtained postmortem hippocampus samples from 12 suicide victims with a history of childhood abuse and compared them with both 12 suicide victims without a history of childhood abuse and 12 controls. They found an increased level of NR3C1 promoter site methylation, along with a decreased expression of overall glucocorticoid receptor mRNA in the suicide victims with a history of childhood abuse compared with the other groups. Recently the authors' group reported that the risk allele of the FKBP5 gene that mediates the risk for PTSD after child abuse or neglect acts via epigenetic regulation (methylation).[13]

There have been inconsistent findings in relation to BDNF and bipolar disorder. A meta-analysis conducted by Lin[26] concluded that peripheral BDNF levels are lower in patients with bipolar disorder during manic and depressed episodes but not in euthymic states. They also reported that BDNF levels increase after treatment of manic episodes. Fernandes and colleagues[27] also carried out a meta-analysis, including 13 case-control studies that measured BDNF levels in depression, mania, or euthymia states. Similar to Lin's findings, BDNF levels were significantly lower in depressed and manic episodes but normal during euthymic states. Fernandes and colleagues[28] suggested that BDNF concentrations may be used to discriminate MDD versus bipolar disorder. More work is clearly indicated.

PREDICTORS OF TREATMENT RESPONSE

There is a pressing need to identify biomarkers, not only to aid in identifying at-risk groups and to aid in diagnosis if depression but to also predict treatment response. In order to be successful, this will require, in the authors' view, a far better understanding of the pathophysiology of these disorders. It is of paramount importance to determine if there are 5, 10, 50, or 200 distinct endophenotypes of MDD. Nevertheless, progress is beginning to be made. McGrath and colleagues[29] randomized a small group of depressed patients to treatment with either escitalopram or cognitive-behavior therapy (CBT). They obtained a brain PET scan to measure brain glucose metabolism at baseline and then repeated the PET scan after the treatment intervention. Insula hypometabolism was associated with a good response to CBT and poor response to escitalopram, whereas insula hypermetabolism was associated with remission to escitalopram and poor response to CBT. Functional MRI (fMRI) has also been used as a biomarker to identify treatment response in MDD. A recent systematic review conducted by Dichter and colleagues[30] examined the use of fMRI in this regard and concluded that there is an association between increased connectivity between the frontal lobe and limbic system and response to antidepressant treatment. They also implicated visual recognition circuits, including the lingual gyrus, middle occipital gyrus, fusiform gyrus, and cuneus, in distinguishing treatment-resistant and treatment-responsive depressed patients. Additionally, the subcallosal cingulate gyrus was implicated in response to treatment with antidepressants and also to transcranial magnetic stimulation. A recent comprehensive review[31] summarizes the practice of neuroimaging in predicting treatment response in MDD.

Etkin and colleagues[32] tested cognitive and emotional capacities in the following domains to test whether or not they can be used as biomarkers for response to antidepressants: psychomotor, executive, memory-attention, processing speed, inhibitory, and emotional functions. In the international study to predict optimized treatment – in depression (iSPOT-D) study, 1008 patients diagnosed with MDD (665 of completed patients were matched to 336 controls) were randomized to escitalopram, sertraline, or venlafaxine. Approximately one-quarter of the cases exhibited cognitive impairment across all domains, and those patients responded very poorly to treatment. Within this same subgroup, the 16-item Quick Inventory of Depressive Symptomatology predicted remission after escitalopram treatment only with a 72% accuracy. Other important emerging areas of predictors of response as well as defining biologically homogenous subtypes of depression include markers of inflammation, subclinical hypothyroidism, and gonadal steroid dysregulation, to name a few.

SUMMARY

Some of the latest advances in personalized psychiatry with future research directions are discussed in this article. As previously indicated, many factors contribute to the phenotypic psychiatric profile in individual patients. These overlapping factors include but are not limited to genetics, epigenetics, central nervous system circuit alterations, family history, past personal history, environmental influences including early life stress, and more recent life stressors. The authors also discuss the role of pharmacogenomics, particularly in the CYP450 enzyme system in relation to treatment response. Despite some promising advances in personalized medicine in psychiatry, it is still in its early phases of development. Further research is required in order to develop tools that will impact clinical practice.

FINANCIAL DISCLOSURES

Dr C.B. Nemeroff discloses the following:

Research/Grants: National Institutes of Health.

Consulting (last 3 years): Xhale, Takeda, SK Pharma, Shire, Roche, Lilly, Allergan, Mitsubishi Tanabe Pharma Development America, Taisho Pharmaceutical Inc, Lundbeck, Prismic Pharmaceuticals, Clintara LLC, Total Pain Solutions, and Gerson Lehrman Group Healthcare & Biomedical Council.

Stockholder: Xhale, Celgene, Seattle Genetics, Abbvie, and Titan Pharmaceuticals.

Scientific advisory boards: American Foundation for Suicide Prevention, Brain and Behavior Research Foundation (formerly named National Alliance for Research on Schizophrenia and Depression), Xhale, Anxiety Disorders Association of America, Skyland Trail, Clintara LLC, and RiverMend Health LLC.

Board of directors: American Foundation for Suicide Prevention, Gratitude America, and Anxiety Disorders Association of America.

Income sources or equity of $10,000 or more: American Psychiatric Publishing, Inc, Xhale, Clintara, CME Outfitters, and Takeda.

Patents: Method and devices for transdermal delivery of lithium (US 6,375,990B1); method of assessing antidepressant drug therapy via transport inhibition of monoamine neurotransmitters by ex vivo assay (US 7,148,027B2).

Speakers Bureau: None.

REFERENCES

1. Kessler RC, McGonagle KA, Zhao S, et al. Lifetime and 12-month prevalence of DSM-III-R psychiatric disorders in the United States. Results from the National Comorbidity Survey. Arch Gen Psychiatry 1994;51:8–19.
2. Pratt LA, Brody DJ, Gu Q. Antidepressant use in persons aged 12 and over: United States, 2005–2006. NCHS data brief, no 76. Hyattsville (MD): National Center for Health Statistics; 2011.
3. Trivedi MH, Rush AJ, Wisniewski SR, et al, STAR*D Study Team. Evaluation of outcomes with citalopram for depression using measurement-based care in STAR*D: implications for clinical practice. Am J Psychiatry 2006;163:28–40.
4. Smoller JW, Finn CT. Family, twin, and adoption studies of bipolar disorder. Am J Med Genet C Semin Med Genet 2003;123C(1):48–58.
5. Thakur M, Grossman I, McCroy DC, et al. Review of evidence for genetic testing for CYP450 polymorphisms in management of patients with nonpsychotic depression with selective serotonin reuptake inhibitors. Genet Med 2007;9:826–35.
6. Hoefgen B, Schulze TG, Ohlraun S, et al. The power of sample size and homogenous sampling: association between the 5-HTTLPR serotonin transporter polymorphism and major depressive disorder. Biol Psychiatry 2005;57(3):247–51.
7. Caspi A, Sugdon K, Moffitt TE, et al. Influence of life stress on depression: moderation by a polymorphism in the 5-HTT gene. Science 2003;301:386–9.

8. Gatt JM, Williams LM, Schofield PR, et al. Impact of the HTR3A gene with early life trauma on emotional brain networks and depressed mood. Depress Anxiety 2010;27(8):752–9.

9. Gatt JM, Nemeroff CB, Schofield PR, et al. Early life stress combined with serotonin 3A receptor and brain-derived neurotrophic factor valine 66 to methionine genotypes impacts emotional brain and arousal correlates of risk for depression. Biol Psychiatry 2010;68(9):818–24.

10. Myers AJ, Nemeroff CB. New vistas in the management of treatment refractory psychiatric disorders: genomics and personalized medicine. Focus 2010;8: 525–35.

11. Binder E, Salyakina D, Lichtner P, et al. Polymorphisms in FKBP5 are associated with increased recurrence of depressive episodes and rapid response to antidepressant treatment. Nat Genet 2004;36:1319–25.

12. Brent D, Melhem N, Ferrell R, et al. Association of FKBP5 polymorphisms with suicidal events in the treatment of resistant depression in adolescents (TORDIA) study. Am J Psychiatry 2010;167(2):190–7.

13. Klengal T, Mehta D, Anacker C, et al. Allele-specific FKBP5 DNA demethylation mediates gene-childhood trauma interactions. Nat Neurosci 2013;16:33–41.

14. Liu Z, Zhu F, Wang G, et al. Association of corticotropin-releasing hormone receptor1 gene SNP and haplotype with major depression. Neurosci Lett 2006;404(3): 358–62.

15. Bradley R, Binder E, Epstein MP, et al. Influence of child abuse on adult depression: moderation by the corticotropin-releasing hormone receptor gene. Arch Gen Psychiatry 2008;65(2):190–200.

16. Claes S, Villafuerte S, Forsgen T, et al. The corticotropin-releasing hormone binding protein is associated with major depression in a population from Northern Sweden. Biol Psychiatry 2003;54:867–72.

17. Van Den Eede F, Venken T, Del-Favero J, et al. Single nucleotide polymorphism analysis of corticotropin-releasing factor-binding protein gene in recurrent major depressive disorder. Psychiatry Res 2007;153(1):17–25.

18. Binder EB, Owens MJ, Liu W, et al. Association of polymorphisms in genes regulating the corticotropin-releasing factor system with antidepressant treatment response. Arch Gen Psychiatry 2010;67(4):369–79.

19. Ellenbogen MA, Hodgins S, Walker CD, et al. Daytime cortisol and stress reactivity in the offspring of parent with bipolar disorder. Psychoneuroendocrinology 2006;31(10):1164–80.

20. Willour VL, Chen H, Toolan J, et al. Family-based association of FKBP5 in bipolar disorder. Mol Psychiatry 2009;14:261–8.

21. Mansour HA, Wood J, Logue T, et al. Association study of eight circadian genes with bipolar I disorder, schizoaffective disorder and schizophrenia. Genes Brain Behav 2006;5(2):150–7.

22. Shi J, Wittke-Thompson JK, Badner JA, et al. Clock genes may influence bipolar disorder susceptibility and dysfunctional circadian rhythm. Am J Med Genet B Neuropsychiatr Genet 2008;147B(7):1047–55.

23. Benedetti F, Dallaspezia S, Fulgosi MC, et al. Actimetric evidence that CLOCK 3111 T/C SNP influences sleep and activity patterns in patients affected by bipolar depression. Am J Med Genet B Neuropsychiatr Genet 2007;144B(5): 631–5.

24. Tsankova NM, Berton O, Renthal W, et al. Sustained hippocampal chromatin regulation in a mouse model of depression and antidepressant action. Nat Neurosci 2006;9:519–25.

25. McGowan PO, Sasaki A, D'Alessio AC, et al. Epigenetic regulation of the gluco-corticoid receptor in human brain associated with childhood abuse. Nat Neurosci 2009;12(3):342–8.
26. Lin PY. State-dependent decrease in levels of brain-derived neurotrophic factor in bipolar disorders: a meta-analytic study. Neurosci Lett 2009;466:139–43.
27. Fernandes BS, Gama CS, Ceresér KM, et al. Brain-derived neurotrophic factor as a state-marker of mood episodes in bipolar disorders: a systematic review and meta-regression analysis. J Psychiatr Res 2011;45:995–1004.
28. Fernandes BS, Gama CS, Kauer-Sant'Anna M, et al. Serum brain-derived neuro-trophic factor in bipolar and unipolar depression: a potential adjunctive tool for differential diagnosis. J Psychiatr Res 2009;43:1200–4.
29. McGrath CL, Kelley ME, Holtzheimer PE, et al. Toward a neuroimaging treatment selection biomarker for major depressive disorder. JAMA Psychiatry 2013;70(8): 821–9.
30. Dichter GS, Gibbs D, Smoski MJ. A systematic review of relations between resting-state functional-MRI and treatment response in major depressive disor-der. J Affect Disord 2014;172C:8–17.
31. Phillips ML, Chase HW, Sheline YI, et al. Identifying predictors, moderators, and mediators of antidepressant response in major depressive disorder: neuroimag-ing approaches. Am J Psychiatry 2015;172:124–38.
32. Etkin A, Patenaude B, Song YJ, et al. A cognitive-emotional biomarker for predict-ing remission with antidepressant medications: a report from the iSPOT-D trial. Neuropsychopharmacology 2015;40(6):1332–42.

Psychotherapy and Psychosocial Treatment

Recent Advances and Future Directions

Eric M. Plakun, MD

KEYWORDS

- Psychotherapy • Psychosocial treatment • Treatment resistance • Epigenetics
- Comorbidity • Early adversity • Personality disorders • Parity

KEY POINTS

- Psychiatry has become increasingly biologically focused.
- Psychotherapy and psychosocial treatment are effective forms of treatment of a range of individual and complex comorbid disorders.
- The future role of psychotherapy and psychosocial treatment depends on the unfolding of policy and legal issues and on the field's ability to address the following 3 false assumptions related to biological reductionism:
  - Genes = disease.
  - Patients present with single disorders that respond to single evidence-based treatments.
  - The best treatments are pills.

Hundreds of studies suggest that behavioral, psychodynamic, and other forms of psychotherapy and psychosocial treatment are effective for numerous individual and complex comorbid disorders; that the combination of medications and therapy is often better than either alone; and that brain changes associated with psychotherapy allow therapy responders to be differentiated from nonresponders based on imaging.[1–5] In spite of evidence of effectiveness, current trends in psychiatry have tended to minimize the role of psychotherapy and psychosocial treatment in psychiatry. Psychiatrists increasingly focus their practice on diagnosis and psychopharmacological treatment. This focus is a response to several forces, including discovery of neurobiological correlates of mental disorders, a shift toward the medical model as the dominant paradigm for understanding and treating patients and away from the biopsychosocial model, the effectiveness of contemporary psychotropic drugs, the hope that research will reveal genes that underlie major mental disorders, the considerable influence and

No disclosures.
Austen Riggs Center, 25 Main Street, Stockbridge, MA 01262-0962, USA
E-mail address: Eric.Plakun@AustenRiggs.net

Psychiatr Clin N Am 38 (2015) 405–418
http://dx.doi.org/10.1016/j.psc.2015.05.012
0193-953X/15/$ – see front matter

financial power of the pharmaceutical industry, and the transformation of much of reimbursement for psychiatric services into a managed care model.

Forces shaping contemporary psychiatry

- Discovery of neurobiological correlates of mental disorders
- The medical model as dominant paradigm
- Effectiveness of contemporary psychotropic drugs
- Hope that research will reveal genes that underlie major mental disorders
- Influence and financial power of the pharmaceutical industry
- Transformation of reimbursement to a managed care model

Concurrently there has been a decline in provision of psychotherapy by psychiatrists. Mojtabai and Olfson[6] reported that in 1996, almost 44% of psychiatric office visits included psychotherapy, whereas 10 years later in 2004–2005, only 29% of office visits included therapy. A 2010 APIRE (American Psychiatric Institute for Research and Education) survey carried out in collaboration with the American Psychiatric Association (APA) Committee on Psychotherapy by Psychiatrists showed a 20% decline in therapy by psychiatrists among 394 respondents to an online survey.[7] In 2002, about 68% of psychiatric sessions involved therapy with or without medications, whereas in 2010, this was down to 48%. Psychiatrists who administered therapy tended to be older than 65 years, white, and US medical school graduates. Almost 50% or more of their patients were self-pay or privately insured patients, and these psychiatrists were reimbursed comparably for psychotherapy and pharmacotherapy and freer of utilization review burdens. These psychiatrists were also less likely to report that medical debt affected their practice choices than those who practiced less psychotherapy.

Even before these studies documented the decline in provision of psychotherapy by psychiatrists, organized psychiatry recognized these trends. In 1996, the APA established a Committee on Psychotherapy by Psychiatrists, although this group was terminated in 2009 along with most other APA components because of financial constraints. Outside the APA, the Psychiatry Residency Review Committee (RRC) of the Accreditation Council for Graduate Medical Education (ACGME) declared psychotherapy an area of critical concern in residency training, requiring that 3 distinct schools of psychotherapy (supportive therapy, cognitive behavioral therapy [CBT], and psychodynamic therapy) be taught to residents to a measurable level of competence.

Despite evidence of the effectiveness of psychotherapy and psychosocial treatment, the place of psychotherapy and psychosocial treatment in psychiatry is endangered. The future of psychotherapy and psychosocial treatment in psychiatry depends on matters of social policy and law and on whether psychiatry broadens its biological, medical model focus to a "both/and" biopsychosocial perspective. Should psychiatry's future direction continue to focus on a reductionistic "bio-bio-bio" model, as former APA president Steven Sharfstein provocatively called it in his inaugural address, then the practice of psychotherapy and psychosocial treatment may be forfeited to other professional disciplines. However, given the effectiveness and cost-effectiveness of psychotherapy and psychosocial treatment and the unique medical training of psychiatrists, this version of the future would be a serious loss for the field of psychiatry and for patients.[1]

POLICY AND LAW

The Affordable Care Act (ACA), with its focus on medical homes and the creation of large accountable care organizations, will transform the practice of medicine and the treatment of mental disorders—assuming the ACA survives Supreme Court challenges and a Republican Congress. The ACA, which is linked to the Mental Health Parity and Addiction Equity Act of 2008 (or parity law), requires that insurance policies purchased through ACA insurance exchanges include mental health and substance abuse coverage as part of the essential benefit package.

Parity requires that coverage for the treatment of mental disorders be comparable to that for medical disorders. Any treatment limitations imposed on mental health or substance abuse benefits that are not comparable to or are more stringent than those applied to medical and surgical benefits are impermissible. Such impermissible treatment limitations may be quantitative (eg, arbitrarily limiting dollar amounts or numbers of sessions) or nonquantitative (eg, requiring prior authorization for mental health but not for medical benefits). Parity should put an end to disparate annual or lifetime dollar limits for mental health coverage, annual caps on numbers of visits or visit frequencies, medical management techniques (including prior authorization and concurrent utilization review procedures) not required for authorization of medical care, and blanket exclusions of medically necessary services and levels of care (like residential treatment) for covered conditions. Yet, although parity has been the law of the land since 2008, it has not been fully implemented by insurers.

Several class action lawsuits have been filed that are relevant to implementation of parity and thus to future directions in reimbursement for psychotherapy and psychosocial treatment. Among the allegations these suits make concerning access to psychotherapy and psychosocial treatment are that, in a way not comparable to medical or surgical benefits, insurance companies impose arbitrary and excessively stringent medical necessity guidelines, impose arbitrary limits in session numbers and high-utilization review burdens, and exclude coverage for personality disorders—when these are disorders listed in *Diagnostic and Statistical Manual of Mental Disorders* (DSM), have a practice guideline identifying psychotherapy as the mainstay of treatment, are known to carry a substantial risk of suicide, and robustly predicted that comorbid disorders such as major depression will be refractory to treatment.[8]

A legal analysis of the lawsuits and their likely impact on implementation of full mental health parity is beyond the scope of this article, but their outcome will have a profound effect on the future availability of and reimbursement for psychotherapy and psychosocial treatment.

Anticipating greater access to psychosocial treatment under parity, in 2014, the Institute of Medicine established a committee to study psychosocial interventions for the treatment of mental disorders. In 2015, this committee will issue a report that will address supraordinate problems of interest to Medicare, Medicaid, and the insurance industry, as well as the mental health disciplines, including defining quality measures for monitoring provision of psychosocial treatment to large populations.

A comprehensive overview of issues relevant to the practice of psychotherapy and psychiatry under the ACA and parity legislation was the subject of a special issue of *Psychodynamic Psychiatry*, and includes articles written by members of the Group for the Advancement of Psychiatry Psychotherapy Committee, with a preface by former Congressman Patrick Kennedy, author of the parity law.[9]

PSYCHIATRY'S FALSE ASSUMPTIONS

The future of psychotherapy and psychosocial treatment depends in part on psychiatry's ability to notice and correct its often biologically reductionistic stance and move toward a "both/and" biopsychosocial model. Part of psychiatry's drift away from a biopsychosocial stance has been the result of 3 false assumptions that often remain unquestioned, although emerging evidence reveals their inaccuracy. Noticing and naming them is not offered as an antipsychiatry perspective, but rather as a call from within psychiatry to notice where there is a drift away from a model that optimally serves patients. The false assumptions are that (1) genes = disease or that genes are more important than environmental factors in causing mental disorders, (2) most patients present with single disorders that respond to specific, evidence-based treatments, and (3) the best treatments are pills. These assumptions play an important role in the future of psychotherapy and psychosocial treatment in psychiatry.

Contemporary psychiatry has tended to make 3 false assumptions

- Genes = disease
- Patients present with single disorders that respond to specific, evidence-based treatments
- The best treatments are pills

False Assumption #1: Genes = Disease

Mental disorders are clearly heritable. Genetics teaches that there are 2 kinds of genes: those that make proteins and those that regulate other genes—often in response to the environment. Although it was hoped that the sequencing of the human genome would reveal the genetic underpinnings of common mental disorders, the human genome instead is a set of rough plans rather than detailed blueprints for a person or for a disorder.

Over a hundred relevant genetic loci have been identified in schizophrenia, indicating that the heritability of this and other psychotic disorders is far more complex and multifactorial than was expected. Single nucleotide polymorphisms (SNPs) have been found that are associated with medical disorders, such as some cancers, inflammatory bowel disease, and type 2 diabetes. However, even in large samples, genome-wide association studies (GWAS) of depression and depressive symptoms do not reveal meaningful SNPs that illuminate the genetic underpinnings of this common disorder.[10,11] No biomarkers for depression have been found to date, and some have likened the search to that for the Holy Grail.

Meanwhile, Tully and colleagues[12] report that the presence of maternal major depressive disorder during childrearing increased the risk of major depressive disorder in both adopted and nonadopted adolescents. Other studies of early adversity provide support for the notion that early adversity is an "enviromarker," associated with high risk of mental, substance use and medical disorders.[13,14] Clearly, environmental factors matter a great deal in the cause of depression. Also, it is reasonable to extend this to the importance of environmental factors such as psychotherapy and psychosocial treatment used in the treatment of depression.

Maternal major depressive disorder during childrearing significantly increased the risk of major depressive disorder in both adopted and nonadopted adolescents.

Although the issue is not fully settled and the amount of variance in the presence of depression accounted for is small, research into polymorphisms of the serotonin transporter promoter gene are heuristically important.[15–18] The first such study by Caspi and colleagues[15] suggests that homozygous short alleles are associated with not only an increased risk of depression under early adverse environmental conditions but also the best outcomes overall in the absence of early adversity.[16] Belsky and colleagues[16] offer a potentially paradigm shifting observation that what are thought of as "vulnerability genes may actually function more like plasticity genes, resulting in certain individuals being more responsive than others to both positive and negative environmental experiences." The determined medical model focus on a vulnerability model of disease, rather than a plasticity model, seems to be a genuine blind spot in psychiatry. A plasticity model, with its links to concepts such as resilience, makes room for the importance of remote and recent beneficial environments and relationships and thus highlights the potential value of psychosocial treatment.

The heuristic value of attending to plasticity versus vulnerability in the thinking about mental disorders provides a link to concepts such as resilience.

Environmental factors interact with genes to shape individuals by turning genes on and off, so it is more gene-by-environment (G × E) or epigenetics than genes alone. And epigenetic, the author proposes, is another way to say biopsychosocial. As British psychotherapy researcher Holmes[19] puts it, phenotype does not come just from genes, but, rather, $Phe = GE^2$. Here, the researcher mirrors Einstein's transformative $E = mc^2$ equation that taught that energy and matter are different manifestations of the same thing and that even a small amount of matter can produce a huge amount of energy. In his transformative $Phe = GE^2$ equation, Holmes[19] suggests that phenotype is a function not only of genes but also of the environment squared (ie, a function of both the early and recent environments).

According to Holmes:

- $Phe = GE^2$
- Phenotype is a function of genes and of the environment squared (ie, both the early and recent environments)

Recently, there has been an effort to include environmental factors in the search for biomarkers. In the Biomarkers of Intergenerational Risk for Depression model, biological and environmental factors are tallied together to create a predictive score for the risk of depression.[20] The future of psychotherapy and psychosocial research in psychiatry will depend on efforts like this that correct false assumptions and refocus on the important contribution of environmental factors in a biopsychosocial model.

- Multiple, large GWAS studies have not found relevant SNPs associated with depression
- Although it is an important effort, no biomarkers for depression have been identified
- Early adversity seems to be an enviromarker of mental disorders
- Epigenetic is another way of saying biopsychosocial

False Assumption #2: Patients Present with Single Disorders that Respond to Specific, Evidence-Based Treatments

Practice guidelines and randomized trials generally assume that most patients have single disorders that respond to evidenced-based treatments, which are tested in carefully selected noncomorbid samples. How well does this assumption fit the data in, for example, mood disorders?

In the case of bipolar disorder, prescription of a mood stabilizer and/or neuroleptic is not associated with straightforward recovery of functioning—anymore than prescription of insulin in type 1 diabetes mellitus is all that is required to control this disorder. In fact, in the Systematic Treatment Enhancement Program for Bipolar Disorder, only 58% of index mood cases recovered within 6 months and half had recurrences within 2 years.[21] There is something more to bipolar disorder than the need for a medication.

Similarly, in major depressive disorder, the Sequenced Treatment Alternatives to Relieve Depression (STAR*D) study shows that many patients fail to respond to initial treatment of depression or to switch or augmentation strategies, including CBT.[22] The analysis by Wisniewski and colleagues[23] of the STAR*D sample revealed that 78% had comorbid conditions or suicidal ideation that would have excluded them from randomized trials. These comorbid patients were more intolerant of medication, had lower rates of treatment response (39% vs 52%), and had lower remission rates from depressive symptoms (25% vs 34%). This experience matches that of many clinicians that real-world patients who present to clinicians for treatment have more comorbidity and show less response to evidence-based treatments than those on whom the treatments were tested.

A close look at the STAR*D sample suggests the following facts

- Almost 78% had comorbid conditions or suicidal ideation that would exclude them from randomized trials
- This group was more intolerant of medication
- There were lower rates of treatment response (39% vs 52%)
- There were lower remission rates from depressive symptoms (25% vs 34%)

Other evidence highlights the importance of personality disorder comorbidity in mood disorders. In the Collaborative Longitudinal Personality Disorders Study (CLPS), personality disorders were found to adversely affect major depressive disorder outcome, to cause persistent functional impairment, to cause extensive treatment utilization, and to be associated with significant suicide risk.[8,24,25] Personality disorders, especially borderline personality disorder, "robustly predicted persistence" of major depressive disorder.[8] Skodol and colleagues[8] suggest that assessment and treatment of personality disorders is essential in patients with major depressive disorder. The mainstay of treatment of personality disorders is psychotherapy. However, in a field focused on single disorders, the most frequent personality disorder diagnosis made with DSM (Fourth Edition) was deferred. It is unlikely that DSM (Fifth Edition), with its removal of Axis II specifically addressing the presence of personality disorders, will fare any better when it comes to recognition of comorbid personality disorders.

A perspective from the CLPS

- Personality disorders, especially borderline personality disorder, robustly predicted persistence of major depressive disorder
- Assessment and treatment of personality disorders is essential in patients with major depressive disorder
- The mainstay of treatment of personality disorders is psychotherapy

Hence, there is substantial evidence that most patients present with multiple disorders and that comorbidity, especially personality disorder comorbidity, compromises response to evidence-based treatments designed and tested for single disorders. The future of psychotherapy and psychosocial treatment in psychiatry—and the outcomes of patients—will depend on psychiatrists' ability to make a midcourse correction of this false assumption about patients and the treatment they need.

False Assumption #3: The Best Treatments Are Pills

Contemporary psychotropic medications are undoubtedly effective and powerful treatment agents, but knowledge is being gained about their limitations. The efficacy of antidepressants has been overestimated by about a third when all studies are considered, and antidepressant efficacy studies are confounded by high placebo response rates.[26,27] Even when effective, antidepressants may leave patients symptomatic and understandably seeking more treatment.[28] Shedler[29] notes that the effect sizes of psychotherapy are greater than the effect sizes of medications. There is certainly an "apples to oranges" quality to Shedler's[29] comparison, because medication trials generally had larger samples, but the direction of the difference interestingly favors psychotherapy over medications. In schizophrenia, the Clinical Antipsychotic Trials of Intervention Effectiveness (CATIE) study demonstrates that many patients do not find the benefits of medications worth their side effects.[30]

Studies suggest the limits of medications

- Efficacy of antidepressants has been overestimated by a third when unpublished trials are considered
- Antidepressant efficacy studies are confounded by high placebo response rates
- Effect sizes of psychotherapy are greater than the effect sizes of medications
- In schizophrenia, the CATIE study demonstrates that many patients do not find the benefits of medications worth their side effects

Meanwhile, there is evidence that patients with chronic and complex comorbid depression, perhaps especially those with histories of early adversity, respond well to CBT and long-term psychodynamic psychotherapy.[31–33] Nemeroff and colleagues[33] conclude, "Our findings suggest that psychotherapy may be an essential element in the treatment of patients with chronic forms of major depression and a history of childhood trauma."

HOW FALSE ASSUMPTIONS SHAPE THE FUTURE OF PSYCHOTHERAPY AND PSYCHOSOCIAL TREATMENT

Each of the false assumptions risks blinding psychiatrists to the implications of emerging research and depriving patients of what they need, which is treatment that attends to biology as well as to psychosocial factors in the causation and treatment of mental disorders. The future of psychotherapy and psychosocial treatment in psychiatry will depend on the extent to which there is a return to an authentic "both/and" biopsychosocial perspective.

Psychiatrists as a profession, their patients, their families, and society all pay a price for these false assumptions that shape contemporary psychiatry. As a profession, the price that psychiatrists pay for the false assumptions is heuristic blindness, the emergence of treatment resistance, and loss of psychotherapy and psychosocial treatment as part of the training, identity, and practice of psychiatrists.

The price that psychiatrists pay as a profession for the false assumptions

- The heuristic blindness of biological reductionism
- Treatment resistance
- Loss of psychotherapy and psychosocial treatment as part of the training, identity, and practice of psychiatrists

---

Heuristic blindness focuses psychiatrists on vulnerability rather than on plasticity. Biological reductionism can blind them to the implications of emerging data because the false assumptions limit their thinking about cause and treatment. There is an apt old aphorism that, "If all you have is a hammer, everything looks like a nail."

An example of psychiatry's heuristic blindness is avoidance of expert consensus in thinking about clinical issues, preferring reliance on randomized controlled trials as the gold standard of research. While it is far easier to do randomized trials of medications than of psychosocial treatments, this preference is part of a longing to make psychiatry a robustly evidence-based medical specialty. However, the desire to be as solidly evidence-based as other medical specialties risks missing an important reality about them. Tricoci and colleagues[34] studied the 2711 cardiovascular practice guidelines of the American College of Cardiology and the American Heart Association.[34] Only 11% of the cardiology treatment recommendations were supported by the highest level of statistical evidence and 48% were based on expert consensus.

Another price that psychiatrists pay for biological reductionism is the contribution of a narrow unimodal perspective on treatment to the growth of treatment resistant disorders. Mintz and Belnap[35,36] report that during a recent 20-year period there was a 25% increase in the number of Medline citations throughout psychiatry. During the same period, there was an 800% increase in citations on treatment-resistant psychiatric disorders. Since 2011, three books have been published on treatment resistant disorders.[37–39] Substantial percentages of all mental disorders fail to respond to treatment, so it is notable that APA practice guidelines do not systematically address treatment resistance. We are also learning about the costs of treatment resistance, with overall medical costs 19 times higher for treatment resistant depression than for more treatment responsive depression.[40] These costs do not take into account lost economic productivity, the suffering associated with lost quality of life, or premature death due to suicide and heart disease that are associated with treatment-resistant depression. Psychiatrists are learning that contributions to treatment resistance in mood disorders come from comorbidity, especially personality disorder comorbidity, and from the impact of early adverse experiences.

To be sure, correcting these false assumptions would not lead to the end of treatment resistance, but the limited scope of a biologically reductionistic stance increases the likelihood that patients will receive and fail a limited treatment approach. In this way, the resistance in treatment resistance can be located in the stance and in the limitations of treatments—and not in patients.[37] Algorithms for treatment-resistant depression, for example, may offer a rational sequence of trials of medications and other biological treatments, without addressing research that psychosocial factors such as early adversity contribute to treatment resistance and likely need a psychosocial intervention, or that personality disorder comorbidity increases the likelihood of treatment resistance, while the mainstay of treatment of personality disorders is psychotherapy rather than medication.

> The resistance in treatment resistance may be located in the biologically reductionistic stance and in the limitations of treatments—and not in patients.

In addition, if psychiatrists lose psychotherapy skills and drift toward a view of patients as passive receptor sites for molecules, they will risk losing the capacity to engage with patients and their families in nuanced ways that foster an optimal therapeutic alliance and that mobilize the patient's agency and authority in treatment. Readiness to change[41] and the strength of the alliance[42] are key factors in how and whether patients will respond to treatment. Recognition of the important role of relationships and of meaning in psychotropic drug efficacy has led to the emergence of a psychodynamic psychopharmacology that attends not only to the biochemical effects of medications but also to their meaning to patients and treaters—an example of a "both/and" biopsychosocial perspective on treatment.[35,36]

> If psychiatrists lose psychotherapy skills, they risk losing the capacity to engage with patients and their families in nuanced ways that foster an optimal therapeutic alliance and that mobilize the patient's agency and authority in treatment.

Patients and their families also pay a price for the false assumptions. This price includes worse outcomes, wasted lives, and suicide. Society pays the price of squandered resources for treatment and squandered opportunity to study and use psychosocial treatments. The National Institute of Mental Health focus on brain research often seems far removed from offering direct benefit to patients, although its effort to define Research Domain Criteria is a helpful reframing of diagnosis that may be useful in understanding gene-by-environment interactions.

If the false assumptions and the prices that psychiatrists pay for them are taken seriously, and appropriate midcourse corrections are made, the future of psychiatry will include a greater openness to the implications of psychosocial factors on the causation and in the treatment of psychiatric disorders. To the extent this happens, parts of psychiatry that have long focused on environmental factors in complex and nuanced ways may return to the mainstream of psychiatric treatment, including that intersection between psychoanalytic theory and psychiatry known as psychodynamic psychiatry.

> If these false assumptions and the prices that psychiatrists pay for them are taken seriously, and appropriate midcourse corrections are made, the future of psychiatry will include a greater openness to the implications of psychosocial factors on the causation and in the treatment of psychiatric disorders.

Perhaps there are some reasons for optimism. Although the APA terminated its Committee on Psychotherapy by Psychiatrists, APA member psychiatrists have used the APA bylaws to establish a Psychotherapy Caucus from the grass roots up that has grown from 10 initial members to over 250 members by mid-2015. Although some psychiatrists with a biopsychosocial perspective have worried that, in its focus on the brain, psychiatry has lost its mind, this may be shifting. For example, APA's "New Look," introduced at the 2015 annual meeting, is "American Psychiatric Association—Medical leadership for mind, brain, and body," and the theme of the 2015 annual meeting was "Psychiatry: Integrating Body and Mind, Heart and Soul." Mind seems to be back in psychiatry!

Whether the future will include greater recognition of the importance and value of psychotherapy and psychosocial treatment will depend, too, on whether those interested in practicing and researching psychotherapy and psychosocial treatment can put aside internecine rivalries between schools of therapy to attend to common factors across schools of therapy that are associated with desired outcomes. While manualized therapies with evidence of efficacy proliferate, including dialectical behavior therapy (DBT), CBT, schema therapy, transference-focused psychotherapy, panic-focused psychodynamic psychotherapy, mentalization-based therapy, and others, few clinicians will become competent in providing any one of these, while the number of patients needing treatment is great.

One practical solution has been the delineation of common factors shared by therapies, while also recognizing differentiating features. A common factors approach is arguably a crucial part of evidence-based practice, along with empirically supported treatment.[43] Approaches to delineating common factors across forms of therapy have begun to make useful contributions to clinicians struggling to treat difficult patients, such as those with borderline personality disorder who struggle with suicide.[44–46] It may be easier to teach common factors to residents and practicing clinicians than to have them master a manualized therapy.

Helping the pendulum swing back toward recognition of the importance of psychosocial treatment and a biopsychosocial perspective will require those committed to such treatment to speak a common language rather than focus on competition between schools of therapy. A big tent model is needed that allows us to engage in conversation with colleagues who have focused nearly exclusively on the biology of disorders.

EDUCATION AND THE FUTURE OF PSYCHOTHERAPY AND PSYCHOSOCIAL TREATMENT

Psychotherapy and psychosocial treatment face formidable educational challenges. Despite ACGME RRC psychotherapy training requirements, psychotherapy training is quite variable around the nation. In some major cities, there are many psychotherapeutically sophisticated faculty, but other residency programs lack such faculty. In these programs, the teaching faculty often represents a lost generation of psychiatrists who trained at the height of biological reductionism and before psychotherapy training was identified as an area of critical concern.[47] With some exceptions, then, there is a scarcity of sophisticated teachers, mentors, or role models in psychotherapy in residency programs across the country.[48,49] One cannot teach what one does not know, and one cannot practice what one has not been taught.

One challenge in teaching psychotherapy is the previously referenced competition between teaching faculty representing different schools of therapy. Such internecine struggles can prove confusing to residents. One solution to this problem from a common factors approach is the Y model.[50,51] This psychotherapy teaching model conceptualizes common factors across schools of psychotherapy as located on the stem of a Y and then compares and contrasts the psychodynamic therapy and CBT forks of the Y based on their evidence-based, core distinguishing features.

The future of psychotherapy training will depend on the ability to develop innovative approaches that can supplement on-site psychotherapy training. One such approach is visiting psychotherapy scholar programs such as the Eugene Pumpian-Mindlin Seminar at the University of Oklahoma Health Sciences Center or the Teichner Visiting Psychoanalytic Scholar program funded by the American Academy of Psychoanalysis and Dynamic Psychiatry (AAPDP) and administered by American Association of Directors of Psychiatric Residency Training (AADPRT). Both AAPDP and the Austen Riggs Center offer menus of psychodynamic grand rounds speakers, while leading CBT, DBT, and other therapists often provide grand rounds presentations as well.

New online technologies can also help supplement psychotherapy teaching where a residency program may lack adequate resources. For example, the Psychotherapy Training e-Resources of McMaster University is an online program intended to supplement other psychotherapy training through 11 separate modules representing a range of schools of psychotherapy.[52] For those who are in residency or postresidency and seeking additional training, online programs are available, such as those provided by the Austen Riggs Center, offering free online CME courses focused specifically on psychodynamic psychiatry and psychotherapy.

Innovations in teaching psychotherapy

- Individual residency program support for visiting psychotherapy scholars
- Psychotherapy-focused grand rounds
- AAPDP/AADPRT Teichner Visiting Psychoanalytic Scholar program
- Online resources (eg, psychotherapy training e-resources)

SUMMARY

Psychotherapy and psychosocial treatment are effective forms of treatment of patients with a range of individual and comorbid disorders, and emerging evidence from molecular genetics, psychiatric epidemiology, and clinical research suggests that psychosocial factors are far more important than realized in the causation and treatment of mental disorders. Despite this, psychiatry has drifted away from a biopsychosocial perspective and has tended to minimize psychotherapy and psychosocial treatment; this has an adverse effect on psychiatrist's profession, their patients and their families, and the society.

The future role of psychotherapy and psychosocial treatment depends on several factors. These factors include full implementation of mental health parity, correction of underlying false assumptions that shape treatment, payment priorities, and research. Educational issues include identification and teaching of common factors shared by effective psychosocial therapies, adequate teaching of psychotherapy and psychosocial treatment to trainees and practicing psychiatrists, and reaffirmation by the profession of an authentically biopsychosocial model.

REFERENCES

1. Lazar SG, editor. Psychotherapy is worth it: a comprehensive review of its cost-effectiveness. Washington, DC: American Psychiatric Publishing, Inc; 2010.

2. Butler AC, Chapman JE, Forman EM, et al. The empirical status of cognitive-behavioral therapy: a review of meta-analyses. Clin Psychol Rev 2006;26(1): 17–31.

3. Levy KN, Ehrenthal JC, Yeomans FE, et al. The efficacy of psychotherapy: focus on psychodynamic psychotherapy as an example. Psychodyn Psychiatry 2014; 43(3):377–421.

4. Schwartz JM, Stoessel PW, Baxter LR, et al. Systematic changes in cerebral glucose metabolic rate after successful behavior modification treatment of obsessive-compulsive disorder. Arch Gen Psychiatry 1996;53:109–13.

5. Roffman JL, Witte JM, Tanner AS, et al. Neural predictors of successful brief psychodynamic psychotherapy for persistent depression. Psychother Psychosom 2014;83:364–70.

6. Mojtabai R, Olfson M. National trends in psychotherapy by office-based psychiatrists. Arch Gen Psychiatry 2008;65(8):962–70.

7. Perry JC, West J and Plakun, EM. Why psychiatrists don't do therapy even though it works. Workshop Presentation at APA Institute on Psychiatric Services. New York, October 7, 2012.

8. Skodol AE, Grilo CM, Keyes KM, et al. Relationship of personality disorders to the course of major depressive disorder in a nationally representative sample. Am J Psychiatry 2011;168:257–64.

9. Committee on Psychotherapy of the Group for the Advancement of Psychiatry. Psychotherapy, the Affordable Care Act, and Mental Health Parity: obstacles to implementation. Psychodynamic Psychiatry 2014;42(3):339–551.

10. Major Depressive Disorder Working Group of the Psychiatric GWAS Consortium. A mega-analysis of genome-wide association studies for major depressive disorder. Mol Psychiatry 2012;3:1–15.

11. Hek K, Demirkan A, Lahti J, et al. A genome-wide association study of depressive symptoms. Biol Psychiatry 2013;73:667–78.

12. Tully EC, Iacono WG, McGue M. An adoption study of parental depression as an environmental liability for adolescent depression and childhood disruptive disorders. Am J Psychiatry 2008;165(9):1148–54.

13. Molnar BE, Buka SL, Kessler RC. Child sexual abuse and subsequent results from the National Comorbidity Survey. Am J Public Health 2001;91(5):753–60.

14. Kendler KS, Bulik CM, Silberg J, et al. Childhood sexual abuse and adult psychiatric and substance use disorders in women: an epidemiological and co-twin control analysis. Arch Gen Psychiatry 2000;57:953–9.

15. Caspi A, Sugden K, Moffitt TE, et al. Influence of life stress on depression: moderation by a polymorphism in the 5-HTT gene. Science 2003;301(5631):291–3.

16. Belsky J, Jonassaint C, Pluess M, et al. Vulnerability genes or plasticity genes? Mol Psychiatry 2009;14:746–54.

17. Duncan LE, Keller MC. A critical review of the first ten years of candidate gene-by-environment interaction research in psychiatry. Am J Psychiatry 2011;168: 1041–9.

18. Karg K, Burmeister M, Shedden K, et al. The serotonin transporter promoter variant (5-HTTLPR), stress and depression meta-analysis revisited: evidence of genetic moderation. Arch Gen Psychiatry 2011;68(5):444–54.

19. Holmes J. An attachment model of depression: integrating findings from the mood disorder laboratory. Psychiatry 2013;76(1):68–86.

20. Jacobs RH. Biomarkers for Intergenerational risk for depression: a review of mechanisms in longitudinal high-risk studies. J Affect Disord 2015;175: 494–506.

21. Perlis RH, Ostacher MJ, Patel JK, et al. Predictors of recurrence in bipolar disorder: primary outcomes from the Systematic Treatment Enhancement Program for Bipolar Disorder (STEP-BD). Am J Psychiatry 2006;163:217–24.
22. Thase ME, Friedman ES, Biggs MM, et al. Cognitive therapy versus medication in augmentation and switch strategies as second-step treatments: a STAR*D report. Am J Psychiatry 2007;164:739–52.
23. Wisniewski SR, Rush AJ, Nierenberg AA, et al. Can phase III trial results of antidepressant medications be generalized to clinical practice? A STAR*D report. Am J Psychiatry 2009;166:599–607.
24. Bender DS, Skodol AE, Pagano ME, et al. Prospective assessment of treatment use by patients with personality disorders. Psychiatr Serv 2006;57(2):254–7.
25. Skodol AE, Gunderson JG, Shea MT, et al. The Collaborative Longitudinal Personality Disorders Study (CLPS): overview and implications. J Personal Disord 2005; 19:487–504.
26. Turner EH, Matthews AM, Linardatos E, et al. Selective publication of antidepressant trials and its influence on apparent efficacy. N Engl J Med 2008;358(3): 252–60.
27. Kirsch I, Deacon BJ, Huedo-Medina TB, et al. Initial severity and antidepressant benefits: a meta-analysis of data submitted to the Food and Drug Administration. PLoS Med 2008;5(2):e45.
28. Westen D, Morrison K. A multidimensional meta-analysis of treatments for depression, panic, generalized anxiety disorder: an empirical examination of the status of empirically supported treatments. J Consult Clin Psychol 2001;69: 875–99.
29. Shedler J. The efficacy of psychodynamic therapy. Am Psychol 2010;65(2): 98–109.
30. Lieberman JA, Stroup TS, McEvoy JP, et al. Effectiveness of anti-psychotic drugs in patients with chronic schizophrenia. N Engl J Med 2005;353:1209–23.
31. Leichsenring F, Rabung S. Effectiveness of long-term psychodynamic psychotherapy: a meta-analysis. J Am Med Assoc 2008;300(13):1551–65.
32. Leichsenring F, Rabung S. Long-term psychodynamic psychotherapy in complex mental disorders: update of a meta-analysis. Br J Psychiatry 2011;199:15–22.
33. Nemeroff CB, Heim CM, Thase ME, et al. Differential response to psychotherapy versus pharmacotherapy in patients with chronic forms of major depression and childhood trauma. Proc Natl Acad Sci U S A 2003;100:14293–6.
34. Tricoci P, Allen JM, Kramer JM, et al. Scientific evidence underlying the ACC/AHA clinical practice guidelines. JAMA 2009;301(8):831–41 [Erratum appears in JAMA 2009;301(15):1544].
35. Mintz D, Belnap BA. A view from Riggs: treatment resistance and patient authority. III. What is psychodynamic psychopharmacology? An approach to pharmacologic treatment resistance. J Am Acad Psychoanal Dyn Psychiatry 2006;34: 581–601.
36. Mintz D, Belnap BA. What is psychodynamic psychopharmacology? An approach to pharmacologic treatment resistance. In: Plakun EM, editor. Treatment resistance and patient authority: the Austen Riggs reader. New York; London: Norton Professional Books; 2011. p. 42–65.
37. Plakun EM, editor. Treatment resistance and patient authority: the Austen Riggs reader. New York: Norton Professional Books; 2011.
38. Greden JS, Riba MB, McInnis MG, editors. Treatment resistant depression: a roadmap for effective care. Arlington (VA): American Psychiatric Publishing; 2011.

39. Nemeroff CB. Management of treatment–resistant major psychiatric disorders. New York: Oxford University Press; 2012.

40. Crown WH, Finkelstein S, Berndt ER, et al. The impact of treatment-resistant depression on health care utilization and costs. J Clin Psychiatry 2002;63:963–71.

41. Beitman BD, Beck NC, Denser WE, et al. Patent stage of change predicts outcome in a panic disorder medication trial. Anxiety 1994;1(2):64–9.

42. Horvath AO, Del Re AC, Fluckiger C, et al. Alliance in individual psychotherapy. Psychotherapy 2011;48:9–16.

43. Laska KM, Gurman AS, Wampold BE. Expanding the lens of evidence-based practice in psychotherapy: a common factors perspective. Psychotherapy 2014;51(4):467–81.

44. Weinberg I, Ronningstam E, Goldblatt MJ, et al. Strategies in treatment of suicidality: identification of common and treatment-specific interventions in empirically supported treatment manuals. J Clin Psychiatry 2010;71:699–706.

45. Gunderson J, Links P. Good psychiatric management for borderline personality disorder. Arlington (VA): American Psychiatric Publishing; 2014.

46. Sledge W, Plakun EM, Bauer S, et al, Group for the Advancement of Psychiatry Psychotherapy Committee. Psychotherapy for suicidal patients with borderline personality disorder: an expert consensus review of common factors across five therapies. Borderline Personal Disord Emot Dysregul 2014;1:16. Available at: http://www.bpded.com/content/1/1/16.

47. Plakun EM. Finding psychodynamic psychiatry's lost generation. J Am Acad Psychoanal Dyn Psychiatry 2006;34(1):135–50.

48. Kay J, Myers MF. Current state of psychotherapy training: preparing for the future. Psychodyn Psychiatry 2014;42(3):535–51.

49. Clemens NA, Plakun EM, Lazar SG, et al. Obstacles to early career psychiatrists practicing psychotherapy. Psychodyn Psychiatry 2014;42(3):479–95.

50. Plakun EM, Sudak DM, Goldberg D. The Y model: an integrated, evidence-based approach to teaching psychotherapy competencies. J Psychiatr Pract 2009; 15(1):5–11.

51. Goldberg D, Plakun EM. Teaching psychodynamic psychotherapy with the Y model. Psychodyn Psychiatry 2013;41(1):111–25.

52. Weerasekera P. Psychotherapy Training e-Resources (PTeR): on-line psychotherapy education. Acad Psychiatry 2013;37(1):51–4.

A Shared Molecular and Genetic Basis for Food and Drug Addiction

Overcoming Hypodopaminergic Trait/State by Incorporating Dopamine Agonistic Therapy in Psychiatry

Mark S. Gold, MD[a,b,c,d,*], Rajendra D. Badgaiyan, MD[e],
Kenneth Blum, PhD[f,g,h,i]

KEYWORDS

- Molecular basis • Genetic basis • Food addiction • Drug addiction
- Hypodopaminergic state • Dopamine agonistic therapy • Psychiatry

KEY POINTS

- A brief history is presented of the importance of the molecular neurobiology and neurogenetics of reward brain circuitry in addiction.

Continued

Funding Sources: Funded by NINDS Grant R01NS073884 and the VA Merit Review Grants CX000479 and CX000780 (Dr R.D. Badgaiyan).
Conflict of Interest: Dr K. Blum holds US and foreign patents on a nutraceutical complex and nutrigenomics. He is the owner of IGENE, LLC. He serves as the Chief Scientific Advisor of Dominion Diagnostics, LLC. He is a paid consultant of Malibu Beach Recovery Center, Malibu Beach, CA (owned by Rivermend Health); RDSolutions, Salt Lake City, UT; and Victory Nutrition International, Lederach, PA. Dr M.S. Gold is the Chairman of the Scientific Advisory Board of Rivermend Health, Atlanta, GA. Dr R.D. Badgaiyan has no conflicts of interest.
Author Contributions: The authors contributed equally.

[a] Departments of Psychiatry & Behavioral Sciences, Keck School of Medicine, University of Southern California, 1975 Zonal Avenue, Los Angeles, CA 90033, USA; [b] Department of Psychiatry, Washington University School of Medicine, 660 South Euclid Avenue, St. Louis, MO 63110, USA; [c] Rivermend Health Scientific Advisory Board, 2300 Windy Ridge Parkway South East, Suite 210S, Atlanta, GA 30339, USA; [d] Drug Enforcement Administration (DEA) Educational Foundation, Washington, DC, USA; [e] Laboratory of Advanced Radiochemistry and Molecular and Functioning Imaging, Department of Psychiatry, College of Medicine, University of Minnesota, Minneapolis, MN, USA; [f] Department of Psychiatry, McKnight Brain Institute, University of Florida College of Medicine, Gainesville, FL, USA; [g] Department of Psychiatry, Center for Clinical & Translational Science, Community Mental Health Institute, University of Vermont College of Medicine, University of Vermont, Burlington, VT, USA; [h] Division of Applied Clinical Research, Dominion Diagnostics, LLC, 211 Circuit Drive, North Kingstown, RI 02852, USA; [i] Rivermend Health Scientific Advisory Board, Atlanta, GA, USA
* Corresponding author. Department of Psychiatry, Washington University School of Medicine, 660 South Euclid Avenue, St. Louis, MO 63110.
E-mail address: drmarkgold@gmail.com

Psychiatr Clin N Am 38 (2015) 419–462
http://dx.doi.org/10.1016/j.psc.2015.05.011
0193-953X/15/$ – see front matter © 2015 Elsevier Inc. All rights reserved.

Continued

- Shared common mechanisms exist between food and drug addiction with emphasis on similar neurochemical brain changes in acute and chronic conditions.
- Treatment approaches are listed arguing for dopaminergic agonistic therapy rather than dopaminergic antagonistic therapy.
- A genetic addiction risk score needs to be developed for early age identification of food and or drug addiction risk.
- Policymakers should be convinced that they must develop public health messages like they did with tobacco and use other tactics including taxation to find new treatments that target our youth as preventive measures.

INTRODUCTION

How we feel when we are starving or miss a meal, or two, may be linked to the brain's complex role in controlling appetite. This understanding may be crucial in efforts to develop better ways of helping the millions of Americans afflicted with obesity.[1]

There may be useful ways to identify the role of food addiction in the obesity pandemic. Obesity is rapidly surpassing smoking as the number one killer in the industrialized world. The cost is an estimated $117 billion annually in related illnesses and loss of productivity.[2,3] Food addiction does not explain all cases of obesity, and as the number of persons diagnosed with obesity continues to increase, many people are seeking answers. The increased number of people who eat more food than is required for the basic energetic needs suggests that food intake is no longer simply for purposes of survival.[4] Behavioral and brain changes resembling the effects of drugs of abuse have been observed in rats trained to overeat sugar solution.[5–7] Another similarity was observed in that the dopaminergic reward circuitry of the brain system was involved in animals overfed highly palatable foods.[8–13]

The Molecular Aspects of Dopamine in Reward Circuitry

Feelings of well-being are controlled by dopamine (DA), a neurotransmitter in the brain. The healthy interaction of neurotransmitters, such as serotonin, the opioids, and other brain chemicals, with DA results in feeling well and happy. Depression in contrast has been associated with low serotonin levels.[14] Drug development for the treatment of neurologic, psychiatric, and ocular disorders has targeted DA receptors, a class of G-protein-coupled receptors.[15]

Recently, Salamone and Correa,[16] Sinha,[17] and Nutt and colleagues[18] have debated the claim that DA is the "antistress" or "pleasure" molecule. Nutt and colleagues[18] argue that although addiction is viewed as a disorder of the DA neurotransmitter system, this view has not led to new treatments. Although true, it is not because DA is not a key neurotransmitter in the addiction process requiring not only release in the human striatum but also appropriate responsivity in terms of receptor function. Nutt suggests that only stimulants like cocaine and alcohol require dopaminergic function not cannabis, heroin or nicotine.

The authors do not agree with this oversimplification and intend to show the relationship between glucose cravings and other drugs of abuse. Accordingly, they have argued[19–21] that of depression and other disorders.[22] According to Salamone and Correa, labeling DA neurons as reward neurons may be an overgeneralization;

however, they talk about how different aspects of motivation are affected by dopaminergic manipulations. For example, although nucleus accumbens (NAc) DA does not mediate initial hunger, motivation to eat or appetite it is involved in Pavlovian processes. These Pavlovian processes are instrumental learning appetitive-approach behavior, aversive motivation, behavioral activation processes, sustained task engagement, and exertion of effort.[14,19–21,23,24] Even if this is correct that appetite is tied to motivation, the process does involve a dopaminergic trait, whereas low DA increases craving, especially for glucose.

Although in agreement that NAc DA is involved in appetitive and aversive motivational processes, the authors argue that, similar to drugs of abuse, DA is also involved as an important mediator in appetite, a primary food motivation. The importance of DA in food craving behavior and appetite mediation has been argued in the literature.[23,24] The concept of food addiction was pioneered by Gold and colleagues.[25,26] Avena and colleagues[5–7] correctly argue that addiction to food seems plausible because addictive drugs activate the same neurologic pathways that evolved to respond to natural rewards. Moreover, sugar per se is noteworthy as a substance that releases enkephalins and DA and thus might be expected to have addictive potential. Specifically, neural adaptations occur that include changes in DA and opioid receptor binding, enkephalin mRNA expression, and DA and acetylcholine release in the NAc. The evidence supports the hypothesis that rats can become sugar-dependent and repetitive uncontrollable human consumption is considered an addictive behavior.[27]

Using brain imaging studies in humans, Wang and colleagues[28] implicated DA-modulated circuits in pathologic eating behavior. Their studies suggest that the DA in the extracellular space of the striatum is increased by food cues; this is evidence that DA is potentially involved in the nonhedonic motivational properties of food. They also found that orbitofrontal cortex metabolism is increased by food cues, indicating that this region is associated with motivation for the mediation of food consumption. There is an observed reduction in striatal DA D2 receptor availability in obese subjects, similar to the reduction in drug-addicted subjects. Obese subjects, like addicted subjects, may be predisposed to use food to compensate temporarily for understimulated reward circuits.[29] Along these lines, Chen and colleagues[30] showed that the DA D2 receptor gene A1 allele is associated with obesity, and the prevalence of this allele is increased in obesity with comorbid substance use disorder (SUD). In fact, they found that compared with 23.5% in obese subjects without comorbid SUD, the DRD2 A1 allele was present in 73.9% of the obese subjects with comorbid SUD. Other studies by the same group[29] showed the association of DRD2 genotypes and the percentage fat phenotype. In their study, the DRD2 *Taq*1 A1 allele was present in 67% of the obese/overweight subjects compared with 3.3% of super controls, 33.3% of screened (for drug abuse and obesity) controls, and unscreened literature controls 29.4% ($P \leq .001$). Using logistic regression analysis, in a comparison of all cases with more than 34% body fat, the DRD2 A1 allele accounts for 45.9% of the variance, which is statistically significant ($P < .0001$). There is consistency in the role for the DRD2 gene in obesity, as measured by percentage body fat as well as by weight and body mass index (BMI).[31]

Essentially, the powerful reinforcing effects of both food and drugs are in part mediated by abrupt DA increases in the mesolimbic brain reward centers. Volkow and colleagues[32] point out that abrupt DA increases can override homeostatic control mechanisms in the brains of vulnerable individuals. The neurologic dysfunction that generates the shared features of food and drug addictions has been identified in brain imaging studies. The commonality of root causes of addiction is shared impairments in the dopaminergic pathways that regulate the neuronal systems associated also with self-control, conditioning, stress reactivity, reward sensitivity, and incentive motivation.[33] In obese subjects, decreased DA D2 receptors are associated with decreased prefrontal metabolism, which involves ghrelin and its subsequent effects related to inhibitory control of the ability to limit food intake.[34,35] Gastric stimulation in obese subjects activates the same limbic and cortical regions involved with motivation, memory, and self-control[36] as are activated by drug craving in drug-addicted subjects. An enhanced sensitivity to the sensory properties of food is suggested by increased neurometabolism in the somatosensory cortex of obese subjects. This enhanced sensitivity to food palatability coupled with reduced DA D2 receptors could make food the salient reinforcer for compulsive eating and obesity risk.[37–39] The prevention and treatment of obesity may in accordance with this research benefit from strategies that target improved DA function.

Lindblom and colleagues[40] reported that as a strategy dieting to reduce body weight often fails because it causes food cravings that lead to bingeing and weight regain. They also agree that evidence from several lines of research suggests the presence of shared elements in the neural regulation of food and drug craving. Lindblom and colleagues[40] quantified the expression of 8 genes involved in DA signaling in brain regions related to the mesolimbic and nigrostriatal DA system in male rats. The rats were subjected to chronic food restriction using quantitative real-time polymerase chain reaction. Lindblom and colleagues found that mRNA levels of tyrosine hydroxylase and the DA transporter in the ventral tegmental area (VTA) were strongly increased by food restriction. Concurrent Dopamine Transporter (DAT) upregulation at the protein level in the shell of the NAc was also observed via quantitative autoradiography. That these effects were observed after chronic rather than acute food restriction suggests that sensitization of the mesolimbic DA pathway may have occurred. Thus, sensitization possibly due to increased clearance of extracellular DA from the NAc shell may be one of the underlying causes for the food cravings that hinder dietary compliance.

These findings are in agreement with earlier findings by Patterson and colleagues,[41] who demonstrated that direct intracerebroventricular infusion of insulin results in an increase in mRNA levels for the DA reuptake transporter DAT. In a 24- to 36-hour food deprivation study, hybridization was used in situ to assess DAT mRNA levels in food-deprived (hypoinsulinemic) rats. Levels were in the VTA/substantia nigra pars compacta significantly decreased, suggesting that moderation of striatal DAT function can be affected by nutritional status, fasting, and insulin. Ifland and colleagues[42] advanced the hypothesis that processed foods with high concentrations of sugar and other refined sweeteners, refined carbohydrates, fat, salt, and caffeine are addictive substances. Other studies have evaluated salt as an important factor in food-seeking behavior. Roitman and colleagues[43] point out that increased DA transmission in the NAc is correlated with motivated behaviors, including salt appetite. DA transmission is modulated by DAT and may play a role in motivated behaviors. In their studies in vivo, robust decreases in DA uptake via DAT in the rat NAc were correlated with salt appetite induced by salt depletion. Decreased DAT activity in the NAc was observed after in vitro aldosterone treatment. Thus, a reduction in DAT activity, in the NAc, may be the consequence of a direct action of aldosterone and may be a mechanism by which salt depletion induces generation of increased NAc DA transmission during salt appetite. Increased NAc DA may be the motivating property for the salt-depleted rat. Further support for the role of salted food as possible substance (food) of abuse has resulted in the "The Salted Food Addiction Hypothesis" as proposed by Cocores and Gold,[44] who did a pilot study to determine if salted foods act like a mild opiate agonist that drives overeating and weight gain. They found that an opiate-dependent group developed a 6.6% increase in weight during opiate withdrawal, showing a strong preference for salted food. Based on this and other literature,[45] they suggest that salted food may be an addictive substance that can stimulate opiate and DA receptors in the reward and pleasure center of the brain. Alternately, preference, hunger, urge, and craving for tasty salted food and the opiatelike effect of salty food may be symptoms of opiate withdrawal. Both salty foods and opiate withdrawal stimulate the salt appetite and result in increased calorie intake, overeating, and disease related to obesity.

Currently, not all foods are implicated in the development of food addictions.[15] Foods that are thought to be addictive tend to be highly palatable, are rich in fats, sugars, and salt, and are calorie dense.[5] These foods that may potentially be more addictive than traditional foods are often composed of synthetic combinations of ingredients. Recent research has demonstrated that each of these nutrient elements affects specific neurotransmitter systems in the brain,[6,46] providing the potential for targeted pharmacologic treatments.[47] With the numbers of individuals affected with obesity soaring and many children being affected, it is important to seriously evaluate some of these new treatment modalities and early genetic testing for addiction risk.[19,48–51]

Food Intake and Reward

Changes in the mesocorticolimbic system of the brain have been linked with motivational abnormalities such as excessive overeating. The mesocorticolimbic system is a complex and interrelated network with many functions, including food addiction.[52] The mesocorticolimbic reward circuit consists of the amygdala, hippocampus, nucleus accumbens (ventral striatum), and ventral diencephalon (including the basal forebrain, ventral tegmentum, and hypothalamus). In addition, the cortical areas, such as the dorsolateral prefrontal, orbitofrontal, temporal pole, subcallosal, and cingulate cortices, parahippocampal gyri, and the insula, provide modulating and oversight functions. Dysfunctional eating may reflect an underlying addictive state. Interestingly, a common mechanism for food and drug addiction as encompassed by the reward deficiency syndrome (RDS) concept has been supported by the work of Robinson and colleagues,[52] showing that central nucleus of photo-excitation specifically enhances and narrows incentive motivation to pursue an associated external reward at the expense of another reward.

Eating is essential for the survival of all living organisms,[53] and detrimental physical and psychological changes can occur with even relatively brief durations of starvation.[54] Therefore, eating behaviors are programmed in the brain by powerful neural systems to ensure food intake and to regulate caloric balance. These feeding behaviors are, however, controlled by more than homeostatic mechanisms. As it has been pointed out, "If feeding were controlled solely by homeostatic mechanisms, most of us would be at our ideal body weight, and people would consider feeding like breathing or elimination, a necessary but unexciting part of existence."[55] A role for the reward systems in the brain to promote motivational, hedonically driven feeding is suggested by the fact that this is not the case. Thus, excessive food intake may be explained more by dysfunction in the reward circuitry than by dysfunction in the homeostatic mechanisms controlling feeding habits. Both human and nonhuman studies have supported the hypothesis that the brain's reward circuitry may be dysregulated in cases of obesity, disordered eating, anorexia nervosa, and, more recently, food addiction.[5–7,13,56]

In fact, Avena and colleagues[57] suggested based on a literature review that brain imaging may provide insights into understanding some differences in the neuroanatomy of individuals having anorexia nervosa compared with bulimia nervosa and obesity. Studies suggest that ill adult and adolescent anorexia nervosa after recovery, and those with adult bulimia nervosa, have larger volume in the left medial orbitofrontal gyrus rectus. In ill adult and adolescent anorexia nervosa, as well as recovered adults, the right insula, which processes taste but also interoception, was enlarged. A few studies investigated white matter integrity. The most consistent finding was of reduced fornix integrity, a limbic pathway that is important in emotion but also food intake regulation in both anorexia and bulimia nervosa. Functional brain imaging using basic sweet taste stimuli in eating disorders during the ill state or after recovery repeatedly implicated reward pathways, including insula and striatum. Importantly, brain imaging targeting DA-related brain activity using taste-reward conditioning tasks suggested that this circuitry is hypersensitive in anorexia nervosa, but hyporesponsive in bulimia nervosa and obesity. Those results are in-line with basic research, and as proposed by Avena and Brown and colleagues,[57,58] suggest adaptive reward system changes in the human brain in response to extremes of food intake changes that could interfere with normalization of eating behavior.

Genetics may play a role in the underlying addictive feeding. As not everyone who is exposed to drugs becomes an addict (possibly due to epigenetic effects), similarly, exposure to high-risk foods does not necessarily result in compulsive overeating. The difference in susceptibility can be attributed, at least in part, to underlying genetic predispositions, specifically, downregulation of DA D2 receptors.[59–61] As discussed earlier, the *TaqIA* A1 allele has been implicated specifically in obesity and SUDs through increases in reward sensitivity in the striatum by elevated DA activity levels.[10,14,19,30,62] New forms of treatment, largely pharmaceutical, would potentially target these genetic predispositions as a means of intervention. However, it might be possible to develop nutrigenomic approaches as well with the chance of elimination of DR2 downregulation by using powerful D2 agonists like bromocriptine.[63] In fact, its use has been considered in the treatment of anorexia nervosa with negative outcome.[64]

There is a plethora of research on the molecular neurobiological aspects of both food and drug addiction, suggesting shared mechanisms, and as such, possible therapeutic targets.[65–79]

Neurogenetics of Genes Relates to Eating Disorders

Based on association and linkage studies implicating the alleles of the genes listed in later discussion, individuals possessing dopaminergic regulatory gene variants of, for example, the DRD2, DRD3, DRD4, DAT1, COMT, MOA-A, SLC6A4, Mu, and GABA$_B$, are at genetic risk for drug-seeking behaviors. Support is derived from several important studies illustrating an association of these risk antecedents that have an impact on the mesocorticolimbic system (**Table 1**). There are many more genes involved in obesity and subtypes like anorexia nervosa, bulimia, and binge-eating behavior.

Along these lines, Do and colleagues[130] used genome-wide association studies to reveal potential genetic polymorphisms that may influence eating behaviors pertinent to the human condition. Observation of eating behaviors in pigs and the use of comparative mapping were accomplished to discern the implications for human obesity and metabolic syndrome. Specifically, they found 16 single-nucleotide polymorphisms (SNPs) to have moderate genomewide significance, and 76 SNPs were suggestive of an association with feeding behavioral traits. Eating frequency was very strongly associated with the MSI2 gene on chromosome SSC 14. Thirty-six SNPs were located in the same genome regions where quantitative trait loci (QTL) have previously been reported for food intake or feeding behavior traits in pigs.

Several significant SNPs were found in the regions: 64–65 Mb on SSC 1, 124–130 Mb on SSC 8, 63–68 Mb on SSC 11, 32–39 Mb and 59–60 Mb on SSC 12. Genes that were associated very significantly with feeding behavior traits included synapse genes (GABRR2, PPP1R9B, SYT1, GABRR1, CADPS2, DLGAP2, and GOPC), the positive regulation of peptide secretion genes (GHRH, NNAT, and TCF7L2), and the dephosphorylation genes (PPM1E, DAPP1, PTPN18, PTPRZ1, PTPN4, MTMR4, and RNGTT).

Most recently, Locke and colleagues[131] presented an update of the human obesity gene map (http://obesitygene.pbrc.edu), extending the number of genes involved in obesity. In summary, they reported that, as of 2005, 176 human obesity cases due to single-gene mutations in 11 different genes have been reported. In addition, 50 genomic regions related to human obesity have been mapped, and strong candidates or causal genes have been identified for most of the Mendelian syndromes. There are 244 mouse genes that, when mutated or expressed as transgenes, result in phenotypes that affect adiposity and body weight. There are presently 408 QTLs reported from animal models. There is also a growing number of obesity QTLs derived from human genome scans. From 61 genome-wide scans, 253 QTLs for obesity-related phenotypes have been found. Two or more studies support a total of 52 genomic regions that harbor QTLs. There are also 426 findings of positive associations with 127 candidate genes reported between DNA sequence variation in specific genes and obesity phenotypes. At least 5 positive studies support associations with 22 genes. The putative loci on all chromosomes except Y are shown on the obesity gene map. Locke and colleagues[131] extended this genetic basis for obesity by conducting a genome-wide association study and metabochip meta-analysis of BMI in 339,224 subjects. The 97 loci account for ~ 2.7% of BMI variation, and genome-wide estimates suggest that common variation accounts for greater than 20% of BMI variation. The most important pathways include synaptic function, glutamate signaling, insulin secretion/action, energy metabolism, lipid biology, and adipogenesis.

Garfield and colleagues,[132] using several innovative techniques to control the brain activity of living mice, identified one particular circuit that seems to switch hunger off and on. The circuit involves a protein called the melanocortin-4 receptor (MC4R) expressed on the surface of a group of neurons. Interestingly, the important role of the gene that codes for MC4R has been known to play in obesity has been known for years. Mutations in *MC4R* are rare, but can cause inherited obesity in humans. Also, mice that lack functional versions of the gene overeat and grow extremely obese, ballooning to double their normal weight. Moreover, Shah and colleagues[133] discovered that MC4R-expressing neurons reside in the paraventricular nucleus of the hypothalamus, a very specific region of the brain known for its role in energy balance and hunger. Krashes' group found that by selectively activating MC4R neurons in genetically engineered mice with either optogenetics (light) or chemicals, the animals lost their appetite when MC4R neurons were switched on (which happens to be the normal, default state). Only when MC4R neurons were switched off did the mice express any interest in eating. They suggest that when the animal's body needs more calories, other types of neurons send a signal that turns the MC4R neurons off.

These findings take on real significance in terms of dopaminergic regulation. It is well-known that chronic stress is a strong diathesis for depression in humans and is used to generate animal models of depression. As such, stress leads to several major symptoms of depression, including dysregulated feeding behavior, anhedonia, and behavioral despair. Lim and colleagues[134] showed that chronic stress in mice decreases the strength of excitatory synapses on D1 DA receptor-expressing nucleus accumbens medium spiny neurons owing to activation of the MC4R. Stress-elicited increases in behavioral measurements of anhedonia are prevented by blocking these

Table 1
Candidate reward genes and RDS: a sampling

Gene	Polymorphism(s)	Study Findings	Reference	Comment
D2 dopamine receptor gene (DRD2)	SNP rs: 1800497	*Taq* A1 allele associates with sever alcoholism	Blum et al,[80] 1990	First study to associate with alcoholism (called reward gene)
	ANKKI-p.Glu713Lys	DRD2 *Taq*1A RFLP is a SNP that causes an amino acid substitution within the 11th ankyrin repeat of ANKK1	Neville et al,[81] 2004	The ANKKI gene is a reflection of DRD2 A_1 allele.
	SNP rs: 1800497	This SNP has been found to predict future RDS behaviors as high as 74%.	Blum et al,[82] 1995	Using Bayesian analysis
	SNP rs: 1800497	Presence of the A1+ genotype (A1/A1, A1/A2), compared with the A− genotype (A2/A2), is associated with reduced density.	Noble et al,[83] 1991	This reduction causes hypodopaminergic functioning in the DA reward pathway.
	SNP rs: 6277 at exon 7	T+ allele associates with alcohol dependence.	Hoffman et al,[84] 2008	Associates with drug-seeking behavior and other RDS behaviors
	SNP rs: 1800497	10-y follow-up that carriers of the DRD2 A1 allele have a higher mortality compared with carriers of the A2 allele in alcohol-dependent individuals.	Dahlgren et al,[85] 2011	*Taq*I A1 allele and a substantially increased relapse rate
	DRD2-haplotypes I-C-G-A2 and I-C-A-A1	Confirmed the hypothesis that haplotypes, which are supposed to induce a low DRD2 expression, are associated with alcohol dependence.	Kraschewski et al,[86] 2009	High frequency of haplotype was associated with Cloninger type 2 and family history of alcoholism.
	SNP rs: 1800497	Genotype analysis showed a significantly higher frequency for the *Taq*IA polymorphism among the addicts (69.9%) compared with control subjects (42.6%; Fisher's exact χ^2, $P<.05$).	Teh et al,[87] 2012	The addicts had higher scores for novelty seeking (NS) and harm avoidance (HA) personality traits

Gene	Polymorphism	Finding	Reference	Comment
D4 dopamine receptor gene (DRD4)	DRD4: The 7R VNTR	The length of the DRD4 exon 3 VNTR affects DRD4 functioning by modulating the expression and efficiency of maturation of the receptor.	Van Tol,[88] 1998	The 7R VNTR requires significantly higher amounts of DA to produce a response of the same magnitude as other size VNTRs. This reduced sensitivity or "dopamine resistance" leads to hypodopaminergic functioning. Thus, 7R VNTR has been associated with substance-seeking behavior.
	120-bp duplication, −616C/G, and −521C/T	Strong finding of −120-bp duplication allele frequencies with schizophrenia ($P = .008$); −521 C/T polymorphism is associated with heroin addiction.	Lai et al,[89] 2010	
	DRD4 7R allele	Several putative risk alleles using survival analysis revealed that by 25 y of age, 76% of subjects with a DRD4 7R allele were estimated to have significantly more persistent ADHD compared with 66% of subjects without the risk allele.	Biederman et al,[90] 2009	Findings suggest that the DRD4 7R allele is associated with a more persistent course of ADHD.
	7R allele of the dopamine D(4) receptor gene (DRD4)	Although the association between ADHD and DRD4 is small, these results suggest that it is real.	Faraone et al,[91] 2001	For both the case-control and the family-based studies, the authors found (1) support for the association between ADHD and DRD4; (2) no evidence that this association was accounted for by any one study; and (3) no evidence for publication bias.
	DRD4 exon 3 polymorphisms (48-bp VNTR)	Found significant differences in the short alleles (2–5 VNTR) frequencies between controls and patients with a history of delirium tremens or alcohol seizures ($P = .043$)	Grzywacz et al,[92] 2008	A trend was also observed in the higher frequency of short alleles among individuals with an early age of onset of alcoholism ($P = .063$).
	DRD4 7R allele	Show that the 7R allele is significantly overrepresented in the opioid-dependent cohort and confers a relative risk of 2.46	Kotler et al,[93] 1997	This is the first report of an association between a specific genetic polymorphism and opioid addiction.

(continued on next page)

Table 1
(continued)

Gene	Polymorphism(s)	Study Findings	Reference	Comment
Dopamine transporter gene (DAT1)	Localized to chromosome 5p15.3. Moreover, within 3 noncoding region of DAT1 lies a VNTR polymorphism 9-repeat (9R) VNTR	The 9-repeat (9R) VNTR has been shown to influence gene expression and to augment transcription of the DA transporter protein	Byerley et al,[94] 1993	Having this variant results in an enhanced clearance of synaptic DA, yielding reduced levels of DA to activate postsynaptic neurons.
	9R VNTR	DAT1, genotype 9/9 was associated with early opiate addiction	Galeeva et al,[95] 2002	The combination of SERT genotype 10/10 with DAT1 genotype 10/10 was shown to be a risk factor of opiate abuse <16 y of age.
	Exon 15 rs27072 and VNTR (DAT), promoter VNTR and rs25531	The haplogenotypes 6-A-10/6-G-10 and 5-G-9/5-G-9 were more often present in type 2 alcoholics than type 1 alcoholics (odds ratio [OR]: 2.8), and controls (OR: 5.8), respectively.	Reese et al,[96] 2010	In a typology proposed by Cloninger on the basis of adoption studies, a subgroup has been classified as type 2 with patients having high genetic loading for alcoholism, an early onset of alcoholism, a severe course, and coexisting psychiatric problems consisting of aggressive tendencies or criminality.
	VNTR polymorphism at the DA transporter locus (DAT1) 480-bp DAT1 allele	Using the haplotype-based haplotype relative risk method revealed significant association between ADHD/undifferentiated attention deficit disorder and the 480-bp DAT1 allele (χ^2 7.51, 1 df, $P = .006$).	Cook et al,[97] 1995	Although there have been some inconsistencies associated with the earlier results, the evidence is mounting in favor of the view that the 10R allele of DAT is associated with high risk for ADHD in children and in adults alike.
	DAT1 variable number tandem repeats (VNTR), genotypes: both 9R and 10R alleles	The nonadditive association for the 10R allele was significant for hyperactivity-impulsivity (HI) symptoms. However, consistent with other studies, exploratory analyses of the nonadditive association of the 9R allele of DAT1 with HI and oppositional defiant disorder symptoms	Lee et al,[98] 2007	The inconsistent association between DAT1 and child behavior problems in this and other samples may reflect joint influence of the 10R and 9R alleles.

COMT	COMT Val158Met and DRD2 Taq1A genotypes	COMT Val158Met and DRD2 Taq1A may affect the intermediate phenotype of central DA receptor sensitivity.	COMT Val158Met and DRD2 Taq1A may confer their risk of alcohol dependence through reduced DA receptor sensitivity in the prefrontal cortex and hindbrain, respectively.	Schellekens et al,[99] 2012
	The functional polymorphism (COMT Val108/158Met) affects COMT activity, with the valine (Val) variant associated with higher and the methionine (Met) variant with lower COMT activity.	Male alcoholic suicide attempters, compared with male nonattempters, had the higher frequency of Met/Met genotype or Met allele, and significantly (Kruskal-Wallis ANOVA on ranks and Mann-Whitney test) higher aggression and depression scores.	These results confirmed the associations between Met allele and aggressive behavior or violent suicide attempts in various psychiatric diagnoses and suggested that Met allele of the COMT Val108/158 Met might be used as an independent biomarker of suicidal behavior across different psychopathologies.	Nedic et al,[100] 2011
	COMT Val(158)Met variation	Both controls and opiate users with Met/Met genotypes showed higher NS scores compared with those with the Val allele.	Association of the COMT polymorphism and NS temperament scale has been shown for heroin-dependent patients and controls regardless of group status.	Demetrovics et al,[101] 2010
	A functional polymorphism (COMT Val158Met) resulting in increased enzyme activity has been associated with polysubstance abuse and addiction to heroin and methamphetamine.	These results suggest a significant association between COMT Val158Met polymorphism and susceptibility to cannabis dependence.	Cannabis stimulates DA release and activates dopaminergic reward neurons in central pathways that lead to enhanced dependence. COMT inactivates extraneuronally amplified extraneuronally released DA.	Baransel Isir et al,[102] 2008

(continued on next page)

Table 1
(continued)

Gene	Polymorphism(s)	Study Findings	Reference	Comment
Serotonin transporter gene	Serotonin transporter promoter polymorphism (5-HT transporter gene-linked polymorphic region [5-HTTLPR])	5-HTTLPR had age-dependent effects on alcohol, tobacco, and drug use: substance use did not differ by genotype at age 9, but at age 15, the participants with the short (s)/s genotype had higher tobacco use, and at age 18, they were more active alcohol, drug, and tobacco users.	Merenäkk et al,[103] 2011	Results reveal that expression of genetic vulnerability for substance use in children and adolescents may depend on age, gender, interaction of genes, and type of substance.
	The short (s), low-activity allele of a polymorphism (5-HTTLPR) in the serotonin transporter gene (SLC6A4) has been related to alcohol dependence.	The 5-HTTLPR short allele predicted adolescent's growth (slope) in alcohol use over time. Adolescents with the 5-HTTLPR short allele showed a larger increase in alcohol consumption than those without the 5-HTTLPR short allele.	van der Zwaluw et al,[104] 2010	5-HTTLPR genotype was not related to the initial level (intercept) of alcohol consumption.
	Triallelic 5-HTTLPR genotype: SA/SA and SA/lG compared with LA/LA	Remifentanil and opioid drugs had a significantly better analgesic effect in individuals with a genotype coding for low 5-HTT expression (SA/SA and SA/lG) as compared with those with high expression (LA/LA), $P < .02$.	Kosek et al,[105] 2009	Previously the 5-HTTLPR s-allele has been associated with higher risk of developing chronic pain conditions, but in this study, the authors show that the genotype coding for low 5-HTT expression is associated with a better analgesic effect of an opioid. The s-allele has been associated with downregulation of 5-HT1 receptors and the authors suggest that individuals with a desensitization of 5-HT1 receptors have an increased analgesic response to opioids during acute pain stimuli, but may still be at increased risk of developing chronic pain conditions.

Mu opiate receptor (MOR)			
A SNP in the human MOR gene (OPRM1 A118G) has been shown to alter receptor protein level in preclinical models and smoking behavior in humans.	Ray et al,[106] 2011	Independent of session, smokers homozygous for the wild-type (WT) OPRM1 A allele exhibited significantly higher levels of MOR BP than smokers carrying the G allele in bilateral amygdala, left thalamus, and left anterior cingulate cortex.	Among G allele carriers, the extent of subjective reward difference (denicotinized vs nicotine cigarette) was associated significantly with MOR BP difference in right amygdala, caudate, anterior cingulate cortex, and thalamus.
Polymorphism in A118G in exon 1 and C1031G in intron 2 of the MOR gene	Szeto et al,[107] 2001	Results showed a significant association for both A118G and C1031G polymorphisms and opioid dependence. The G allele is more common in the heroin-dependent group (39.5% and 30.8% for A118G and C1031G polymorphisms, respectively) when compared with the controls (29.4% and 21.1% for A118G and C1031G polymorphisms, respectively).	This study suggests that the variant G allele of both A118G and C1031G polymorphisms may contribute to the vulnerability to heroin dependence.
A118G SNP in exon 1 of the MOR gene (OPRM1), which encodes an amino acid substitution, is functional, and receptors encoded by the variant 118G allele bind the endogenous opioid peptide β-endorphin with 3-fold greater affinity than prototype receptors. Other groups subsequently reported that this variant alters stress-responsivity in normal volunteers and also increases the therapeutic response to naltrexone (a μ-preferring opioid antagonist) in the treatment of alcohol dependence.	Bart et al,[108] 2005	There was a significant overall association between genotypes with a 118G allele and alcohol dependence (P = .0074). The attributable risk for alcohol dependence in subjects with a 118G allele was 11.1%.	There was no difference in A118G genotype between type 1 and type 2 alcoholics. In central Sweden, the functional variant 118G allele in exon 1 of OPRM1 is associated with an increased attributable risk for alcohol dependence.
MOR gene knockout (KO) were examined in WT (+/+), heterozygote MOR KO (+/−), and homozygote MOR KO (−/−) mice on voluntary ethanol consumption	Hall et al,[109] 2001	Heterozygous and homozygous MOR KO mice consumed less ethanol than WT mice. These effects appeared to be greater in female KO mice than in male KO mice. MOR KO mice, especially female mice, exhibited less ethanol reward in a conditioned place preference paradigm.	These data fit with the reported therapeutic efficacy of MOR antagonists in the treatment of human alcoholism. Allelic variants that confer differing levels of MOR expression could provide different degrees of risk for alcoholism.

(continued on next page)

Table 1
(continued)

Gene	Polymorphism(s)	Study Findings	Reference	Comment
GABA β subunit 3	GABA A receptor β3 subunit gene (GABRB3)	The G1– alleles of the GABRB3 in COAs were significantly higher than non-COAs.	Namkoong et al,[110] 2008	In the same study, the frequency of the A1+ allele at DRD2 in the COAs was significantly higher than non-COAs.
	β3 subunit mRNAs	The levels of the β2 and β3 subunit mRNAs remain elevated at 24 h withdrawal from chronic ethanol. Chronic ethanol treatment increased the levels of both of these polypeptides in cerebral cortex.	Mhatre & Ticku,[111] 1994	Chronic ethanol administration produced an upregulation of the β-subunit mRNA and the polypeptide expression of these subunits in rat cerebral cortex.
	A1+ (A1A1 and A1A2 genotypes) and A1– (A2A2 genotype) alleles of the DRD2 and G1+ (G1G1 and G1 non-G1 genotypes) and G1– (non-G1 non-G1 genotype) alleles of the GABRB3 gene. Study involved mood-related alcohol expectancy (AE) and drinking refusal self-efficacy (DRSE) were assessed using the drinking expectancy profile	Patients with the DRD2 A1+ allele, compared with those with the DRD2 A1– allele, reported significantly lower DRSE in situations of social pressure. Similarly, lower DRSE was reported under social pressure by patients with the GABRB3 G1+ allele when compared with those with the GABRB3 G1– alleles. Patients with the GABRB3 G1+ allele also revealed reduced DRSE in situations characterized by negative affect than those with the GABRB3 G1– alleles. Patients carrying the GABRB3 G1+ allele showed stronger AE relating to negative affective change (for example, increased depression) than their GABRB3 G1– counterparts.	Young et al,[112] 2004	Molecular genetic research has identified promising markers of alcohol dependence, including alleles of the D2 DA receptor (DRD2) and the GABAA receptor β3 subunit (GABRB3) genes.

Dinucleotide repeat polymorphisms of the GABA(A) receptor β-3 subunit gene were compared with scores on the General Health Questionnaire-28 (GHQ).	Analysis of GHQ subscale scores showed that heterozygotes compared with the combined homozygotes had higher scores on the somatic symptoms ($P = .006$), anxiety/insomnia ($P = .003$), social dysfunction ($P = .054$), and depression ($P = .004$) subscales.	Feusner et al,[113] 2001	In conclusion, the present study indicates that in a population of PTSD patients, heterozygosity of the GABRB3 major (G1) allele confers higher levels of somatic symptoms, anxiety/insomnia, social dysfunction, and depression than found in homozygosity.
GABRB3 major (G1) allele & DRD @ A1 allele	A significant progressive increase was observed in DRD2 A1 allelic prevalence ($P = 3.11 \times 10^{-6}$) and frequency ($P = 2.7 \times 10^{-6}$) in the order of nonalcoholics, less severe alcoholics, and severe alcoholics. In severe alcoholics, compared with nonalcoholics, a significant decrease was found in the prevalence ($P = 4.5 \times 10^{-3}$) and frequency ($P = 2.7 \times 10^{-2}$) of the GABRB3 major (G1) allele. Furthermore, a significant progressive decrease was noted in G1 allelic prevalence ($P = 2.4 \times 10^{-3}$) and frequency ($P = 1.9 \times 10^{-2}$) in nonalcoholics, less severe alcoholics, and severe alcoholics, respectively.	Noble et al,[114] 1988	In sum, in the same population of nonalcoholics and alcoholics studied, variants of both the DRD2 and the GABRB3 genes independently contribute to the risk for alcoholism, with the DRD2 variants revealing a stronger effect than the GABRB3 variants. However, when the DRD2 and the GABRB3 variants are combined, the risk for alcoholism is more robust than when these variants are considered separately.

(continued on next page)

Table 1
(continued)

Gene	Polymorphism(s)	Study Findings	Reference	Comment
MOA-A	MAOA genotype	Significant 3-way interactions, MAOA genotype by abuse by sex, predicted dysthymic symptoms. Low-activity MAOA genotype buffered against symptoms of dysthymia in physically abused and multiply-maltreated women. Significant 3-way interactions, MAOA genotype by sexual abuse by race, predicted all outcomes. Low-activity MAOA genotype buffered against symptoms of dysthymia, major depressive disorder, and alcohol abuse for sexually abused white participants. The high-activity genotype was protective in the nonwhite sexually abused group.	Nikulina et al,[115] 2012	This prospective study provides evidence that MAOA interacts with child maltreatment to predict mental health outcomes.
	Low-repeat MAOA allele	Individuals with cocaine use disorders (CUD) had reductions in gray matter volume in the orbitofrontal, dorsolateral prefrontal, and temporal cortex and the hippocampus compared with controls. The orbitofrontal cortex reductions were uniquely driven by CUD with low-MAOA genotype and by lifetime cocaine use.	Alia-Klein et al,[78] 2011	Long-term cocaine users with the low-repeat MAOA allele have enhanced sensitivity to gray matter loss, specifically in the orbitofrontal cortex, indicating that this genotype may exacerbate the deleterious effects of cocaine in the brain.
	MAOA u-VNTR	Girls carrying the long MAOA-uVNTR variant showed a higher risk of being high alcohol consumers, whereas among boys, the short allele was related to higher alcohol consumption.	Nilsson et al,[116] 2011	The present study supports the hypothesis that there is a relation between MAOA-uVNTR and alcohol consumption, and that this relation is modulated by environmental factors.
	30-bp repeat in the promoter region of the MAO-A	Significant associations between cold pain tolerance and DAT-1 ($P = .008$) and MAO-A ($P = .024$) polymorphisms were found. Specifically, tolerance was shorter for carriers of allele 10 and the rarer allele 11, as compared with homozygous for allele 9, and for carriers of allele 4 (MAO) as compared with homozygous for allele 3, respectively.	Treister et al,[117] 2009	These results, together with the known function of the investigated candidate gene polymorphisms, suggest that low dopaminergic activity can be associated with high pain sensitivity and vice versa.

The Revised Psychopathy Checklist (PCL-R) has shown a moderate association with violence and as such studied with MAOA genotyped alcoholic offenders.	The PCL-R total score predicts impulsive reconvictions among high-activity MAOA offenders (6.8% risk increase for every 1-point increase in PCL-R total score, $P = .015$), but not among low-activity MAOA offenders, whereas antisocial behavior and attitudes predicted reconvictions in both genotypes (17% risk increase among high-activity MAOA offenders and 12.8% increase among low-activity MAOA offenders for every 1-point increase in factor 2 score).	Tikkanen et al,[118] 2011	Results suggest that the efficacy of PCL-R is altered by MAOA genotype, alcohol exposure, and age, which seems important to note when PCL-R is used for risk assessments that will have legal or costly preventive work consequences.
Genotyping of 2 functional polymorphisms in the promoter region of the serotonin transporter and monoamine oxidase-A, respectively (5-HTT-LPR and MAOA-VNTR), was performed in a group of women with severe alcohol addiction.	Within the group of alcoholics, when the patients with known comorbid psychiatric disorders were excluded, aggressive antisocial behavior was significantly linked to the presence of the high activity MAOA allele.	Gokturk et al,[119] 2008	The pattern of associations between genotypes of 5-HTT-LPR and MAOA-VNTR in women with severe alcoholism differs from most corresponding studies on men.
The MAOA gene presents several polymorphisms, including a 30-bp VNTR in the promoter region (MAOA-uVNTR). Alleles with 3.5 and 4 repeats are 2–10 times more efficient than the 3-repeat allele.	The results suggest that the 3R allele is associated with (1) alcohol dependence ($P<.05$); (2) an earlier onset of alcoholism ($P<.01$); (3) comorbid drug abuse among alcoholics ($P<.05$); and (4) a higher number of antisocial symptoms ($P<.02$).	Contini et al,[120] 2006	Results confirmed previous reports showing an association of the low-activity 3R allele of MAOA-uVNTR polymorphism with substance dependence and impulsive/antisocial behaviors. These findings in a different culture further support the influence of the MAOA-uVNTR in psychiatric disorders.

(continued on next page)

Table 1
(continued)

Gene	Polymorphism(s)	Study Findings	Reference	Comment
Dopamine D3	The genotypes of the BDNF Val66Met and DRD3 Ser9Gly polymorphisms. BDNF regulates expression of D3.	Logistic regression analysis showed a significant main effect for the Val/Val genotype of the BDNF Val66Met polymorphism ($P = .020$), which predicted bipolar-II patients. Significant interaction effects for the BDNF Val66Met Val/Val genotype and both DRD3 Ser9Gly Ser/Ser and Ser/Gly genotypes were found only in bipolar-II patients ($P = .027$ and .006, respectively).	Lee et al,[121] 2012	Evidence that the BDNF Val66Met and DRD3 Ser9Gly genotypes interact only in bipolar-II disorder (hypomania) and that bipolar-I (mania) and bipolar-II may be genetically distinct.
	D3 receptor (D3R) KO mice	The possible interaction between morphine-induced tolerance and D3Rs has not been investigated. Compared with WT mice, the DA D3R knockout (D3R KO) mice showed pronounced hypoalgesia. The D3R KO mice clearly developed lower morphine-induced tolerance and showed attenuated withdrawal signs compared with the WT mice.	Li et al,[122] 2012	These results suggest that D3Rs regulate basal nociception and are involved in the development of morphine-induced tolerance and withdrawal.
	DNA microarrays of 2 different alcohol-preferring rat lines (HAD [high alcohol drinking] and P [preferring]) and D3Rs.	Data revealed an upregulation of the DA D3R after 1 y of voluntary alcohol consumption in the striatum of alcohol-preferring rats that was confirmed by quantitative real-time-polymerase chain reaction.	Vengeliene et al,[123] 2006	Long-term alcohol consumption leads to an upregulation of the DA D3R that may contribute to alcohol-seeking and relapse. The authors therefore suggest that selective antagonists of this pharmacologic target provide a specific treatment approach to reduce alcohol craving and relapse behavior.
	Gly9 homozygotes in comparison to Ser9 carriers of D3R gene	German descent was found as diminished parietal and increased frontal P300 amplitudes in Gly9 homozygotes in comparison to Ser9 carriers. Further studies should address the direct role of the DRD3 Ser9Gly polymorphism in attenuated P300 amplitudes in psychiatric disorders like schizophrenia or alcoholism.	Mulert et al,[124] 2006	An important reason for the interest in P300 event-related potentials are findings in patients with psychiatric disorders like schizophrenia or alcoholism in which attenuations of the P300 amplitude are common findings.

Dopamine receptor D3 gene *BalI* polymorphism	Patients above the median value for cognitive impulsiveness (1 of the 3 dimensions of the Barratt scale) were more frequently heterozygous than alcohol-dependent patients with lower impulsiveness (OR = 2.51, P = .019) than 71 healthy controls (OR = 2.32, P = .025).	Limosin et al,[125] 2005	The D3R gene has been associated with addictive behaviors, especially impulsiveness.
BalI polymorphism at the DRD3 gene	Patients with a sensation-seeking score >24 were more frequently homozygous for both alleles than patients with a sensation-seeking score <24 (P = .038) or controls (P = .034).	Duaux et al,[126] 1998	These results suggest that the DRD3 gene may have a role in drug dependence susceptibility in individuals with high sensation-seeking scores.
mRNA of both DRD2 and DRD3 gene expression	After a chronic schedule of intermittent bingeing on a sucrose solution, mRNA levels for the D2 DA receptor, and the pre-proenkephalin and pre-protachykinin genes were decreased in DA-receptive regions of the forebrain, whereas D3 DA receptor mRNA was increased. The effects of sugar on mRNA levels were of greater magnitude in the nucleus accumbens than in the caudate-putamen.	Spangler et al,[127] 2004	Striatal regions of sugar-dependent rats show alterations in DA and opioid mRNA levels similar to morphine-dependent rats.
MscI/BalI polymorphism of the DRD3 gene	Significant decrease in the frequency of 12 heterozygotes (increased homozygosity) in subjects with cocaine dependence (29.8%) vs controls (46.9%) (P≤.028). This percentage was still lower in those who had chronically used cocaine for more than 10 y (25%), or more than 15 y (21.5%).	Comings et al,[128] 1999	DRD3 gene accounted for 1.64% of the variance of cocaine dependence. The DRD2 gene had an independent and additive effect on cocaine dependence. These findings support a modest role of the DRD3 gene in susceptibility to cocaine dependence.

Data from Refs.[78,80-129]

MC4R-mediated synaptic changes in vivo. Thus, stress turns on the MC4R that, in turn, reduces DA D1 receptor activation causing anhedonia. The role of anhedonia has been reviewed by Blum and colleagues.[135]

Along with the DA D2 receptor, the melanocortin-3 receptor (MC3R) and MC4R are known to play critical roles in energy homeostasis.[136,137] Interestingly, the VTA is one of the sites of highest MC3R expression. Lippert and colleagues[138] demonstrated that MC3R, but not MC4R, is expressed in up to a third of dopaminergic neurons of the VTA. Total DA in the VTA increases by 42% following global deletion of the MC3R and sucrose preference and intake decreases in female but not male mice. In fact, ovariectomy restores DA levels to normal, but aberrant decreased VTA DA levels are also observed in prepubertal female mice. The arcuate agouti-related peptide/neuropeptide Y neurons that are involved in eating behavior[138] are known to innervate and regulate VTA signaling. The MC3R in dopaminergic neurons provides specific input for communication of a nutritional state within the mesolimbic DA system. This gender-specific effect supports a sexually dimorphic function of MC3R in the regulation of the mesolimbic dopaminergic system and reward and may also involve circulating estrogen. Understanding the role of genetics in obesity and eating disorders provides the impetus to look for potential therapeutic targets by briefly exploring the role of DA genetics in these conditions.

Dopamine D2 Receptor Gene

When stimulated, the DA receptors (D1–D5) release synaptic DA, and individuals experience a reduction in stress and enhanced feelings of well-being.[139] As mentioned earlier, the mesocorticolimbic dopaminergic pathway mediates reinforcement of both unnatural rewards and natural rewards. Natural drives are reinforced physiologic drives, such as hunger and reproduction, whereas unnatural rewards involve the satisfaction of acquired learned pleasures, hedonic sensations like those derived from drugs, alcohol, gambling, and other risk-taking behaviors.[140]

One notable DA gene is the DRD2 gene that is responsible for the synthesis of DA D2 receptors.[83] The allelic form (A1 vs A2) of the DRD2 gene is responsible for the expression of receptors at postjunctional sites. The A1 form results in hypodopaminergic function,[83,141] and in people, a paucity of DA receptors are predisposed to seek any substance or behavior that stimulates the dopaminergic system.[142]

The neurotransmitter DA and the DRD2 gene, despite controversy,[143] have long been associated with reward.[14] Although the *Taq*1 A1 allele of the DRD2 gene has been associated with many neuropsychiatric disorders and initially with severe alcoholism, it also has a genetic association with other substance and process addictions as well as Tourette syndrome, high novelty-seeking behaviors, attention deficit hyperactivity disorder (ADHD), and in children and adults, with comorbid antisocial personality disorder symptoms as denoted in RDS.[144]

Although the focus of this article is on food and drugs and being mutuality addictive, the role and function of DA genetics in addictions and the concept that concerns the genetic antecedents of multiple addictions are reviewed. There may be a common neurobiology, neurocircuitry, and neuroanatomy for several psychiatric disorders and multiple addictions. RDS was first described in 1996 as a theoretic genetic predictor of compulsive, addictive, and impulsive behaviors.[27,144,145] The concept evolved with the realization that the DRD2 A1 genetic variant is associated with these behaviors. RDS involves the pleasure or reward mechanisms that rely on DA. RDS behaviors are manifestations of DA resistance or depletion.[146] Reward deficiency can be the result of overindulgence or stress, or a DA deficiency based on genetic makeup. RDS or antireward pathways help to explain how certain genetic anomalies can give rise to complex aberrant behavior. It is well known that drugs of abuse, alcohol, sex, food, gambling, and aggressive thrills, indeed, most positive reinforcers, cause activation and neuronal release of brain DA and can decrease negative feelings. Abnormal cravings are linked to low DA function[147] (**Fig. 1**).

Complex behaviors can be produced by specific genetic antecedents. For instance, reduced D2 receptors, a consequence of having the A1 variant of the DRD2 gene,[148] may predispose individuals to a high risk for cravings; this deficiency could be compounded if the person had another polymorphism in, for example, the DAT gene that resulted in the excessive removal of DA from the synapse. In addition, substance abuse and aberrant behaviors also deplete DA. RDS can be manifest in severe or mild forms that are a consequence of the inability to derive reward from ordinary, everyday activities. Although many genes and polymorphisms predispose individuals to abnormal DA function, carriers of the *Taq*1 A1 allele of the DRD2 gene lack enough DA receptor sites to achieve adequate DA sensitivity. This DA deficit in the reward site of the brain can result in unhealthy appetites and craving. In essence, they seek substances like alcohol, opiates, cocaine, nicotine, glucose, and behaviors, even abnormally aggressive behaviors that are known to activate dopaminergic pathways and cause the preferential release of DA in the NAc. There is now evidence that rather than the NAc, the anterior cingulate cortex may be involved in operant, effort-based decision-making[85,148] and may be a site for relapse involving DA D2 receptor gene polymorphisms.

Impairment of the DRD2 gene or in other DA receptor genes, such as the DRD1 involved in homeostasis and so-called normal brain function, could ultimately lead to neuropsychiatric disorders, including aberrant drug- and food-seeking behavior. Prenatal drug abuse in the pregnant woman has been shown to have profound effects

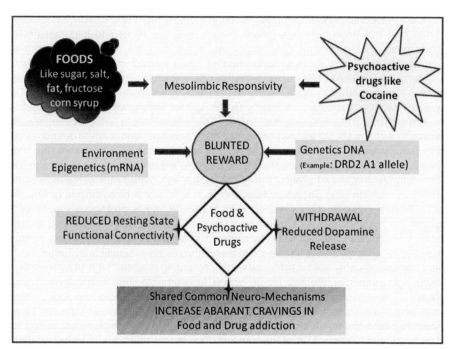

Fig. 1. The common neuro-mechanisms between food and drug addiction.

on the neurochemical state of offspring; these include ethanol,[149] cannabis,[150] heroin,[151] cocaine,[152] and drug abuse in general.[153] Novak and colleagues[154] found strong evidence showing that abnormal development of striatal neurons is part of the pathologic abnormality underlying major psychiatric illnesses. The authors identified an underdeveloped gene network in (early) rat that lacks important striatal receptor pathways (signaling). At 2 postnatal weeks, the network is downregulated and replaced by a network of mature genes expressing striatal-specific genes, including the DA D1 and D2 receptors and providing these neurons with their functional identity and phenotypic characteristics. This developmental switch is potentially a point wherein both the rat and human are susceptible to disruption of growth by epigenetic factors like drug abuse or excessive indulgence in foods, like salt and glucose.

Other Dopamine Genes and Commonality

Sikora and colleagues[155] showed that there is a correlation between mean BMI values and variable number of tandem repeats (VNTR) polymorphisms in SLC6A3 (rs28363170) and DRD4 genes. They found that when the 2 analyzed polymorphisms were combined, the mean BMI values became greater than for single genes. This finding suggests that the effect on body mass of these 2 polymorphisms may combine and cause hypofunctionality of the dopaminergic reward system; this takes on even more importance when the role of the DA transporter gene (SLC6A3) is considered as a factor in drug dependence.[156] van der Zwaluw and colleagues[156] showed that the fast-acting 9 allele of the DAT1 gene resulted in an enhanced withdrawal response in alcoholics.

Can We Explain Relapse via Dopaminergic Genetics?

It is well known that after prolonged abstinence, people who use their drug of choice experience a powerful euphoria that often precipitates relapse. Although a biological explanation for this conundrum has remained elusive, Blum and colleagues[157] suggested that this potentially fatal phenomenon could be related to supersensitivity tied to genetic dopaminergic polymorphisms. In addition, the dopaminergic agonist bromocriptine induces stronger activation of brain reward circuitry in individuals who carry the DRD2 A1 allele compared with DRD2 A2 allele carriers. Because carriers of the A1 allele relative to the A2 allele of the DRD2 gene have significantly lower D2 receptor density, a reduced sensitivity to DA agonist activity would be expected in the former. Thus, it is perplexing that with low D2 density there is an increase in reward sensitivity with the DA D2 agonist bromocriptine. Moreover, under acute but not long-term therapy with D2 agonists, such as bromocriptine, it has been shown in vitro that there is a proliferation of D2 receptors. One possible explanation for this relates to the demonstration that the A1 allele of the DRD2 gene is associated with increased striatal activity of L-amino acid decarboxylase, the final step in the biosynthesis of DA. As such, Blum's group[157] hypothesized that this could be a protective mechanism against low receptor density and would favor the utilization of an amino acid neurotransmitter precursor like L-tyrosine for preferential synthesis of DA. This theory seems to lead to receptor proliferation to normal levels and results in significantly better treatment compliance only in A1 carriers possibly preventing relapse.[85] It is of interest that amino acid precursor therapy as proposed to attenuate drug reinstatement and relapse[158] may involve amino acid inhibition of brain kynurenic acid formation, which could occur with cannabis ingestion. The issue here is that kynurenic acid has been shown to inhibit glutaminergic activity, thereby increasing Gabaergic function, resulting in a reduced release of DA at the NAc loci. Sekine and colleagues[159] most recently showed that precursor neurotransmitter L-amino acids, like phenylalanine, tyrosine, and glutamate for example, inhibit the uptake of kynurenic acid into the rat brain; this seems to be fortuitous when one considers the potential benefit of amino acid nutrient therapy to prevent relapse.

Dopaminergic Agonistic Therapy as a Common Treatment for Food and Drug Addiction

The pharmacologic treatment of obesity may be effective. However, medications may have significant side effects, and the pandemic continues. There is significant evidence to substantiate the existence of RDS in obesity and the role of catecholaminergic pathways in aberrant substance-seeking behavior, in particular, cravings for carbohydrates.[14] Earlier work from Gold's group provided an essential framework for shared common neurochemical mechanisms for both food and drugs.[25,160,161]

In the mid 1970s, it was found that laboratory animals would self-administer drugs of abuse, lose control over the drugs, change behaviors, and make the same choices as human addicts. The realization that laboratory animals will self-administer psychoactive drugs provided the basis for a definition of addiction that involved withdrawal symptoms. Moreover, it was found that self-administration of all abusable drugs, like cocaine, could continue until death or near death, providing compelling evidence that cocaine is a highly addictive drug.[161] This work resulted in the well-known "dopamine depletion hypothesis" first reported by Dackis and Gold.[162] This theory was based on the fact that abusable drugs like cocaine are addicting because they can stimulate the intense release of DA and as such become an acquired drive with a salience equal to food and sex.[21] Certainly, repeated use of psychoactive substances, including glucose, would functionally deplete the brain of DA in the reward circuitry, producing a tremendous drive for repeated use of the psychostimulants, disorder eating, and depressive anhedonia.[163–167]

Gold's group began to consider food as another addiction when they realized that drug-withdrawal states are also associated with overeating and weight gain. Early abstinence is characterized by a rebound hyperphagia-overeating and weight gain during abstinence and recovery. In cigarette smokers, weight gain continued for up to a year after smoking cessation and became a major impediment to successful cessation, which may be due to effects on Ghrelin.[168–170]

It is well-known that even in many treatment centers and 12-step meetings abstinence from drugs and transfer of addictive behaviors that include overeating almost uncontrolled sugar-, carbohydrate-, and fat-seeking can be considered by the uninformed as successful abstinence. These behaviors provided part of the impetus for the development of animal models for drug and food reinforcement. In a series of experiments, it was unequivocally shown that drugs and food have quite similar effects on brain systems. Specifically, it was shown that glucose and fructose corn syrup were avidly self-administered like a drug of abuse and caused brain changes similar to alcohol and other drugs. Drugs, alcohol, and sugar caused DA release and loss of control.[5–8,170–174]

The concept of common mechanisms of action between alcohol and opiates that had its origin in the early 1970s based on several experiments by Blum and associates and others led to the common utilization of narcotic antagonism for not only drugs of abuse like alcohol, heroin, cocaine[175–188] but also even food addiction, including anorexia nervosa, hyperphagia, and binge eating.[57,189–201]

Previous work from the authors' laboratory suggested the importance of early genetic diagnosis of addiction risk, especially in children diagnosed with ADHD.[202–205] Interestingly, Reinblatt and colleagues[206] recently provided evidence that children with ADHD experience pediatric loss of control eating syndrome whereby they are at increased risk for impulsivity linked to eating disorders.

Addiction to psychoactive drugs poses a significant threat to the health and socio-economic fabric of communities, families, and nations. The number of substance users is staggering. The National Institute on Drug Abuse estimates suggest the existence of smokers numbering 1.3 billion, 2 billion alcohol users, and 185 million abusers of other substances[4] (Table 2).

These numbers emphasize the urgent need to develop novel treatments for addiction and advanced methods to evaluate the efficacy of potential therapeutic agents. A major limitation in advancing the development of novel therapeutics for many neuropsychiatric diseases (including substance dependence) is the lack of appropriate methods for analyzing the functional organization of the central nervous system (CNS). The integration of brain regions into transient, and sometimes persistent, functional networks seems to be part of the organizational principles of the brain.[207] Progress in understanding how the in vivo brain is functionally connected during normalcy will likely lead to new understanding of why these functional connections are hampered during disease states. High field functional MRI (fMRI) using well-validated neuroanatomical analysis methods and animal models can provide an understanding of the intrinsic functional organization of the CNS and the ability to test compounds that can alter the brain's connectivity patterns.[208]

Another challenge is the lack of treatment strategies focusing on the well-known, highly characterized biochemical pathways regulating brain DA systems that are involved in mediating rewarding experiences. Because of rapid and prolonged cellular and intracellular adaptations in response to compounds that act selectively (like desensitization, supersensitivity), many pharmacotherapeutics fail at normalizing DA at a neural circuitry level. Normalizing DA is one promising strategy that is consistent with recent animal models of dependence[209] and with previous theories of the role of DA in addiction.[195] Following the discovery of intrinsic oscillations in blood oxygenation levels–dependent signal, there have been several studies reporting evidence of altered functional connectivity induced by or associated with drug use and dependence.[210,211] Healthy correlations in spontaneous resting state activity between specific regions of the cortex and limbic subcortical areas are impacted by drug abuse and are altered in volunteers dependent on alcohol, cocaine, cannabis, or heroin.[212] Similar observations have been reported in adolescents with Internet gaming addiction, in pathologic gamblers, and in persons with bulimia.[213–215]

Despite a growing number of studies applying resting state fMRI to investigate the functional neurocircuitry of human addiction and reward,[216–218] there is a lack of similar studies in laboratory animals. To achieve better treatment outcomes, it is mandatory to

Table 2
Costs of substance abuse

	Health Care	Overall
Tobacco	$130 billion	$295 billion
Alcohol	$25 billion	$224 billion
Illicit drugs	$11 billion	$193 billion

From National Institute on Drug Abuse (NIH). The science of drug abuse & addiction: trends and statistics. Available at: http://www.drugabuse.gov/related-topics/trends-statistics. Accessed May 9, 2015.

maintain steady "dopaminergic homeostasis,"[219] which is essential for achieving plea-surable experiences from ordinary daily activities and for relieving stress. The challenge is to develop nonhazardous, nonaddicting agents with dopaminergic upregulating agonistic properties. Certainly, untreated impairments in the homeostatic balance of the DA signaling can facilitate aberrant substance-related disorders and process addictions including food abuse.

This theory suggests that excessive craving behavior can be attributed to reduced number of DA D_2 receptors, an effect of carrying, for example, the DRD2 A1 allelic genotype, whereas a normal or sufficient density of D_2 receptors results in reduced craving.[220] With the aim of preventing substance abuse, a goal could be to induce a proliferation of D_2 receptors in individuals who are genetically vulnerable. Although, in vivo experiments that used a typical D_2 receptor agonist induce downregulation,[221] in vitro experiments have shown that despite genetic antecedents, constant stimulation with a known D_2 agonist, bromocriptine, results in significant proliferation of D_2 receptors within the DA system. However, the chronic treatment with buprenorphine and methadone results in differential regulation of both D1 and D2 receptors instead of upregulation at different time periods and is a reason for long-term failure in treatment due to mood changes.[222]

Along these lines, Volkow and Baler[223] suggested that balancing behaviors that provide a reward NOW compared with behaviors that provide an advantage LATER is important for survival. They proposed a model in which DA can favor NOW processes through phasic signaling in reward circuits or LATER processes through tonic signaling in control circuits. Under normal physiologic states, DA modulates the orbitofrontal cortex, which processes salience attribution. Moreover, DA also enables shifting from NOW to LATER. In the insula, DA selects NOW versus LATER that influences interoceptive information. Thus, disruptions especially in the balance of D1 versus D2 DA receptors in the brain reward circuitry may contribute to the pathologic abnormality observed in food and drug addiction.

Pharmacologic Treatments

The recognition of addictions as a brain disorder by the American Society of Addiction Medicine (ASAM)[224] indicates that treatments aimed at addressing food addiction must address the dysfunctions at the level of the brain. It follows, then, that pharmaceuticals may be essential adjuncts to the effective treatment of these disordered brain mechanisms. Many excellent reviews have been written outlining the endogenous neurotransmitter involvement in food addiction, including papers on opiates,[225,226] neuropeptide Y and leptin,[227] cannabinoids,[228] and DA.[229,230] Unsurprisingly, the use of pharmaceuticals has been suggested to modulate these brain areas, decrease craving, and negate pathologic drive for overconsumption.[231,232]

Current pharmacologic treatments for obesity have failed to address the problem adequately. Despite the neurobiological linkage with satiety signals and noted elevated levels of leptin in obese individuals and food addicts, trials of pegylated recombinant human leptin that targeted the homeostatic mechanisms of obesity have not succeeded.[227,233–238] Sibutramine, a mixed serotonin, norepinephrine, and DA reuptake inhibitor, had shown some promise of effecting weight loss, but was pulled off the market in 2010 because of concerns about increased risk of stroke and cardiovascular events.[239,240] Orlistat is currently the only pharmacologic therapy for obesity that is approved for long-term use (up to 1 year). It works by inhibiting absorption of fat in the gut and results in modest weight loss, an average of 6.4 pounds in the course of a year.[239] Phentermine and diethylpropion also are commonly provided for obesity and similarly have had limited success.[240] Despite their use, these pharmaceuticals for obesity have failed to produce significant, enduring weight loss[241] and at best have provided only modest, short-term benefit.[242,243]

Given the lack of utility of current treatments, new modalities are currently under investigation. Traditionally, obesity-related treatments have targeted hunger and eating behavior itself. Researchers now are interested in further characterizing the effects of various nutrients and herbals on the neurotransmitter systems of the brain, because these may provide for targeted interventions based on an individual's particular food preference.[244] Researchers also are interested in pharmacotherapeutic interventions aimed at reducing the reinforcing effects of highly palatable nutrients as a means of reducing body mass.[5] Indeed, many new treatments are in both phase II and phase III clinical trials, including Contrave, Qnexa, and Lorcaserin, and other novel pharmaceuticals are being investigated.[47]

Most recently, several combinations are actively being investigated and approved, such as naltrexone and bupropion[245] as well as phentermine and topiramate.[246] Theoretically these combinations in the short term may be useful not only to reduce alcohol intake but also by blocking DA, resulting in attenuated reward, that will make sugar and hedonic foods less pleasurable with potential concomitant weight loss.

Nutrigenomic Treatments

Evidence supports nutrigenomic augmentation using precursor amino acid therapy and enkephalinase, monoamine oxidase (MOA), and catechol-O-methyltransferase (COMT) inhibition as a treatment of brain dysfunctions. Enhanced levels of ASAM neurotransmitters: serotonin, enkephalins, GABA, and DA/norepinephrine, can repair a disrupted dopaminergic homeostasis, including increasing insulin sensitivity (affecting DA neuronal synthesis regulation) is well documented. KB220 and many variants have been researched over the last 40 years[247] in both animal models and humans. This nutrigenomic formula that has a generalized anticraving effect can inhibit carbohydrate bingeing, induce significant healthy fat loss, and prevent relapse.[248] As reported in detailed review and research articles[249–251] on both animals and humans to date, KB220 variants have enhanced brain enkephalin levels in rodents, pharmacogenetically reduced alcohol-seeking behavior in C57/BL mice, and converted ethanol acceptance alcohol in preferring mice to the same levels as found in nonpreferring mice. Human alcohol and drug withdrawal symptoms have been reduced using KB220Z. Benzodiazepine use and days of withdrawal tremor are reduced, and there is no severe depression on the MMPI as well as a lower BUD (building up to drink) score. Patients in recovery had significantly improved physical scores and BESS Scores (behavioral, emotional, social, and spiritual), and reduced stress response was measured by the skin conductance level. When comparing KB220 variant to placebo groups, there was a 6-fold decrease in AMA (against medical advice) rates after detoxification. Healthy volunteers demonstrated an enhanced focus. There are also experiments that show evidence of reduced craving for alcohol, cocaine, heroin, and nicotine. Also, reductions in inappropriate sexual behavior and reduced posttraumatic stress (PTSD) symptoms, such as lucid nightmares, have been reported.[252–258] Quantitative electroencephalography studies have found that KB220Z modulates theta power in anterior cingulate cortex of abstinent psychostimulant addicts.[252,253] In abstinent heroin addicts, a single dose of KB220Z compared with placebo in a pilot study[217] resulted in activation of the nucleus accumbens as well as activation and improvement of the prefrontal-cerebellar-occipital neural network. In addition, it was found that carriers of the DRD2 A1 allele showed a significant Pearson correlation in terms of enhanced compliance to KB220Z treatment relative to carriers of the normal complement of DRD2 receptors in known obese patients.[259] This finding further suggests that improved DA function equates to better treatment outcomes.

Previously, Blum's group theorized that customized nutraceuticals based on DNA individualization may have meaningful effects on whole-body recomposition by off-setting the effects of numerous genetic polymorphisms.[64] Along these lines, obesity and related symptoms significantly aggravate type 2 diabetes, and both obesity and diabetes are influenced by the interaction of genes and environmental factors (epigenetics). Current scientific literature has classified several candidate genes responsible for both of these disorders, especially the DRD2, methylenetetrahydrofolate reductase (MTHFR), serotonin receptor (5-HT2a), peroxisome proliferator-activated receptor gamma (PPAR-γ), and leptin genes.[260]

Here, the authors review the results of several studies[261–263] whereby Blum's Laboratory genotyped 1058 subjects and administered a KB220z variant (LG9939). Formerly called LG9939, Recomposize, and Geno Trim, KB220z is a complex neuro-adaptagen nutraceutical composed of –D,L-phenylalanine, chromium, L-tyrosine and other select amino acids, and adaptogens. Treatment was based on personalized polymorphic genetic outcomes. In a small subset, simple t tests comparing several parameters before treatment and throughout an 80-day treatment period on the nutraceutical were performed.

The significant clinical outcomes are as follows: weight loss ($P<.008$); sugar craving reduction ($P<.008$); appetite suppression ($P<.004$); snack reduction ($P<.005$); reduction of late-night bingeing ($P<.007$); increased perception of overeating ($P<.02$); increased energy ($P<.004$); enhanced quality of sleep ($P<.02$), and increased happiness ($P<.02$). Polymorphic correlates were obtained for a number of genes (PPAR gamma 2, MTHFR, 5-HT2a, and DRD2 genes) with positively tested clinical parameters throughout this study. Importantly, only the DRD2 gene polymorphism (AI allele) had a substantial Pearson correlation regarding number of treatment days ($r = 0.42$, $P = .045$) when compared with all potential outcomes and gene polymorphisms. This 2-fold increase is a very important genotype for compliance in treatment.[261] This work was similarly confirmed in another study.[262]

Although there is still controversy concerning the best approach to treat both drug and food addiction, it seems parsimonious to provide short-term blockade of DA function to attenuate intense pleasure and subsequent substance seeking, but in the long term, the challenge is to find a way to activate DA neuropathways and induce DA homeostasis. The authors are encouraged that based on the work by Willuhn and colleagues[264] that as addictive behaviors like cocaine use and even non-substance-related behaviors increase, dopaminergic function is reduced. This finding highlights that neurologic DA deficit, not a surfeit, is the outcome of addiction. Moreover, in a recent PET study, Tomasi and colleagues[265] found that chronic cocaine exposure has been associated with decreases in D2/D3 receptors and was also associated with lower activation of cues in occipital cortex and cerebellum. Treatment strategies, like DA agonist therapy, that conserve or restore DA function may be an attractive approach to relapse prevention in food, psychoactive drug, and behavioral addictions.

Future Perspectives and Policy

Scientists must recognize that eating disorders, food addiction, and food withdrawal are very similar to drug withdrawal states, especially in terms of concomitant overeating and even weight gain by the addict. Certainly, early abstinence is characterized by a rebound hyperphagia-overeating and weight gain during abstinence from drug abuse. In one known example, cigarette smokers that stopped smoking continued to gain weight.[266] This effect was highlighted by Stice and colleagues[10,59,62] showing that weight gain in subjects that carry the DRD2 A1 allele continues for more than a 1-year period. Simply, drugs of abuse and eating are related for many reasons, not the least of which is that drugs hijack the brain by co-opting existing primary brain reinforcement systems. Understanding the role of tolerance related to excessive DA release in the NAc was indeed a reality observed by the Woodstock generation with a mantra of sex, drugs, and rock and roll,[21] whereby too much of a good thing resulted in the loss of its reinforcement.

The authors are concerned that even today many of the 14,500 treatment centers including 12-step meetings serve cakes, cookies, and coffee as an adjunct to help during recovery. In fact, addicts looking for advice on staying sober are told at Alcohol Anonymous meetings never to get too hungry and carry around sugar or candy for "drug" cravings. Although the authors encourage medical-assisted US Food and Drug Administration–approved drugs during short-term treatment, they also encourage a healthy diet designed by experienced chefs serving up more "dopamine for dinner."[267]

Brownell and Gold summarized the field in their book, *"Food and Addiction,"*[268] Following their pioneering efforts, the book adequately provides the basis for food as a truly addictive substance just like cocaine and other psychoactive licit and illicit abusable substances. Bulimia, anorexia nervosa, bingeing, and hyperphagia as repetitive behaviors share the neurochemical and neurogenetic mechanisms, and all meet the criteria of addiction as espoused by ASAM.[224] It is noteworthy that people with anorexia nervosa are very thin, and with obesity, the opposite is quite true. This phenomenon of opposite effects (anorexia nervosa looks like the opposite of hedonic overeating) seems to be similar in some ways to mania and depression, opposite poles of the same brain system. With this stated, Jung and colleagues[214] recently pointed out that research into addiction prevention and treatment would benefit from patient classification into reproducible categories that have predictive validity and requires the development of better biomarkers. Urine drug testing is a clinically valuable biomarker for relatively recent drug use. Thus, to determine both chronic use and potential high risk, they suggest that more research is required to investigate epitranscriptomics, genetics, epigenetics, and human brain function and neurochemistry (brain imaging tools, including electroencephalography). By doing so, they further suggest that this will enhance the ability to screen and treat patients with SUDs. In fact, Badgaiyan[269] developed a novel neuroimaging method to detect DA across various brain regions from the prefrontal cortices to the hippocampus to the VTA.

In terms of novel therapies, the authors' group recently reviewed the possibility of vaccines[270] and even gene therapy[271] and concluded that addiction medicine due to its complexities and polygenic inheritable factors will not see benefit from these enormous scientific advancements for many years. It is inconceivable that they could attack glucose craving through either a vaccination or gene therapy but they may be able to develop better animal models for anorexia nervosa and bulimia in the future to help formulate new treatments.

Policymakers may consider the model of taxing tobacco products, which has been the single most important prevention tool in reducing smoking. Based on the food addiction hypothesis, higher prices might also reduce soda consumption. A review suggested that for every 10% increase in price, consumption decreases by 7.8%. An industry trade publication reported even larger reductions: as prices of carbonated soft drinks increased by 6.8%, sales dropped by 7.8%, and as Coca-Cola prices increased by

12%, sales decreased by 14.6%. It follows that a tax on sweetened beverages might help consumers switch to water or more healthful beverages. Such a switch would lead to reduced caloric intake and possible weight loss.[272] Moreover, lessons are to be learned from changing public behaviors and attitudes to reduce smoking and smoking-related health care costs and suffering. Changing access to cigarettes by elimination of cigarette vending machines, limiting smoking in public areas, raising the price per pack to decrease numbers of cigarettes or packs per day smoked, training clinicians to reduce smoking initiation, to intervene and not look the other way, all helped reduce smoking. Importantly, aspects of smoking exposure at an early age can induce neuro-epigenetic effects and induce a gateway to harder drugs as researched by Kandel and Kandel.[273] Early exposure in utero or in early life to second-hand tobacco smoke greatly increases the risk of life-long tobacco use and addiction.[272] In the 1990s, sweetened drink intake by children passed that of milk and the per capita caloric intake from sugar/high-fructose corn syrup (HFCS)–sweetened beverages has increased by nearly 30%. Beverages now account for 10% to 15% of the calories consumed by children and adolescents. It is likely that food addiction models can be used to explain early exposure and changes in preference becoming fixed and persistent for life.[272] An extra can or glass of sugar or HFCS-sweetened beverage consumed per day increases the likelihood of a child's becoming obese by 60%.

Although food addiction may explain some, but certainly not all, obesity, understanding shared common brain mechanisms between glucose, for example, and cocaine may lead to newer treatments and better outcomes. With an addiction hypothesis that included DA, the authors discovered the efficacy of bupropion and then Chantix. Thus, rather than a successful short-term treatment rate of less than 20%, they routinely helped 30% of smokers, but there is the potential for mood changes. Still, addiction-inspired public health measures of early intervention and prevention rather than medically assisted treatment were responsible for most of the successful smoking cessation efforts.

Moreover, although the authors treated the lung cancers, stroke, erectile dysfunction, and other diseases caused by smoking, there were 400,000 deaths per year in the United States plus an additional 40,000 deaths due to second-hand smoke. Until recently, little effort was directed at preventing smoking or treating smokers. All of this progress and all of the health savings related to smoking cessation will soon be replaced by obesity-related costs. One must ask, are these 2 events related? As tobacco use and addiction are associated with decreases in eating and weight, a nation detoxifying from smoking addiction should be expected to become overweight. The authors propose that this unwanted side effect of detoxification may be offset by the induction of novel development of modalities that will induce DA homeostasis.[274]

An example of how DA could be regulated may reside in the G-protein-gated inwardly rectifying potassium (GIRK) channels that regulate neuronal excitability and can be activated by ethanol. A recent study by Herman and colleagues[275] showed that genetic ablation of GIRK3, 1 of 4 GIRK subunits, prevents ethanol from activating the mesolimbic dopaminergic pathway. Conversely, increasing GIRK3 expression in the ventral midbrain reduces bingelike drinking. The authors conclude that GIRK3 appears to be a critical gatekeeper of ethanol incentive salience and a potential target for the treatment of excessive ethanol consumption. The authors ask, what about glucose as well?

SUMMARY

Based on experiences with tobacco taxation, proposals for food taxes have been made, and calculations formulated of revenue benefits. Even when these fail, the public and health experts have to think through the idea that fruits and vegetables are more costly than fatty, sweet, fast foods. Using taxes on ingredients such as added sugar and fructose corn syrup would decrease exposure according to addiction models. Coca-Cola and other sodas might return to sucrose as in Mexican or Kosher Coke. Reducing portion size, although supported by cigarette experience with numbers of cigarettes per pack and purchase limits, is a weaker intervention than other approaches. Now food labels and calorie postings are seen that educate everyone as they balance the calories against the time and energy to exercise away the calories ingested. Exercise is necessary and promotes health, but is not a stand-alone in obesity treatment or management strategy. Moreover, stigmatization of the overweight with added health premiums and workplace incentives has not worked well in the past. Blaming the patient, creating shame and guilt, does not do much to inspire treatment efficacy.[272]

Last, obesity has changed the width of the seats in airplanes and dress and trouser sizes. The obesity-related problems: high cholesterol, high blood pressure, high blood sugars, and knee and joint pain, have become routine in medical practice and treatment. Over the past 3 decades, rates of obesity have increased in the United States and elsewhere so that now more people are obese globally and in need of intelligent treatment than ever.

We as authors stay positive in that understanding of both the neurogenetics and the neurobiology of RDS, and as such, addiction medicine and new evidence-based approaches could emerge. Society must embrace novel public health initiatives (as seen in tobacco) and treatment approaches for drug, food, and other behavioral addictions and continue to obtain relevant biomarkers using genomic principles and neuroimaging techniques.

ACKNOWLEDGMENTS

The authors appreciate the expert edits from Margaret A. Madigan.

REFERENCES

1. Budd GM, Peterson JA. The obesity epidemic, part 1: understanding the origins. Am J Nurs 2014;114(12):40–6.
2. Sturm R. The effects of obesity, smoking, and drinking on medical problems and costs. Health Aff (Millwood) 2002;21:245–53.
3. Skidmore PM, Yarnell JW. The obesity epidemic: prospects for prevention. QJM 2004;97:817–25.
4. NIDDK. Overweight and Obesity Statistics WIN: Weight-control Information Network. 2005.
5. Avena NM, Gold MS. Food and addiction - sugars, fats and hedonic overeating. Addiction 2011;106:1214–5.
6. Avena NM, Rada P, Hoebel BG. Evidence for sugar addiction: behavioral and neurochemical effects of intermittent, excessive sugar intake. Neurosci Biobehav Rev 2008;32:20–39.
7. Avena NM, Rada P, Hoebel BG. Sugar and fat bingeing have notable differences in addictive-like behavior. J Nutr 2009;139:623–8.
8. Colantuoni C, Rada P, McCarthy J, et al. Evidence that intermittent, excessive sugar intake causes endogenous opioid dependence. Obes Res 2002;10: 478–88.
9. Johnson PM, Kenny PJ. Dopamine D2 receptors in addiction-like reward dysfunction and compulsive eating in obese rats. Nat Neurosci 2010;13:635–41.

10. Stice E, Yokum S, Blum K, et al. Weight gain is associated with reduced striatal response to palatable food. J Neurosci 2010;30:13105–9.
11. Gearhardt AN, Corbin WR, Brownell KD. Preliminary validation of the Yale food addiction scale. Appetite 2009;52:430–6.
12. Volkow ND, Wang GJ, Fowler JS, et al. Overlapping neuronal circuits in addiction and obesity: evidence of systems pathology. Philos Trans R Soc Lond B Biol Sci 2008;363:3191–200.
13. Volkow ND, Wang GJ, Baler RD. Reward, dopamine and the control of food intake: implications for obesity. Trends Cogn Sci 2011;15:37–46.
14. Blum K, Liu Y, Shriner R, et al. Reward circuitry dopaminergic activation regulates food and drug craving behavior. Curr Pharm Des 2011;17:1158–67.
15. Erlanson-Albertsson C. Appetite regulation and energy balance. Acta Paediatr Suppl 2005;94:40–1.
16. Salamone JD, Correa M. The mysterious motivational functions of mesolimbic dopamine. Neuron 2012;76:470–85.
17. Sinha R. Stress and addiction. In: Brownell Kelly D, Gold Mark S, editors. Food and addiction: a comprehensive handbook. New York: Oxford University Press; 2012. p. 59–66.
18. Nutt DJ, Lingford-Hughes A, Erritzoe D, et al. The dopamine theory of addiction: 40 years of highs and lows. Nat Rev Neurosci 2015;16(5):305–12.
19. Blum K, Oscar-Berman M, Barh D, et al. Dopamine genetics and function in food and substance abuse. J Genet Syndr Gene Ther 2013;4(121) [pii:1000121].
20. Blum K, Payne J. Alcohol & the addictive brain. New York; London: Simon & Schuster Free Press; 1990.
21. Blum K, Werner T, Carnes S, et al. Sex, drugs, and rock 'n' roll: hypothesizing common mesolimbic activation as a function of reward gene polymorphisms. J Psychoactive Drugs 2012;44:38–55.
22. Blum K, Gold MS. Neuro-chemical activation of brain reward meso-limbic circuitry is associated with relapse prevention and drug hunger: a hypothesis. Med Hypotheses 2011;76:576–84.
23. Gunaydin LA, Deisseroth K. Dopaminergic dynamics contributing to social behavior. Cold Spring Harb Symp Quant Biol 2015 [pii:024711].
24. Hart AS, Clark JJ, Phillips PE. Dynamic shaping of dopamine signals during probabilistic Pavlovian conditioning. Neurobiol Learn Mem 2015;17:84–92.
25. Gold MS. From bedside to bench and back again: a 30-year saga. Physiol Behav 2011;104:157–61.
26. Gold MS, Graham NA, Cocores JA, et al. Food addiction? J Addict Med 2009;3: 42–5.
27. Blum K, Sheridan PJ, Wood RC, et al. The D2 dopamine receptor gene as a determinant of reward deficiency syndrome. J R Soc Med 1996;89:396–400.
28. Wang GJ, Volkow ND, Thanos PK, et al. Imaging of brain dopamine pathways: implications for understanding obesity. J Addict Med 2009;3:8–18.
29. Blum K, Braverman ER, Wood RC, et al. Increased prevalence of the Taq I A1 allele of the dopamine receptor gene (DRD2) in obesity with comorbid substance use disorder: a preliminary report. Pharmacogenetics 1996;6: 297–305.
30. Chen AL, Blum K, Chen TJ, et al. Correlation of the Taq1 dopamine D2 receptor gene and percent body fat in obese and screened control subjects: a preliminary report. Food Funct 2012;3:40–8.
31. Shah NR, Braverman ER. Measuring adiposity in patients: the utility of body mass index (BMI), percent body fat, and leptin. PLoS One 2012;7:e33308.

32. Volkow ND, Wang GJ, Tomasi D, et al. The addictive dimensionality of obesity. Biol Psychiatry 2013;73:811–8.

33. Volkow ND, Wang GJ, Tomasi D, et al. Obesity and addiction: neurobiological overlaps. Obes Rev 2013;14:2–18.

34. Savage SW, Zald DH, Cowan RL, et al. Regulation of novelty seeking by midbrain dopamine D2/D3 signaling and ghrelin is altered in obesity. Obesity (Silver Spring) 2014;22:1452–7.

35. Skibicka KP, Shirazi RH, Rabasa-Papio C, et al. Divergent circuitry underlying food reward and intake effects of ghrelin: dopaminergic VTA-accumbens projection mediates ghrelin's effect on food reward but not food intake. Neuropharmacology 2013;73:274–83.

36. Skibicka KP, Hansson C, Alvarez-Crespo M, et al. Ghrelin directly targets the ventral tegmental area to increase food motivation. Neuroscience 2011;180: 129–37.

37. Ahn S, Phillips AG. Dopaminergic correlates of sensory-specific satiety in the medial prefrontal cortex and nucleus accumbens of the rat. J Neurosci 1999; 19:RC29.

38. Martel P, Fantino M. Mesolimbic dopaminergic system activity as a function of food reward: a microdialysis study. Pharmacol Biochem Behav 1996;53:221–6.

39. White NM. Control of sensorimotor function by dopaminergic nigrostriatal neurons: influence on eating and drinking. Neurosci Biobehav Rev 1986; 10:15–36.

40. Lindblom J, Johansson A, Holmgren A, et al. Increased mRNA levels of tyrosine hydroxylase and dopamine transporter in the VTA of male rats after chronic food restriction. Eur J Neurosci 2006;23:180–6.

41. Patterson TA, Brot MD, Zavosh A, et al. Food deprivation decreases mRNA and activity of the rat dopamine transporter. Neuroendocrinology 1998;68:11–20.

42. Ifland JR, Preuss HG, Marcus MT, et al. Refined food addiction: a classic substance use disorder. Med Hypotheses 2009;72:518–26.

43. Roitman MF, Patterson TA, Sakai RR, et al. Sodium depletion and aldosterone decrease dopamine transporter activity in nucleus accumbens but not striatum. Am J Physiol 1999;276:R1339–45.

44. Cocores JA, Gold MS. The Salted Food Addiction Hypothesis may explain overeating and the obesity epidemic. Med Hypotheses 2009;73:892–9.

45. Roitman MF, Schafe GE, Thiele TE, et al. Dopamine and sodium appetite: antagonists suppress sham drinking of NaCl solutions in the rat. Behav Neurosci 1997;111:606–11.

46. Avena NM, Gold MS. Variety and hyperpalatability: are they promoting addictive overeating? Am J Clin Nutr 2011;94:367–8.

47. Blumenthal DM, Gold MS. Neurobiology of food addiction. Curr Opin Clin Nutr Metab Care 2010;13:359–65.

48. Leibowitz SF, Hoebel BG. Behavioral neuroscience and obesity. In: Bray GBC, James P, editors. The handbook of obesity. New York: Marcel Dekker; 2004. p. 301–71.

49. Berner LA, Bocarsly ME, Hoebel BG, et al. Baclofen suppresses binge eating of pure fat but not a sugar-rich or sweet-fat diet. Behav Pharmacol 2009;20:631–4.

50. Corwin RL, Wojnicki FH. Baclofen, raclopride, and naltrexone differentially affect intake of fat and sucrose under limited access conditions. Behav Pharmacol 2009;20:537–48.

51. Volkow ND, Wise RA. How can drug addiction help us understand obesity? Nat Neurosci 2005;8:555–60.

52. Robinson MJ, Warlow SM, Berridge KC. Optogenetic excitation of central amygdala amplifies and narrows incentive motivation to pursue one reward above another. J Neurosci 2014;34:16567–80.

53. Hirano Y, Saitoe M. Hunger-driven modulation in brain functions. Brain Nerve 2014;66:41–8.

54. Uher R, Treasure J, Heining M, et al. Cerebral processing of food-related stimuli: effects of fasting and gender. Behav Brain Res 2006;169:111–9.

55. Saper CB, Chou TC, Elmquist JK. The need to feed: homeostatic and hedonic control of eating. Neuron 2002;36:199–211.

56. Wilson GT. Eating disorders, obesity and addiction. Eur Eat Disord Rev 2010;18: 341–51.

57. Avena NM, Bocarsly ME. Dysregulation of brain reward systems in eating disorders: neurochemical information from animal models of binge eating, bulimia nervosa, and anorexia nervosa. Neuropharmacology 2012;63:87–96.

58. Brown AJ, Avena NM, Hoebel BG. A high-fat diet prevents and reverses the development of activity-based anorexia in rats. Int J Eat Disord 2008;41: 383–9.

59. Stice E, Yokum S, Zald D, et al. Dopamine-based reward circuitry responsivity, genetics, and overeating. Curr Top Behav Neurosci 2011;6:81–93.

60. Comings DE, Flanagan SD, Dietz G, et al. The dopamine D2 receptor (DRD2) as a major gene in obesity and height. Biochem Med Metab Biol 1993;50:176–85.

61. Noble EP, Noble RE, Ritchie T, et al. D2 dopamine receptor gene and obesity. Int J Eat Disord 1994;15:205–17.

62. Stice E, Spoor S, Bohon C, et al. Relation between obesity and blunted striatal response to food is moderated by TaqIA A1 allele. Science 2008;322:449–52.

63. Harrower AD, Yap OL, Nairn IM, et al. Bromocriptine and TRH-induced growth hormone release in anorexia nervosa. PLoS One 2013;8:e71509.

64. Blum K, Chen TJ, Meshkin B, et al. Genotrim, a DNA-customized nutrigenomic product, targets genetic factors of obesity: hypothesizing a dopamine-glucose correlation demonstrating reward deficiency syndrome (RDS). Med Hypotheses 2007;68:844–52.

65. Platania CB, Salomone S, Leggio GM, et al. Homology modeling of dopamine D2 and D3 receptors: molecular dynamics refinement and docking evaluation. PLoS One 2012;7:e44316.

66. Koob G, Kreek MJ. Stress, dysregulation of drug reward pathways, and the transition to drug dependence. Am J Psychiatry 2007;164:1149–59.

67. Olsen CM. Natural rewards, neuroplasticity, and non-drug addictions. Neuropharmacology 2011;61:1109–22.

68. Conrad KL, Ford K, Marinelli M, et al. Dopamine receptor expression and distribution dynamically change in the rat nucleus accumbens after withdrawal from cocaine self-administration. Neuroscience 2010;169:182–94.

69. Bowirrat A, Oscar-Berman M. Relationship between dopaminergic neurotransmission, alcoholism, and reward deficiency syndrome. Am J Med Genet B Neuropsychiatr Genet 2005;132B:29–37.

70. Gardner EL. Addiction and brain reward and anti-reward pathways. Adv Psychosom Med 2011;30:22–60.

71. Walton ME, Groves J, Jennings KA, et al. Comparing the role of the anterior cingulate cortex and 6-hydroxydopamine nucleus accumbens lesions on operant effort-based decision making. Eur J Neurosci 2009;29:1678–91.

72. Rice JP, Suggs LE, Lusk AV, et al. Effects of exposure to moderate levels of ethanol during prenatal brain development on dendritic length, branching,

and spine density in the nucleus accumbens and dorsal striatum of adult rats. Alcohol 2012;46:577–84.

73. Morón JA, Brockington A, Wise RA, et al. Dopamine uptake through the norepinephrine transporter in brain regions with low levels of the dopamine transporter: evidence from knock-out mouse lines. J Neurosci 2002;22:389–95.

74. Schultz W. Predictive reward signal of dopamine neurons. J Neurophysiol 1998; 80:1–27.

75. Derauf C, Kekatpure M, Neyzi N, et al. Neuroimaging of children following prenatal drug exposure. Semin Cell Dev Biol 2009;20:441–54.

76. Di Chiara G. The role of dopamine in drug abuse viewed from the perspective of its role in motivation. Drug Alcohol Depend 1995;38:95–137.

77. Drtilkova I, Sery O, Theiner P, et al. Clinical and molecular-genetic markers of ADHD in children. Neuro Endocrinol Lett 2008;29:320–7.

78. Alia-Klein N, Parvaz MA, Woicik PA, et al. Gene × disease interaction on orbitofrontal gray matter in cocaine addiction. Arch Gen Psychiatry 2011;68:283–94.

79. James GA, Gold MS, Liu Y. Interaction of satiety and reward response to food stimulation. J Addict Dis 2004;23:23–37.

80. Blum K, Noble EP, Sheridan PJ, et al. Allelic association of human dopamine D2 receptor gene in alcoholism. JAMA 1990;263(15):2055–60.

81. Neville MJ, Johnstone EC, Walton RT. Identification and characterization of ANKK1: a novel kinase gene closely linked to DRD2 on chromosome band 11q23.1. Hum Mutat 2004;23(6):540–5.

82. Blum K, Wood RC, Braverman ER, et al. The D2 dopamine receptor gene as a predictor of compulsive disease: Bayes' theorem. Funct Neurol 1995;10(1):37–44.

83. Noble EP, Blum K, Ritchie T, et al. Allelic association of the D2 dopamine receptor gene with receptor-binding characteristics in alcoholism. Arch Gen Psychiatry 1991;48:648–54.

84. Hoffman EK, Zezza N, Thalamuthu A, et al. Dopaminergic mutations: withinfamily association and linkage in multiplex alcohol dependence families. Am J Med Genet B Neuropsychiatr Genet 2008;147B(4):517–26.

85. Dahlgren A, Wargelius HL, Berglund KJ, et al. Do alcohol-dependent individuals with DRD2 A1 allele have an increased risk of relapse? A pilot study. Alcohol Alcohol 2011;46:509–13.

86. Kraschewski A, Reese J, Anghelescu I, et al. Association of the dopamine D2 receptor gene with alcohol dependence: haplotypes and subgroups of alcoholics as key factors for understanding receptor function. Pharmacogenet Genomics 2009;19(7):513–27.

87. Teh LK, Izuddin AF, M H FH, et al. Tridimensional personalities and polymorphism of dopamine D2 receptor among heroin addicts. Biol Res Nurs 2012; 14(2):188–96.

88. Van Tol HH. Structural and functional characteristics of the dopamine D4 receptor. Adv Pharmacol 1998;42:486–9.

89. Lai JH, Zhu YS, Huo ZH, et al. Association study of polymorphisms in the promoter region ofDRD4 with schizophrenia, depression, and heroin addiction. Brain Res 2010;1359:227–32.

90. Biederman J, Petty CR, Ten Haagen KS, et al. Effect of candidate gene polymorphisms on the course of attention deficit hyperactivity disorder. Psychiatry Res 2009;170(2–3):199–203.

91. Faraone SV, Doyle AE, Mick E, et al. Meta-analysis of the association between the 7-repeat allele of the dopamine D(4) receptor gene and attention deficit hyperactivity disorder. Am J Psychiatry 2001;158(7):1052–7.

92. Grzywacz A, Kucharska-Mazur J, Samochowiec J. Association studies of dopamine D4 receptor gene exon 3 in patients with alcohol dependence. Psychiatr Pol 2008;42(3):453–61.
93. Kotler M, Cohen H, Segman R, et al. Excess dopamine D4 receptor (D4DR) exon III seven repeat allele in opioid-dependent subjects. Mol Psychiatry 1997;2(3):251–4.
94. Byerley W, Hoff M, Holik J, et al. VNTR polymorphism for the human dopamine transporter gene (DAT1). Hum Mol Genet 1993;2(3):335.
95. Galeeva AR, Gareeva AE, Iur'ev EB, et al. VNTR polymorphisms of the serotonin transporter and dopamine transporter genes in male opiate addicts. Mol Biol (Mosk) 2002;36(4):593–8.
96. Reese J, Kraschewski A, Anghelescu I, et al. Haplotypes of dopamine and serotonin transporter genes are associated with antisocial personality disorder in alcoholics. Psychiatr Genet 2010;20(4):140–52.
97. Cook EH Jr, Stein MA, Krasowski MD, et al. Association of attention-deficit disorder and the dopamine transporter gene. Am J Hum Genet 1995;56(4):993–8.
98. Lee SS, Lahey BB, Waldman I, et al. Association of dopamine transporter genotype with disruptive behavior disorders in an eight-year longitudinal study of children and adolescents. Am J Med Genet B Neuropsychiatr Genet 2007; 144B(3):310–7.
99. Schellekens AF, Franke B, Ellenbroek B, et al. Reduced dopamine receptor sensitivity as an intermediate phenotype in alcohol dependence and the role of the COMT Val158Met and DRD2 Taq1A genotypes. Arch Gen Psychiatry 2012;69(4):339–48.
100. Nedic G, Nikolac M, Sviglin KN, et al. Association study of a functional catechol-O-methyltransferase (COMT) Val108/158Met polymorphism and suicide attempts in patients with alcohol dependence. Int J Neuropsychopharmacol 2011;4(3):377–88.
101. Demetrovics Z, Varga G, Szekely A, et al. Association between Novelty Seeking of opiate-dependent patients and the catechol-O-methyltransferase Val(158) Met polymorphism. Compr Psychiatry 2010;51(5):510–5.
102. Baransel Isir AB, Oguzkan S, Nacak M, et al. The catechol-O-methyl transferase Val158Met polymorphism and susceptibility to cannabis dependence. Am J Forensic Med Pathol 2008;29(4):320–2.
103. Merenäkk L, Mäestu J, Nordquist N, et al. Effects of the serotonin transporter (5-HTTLPR) and α2A-adrenoceptor (C-1291G) genotypes on substance use in children and adolescents: a longitudinal study. Psychopharmacology (Berl) 2011;215(1):13–22.
104. van der Zwaluw CS, Engels RC, Vermulst AA, et al. A serotonin transporter polymorphism (5-HTTLPR) predicts the development of adolescent alcohol use. Drug Alcohol Depend 2010;112(1–2):134–9.
105. Kosek E, Jensen KB, Lonsdorf TB, et al. Genetic variation in the serotonin transporter gene (5-HTTLPR, rs25531) influences the analgesic response to the short acting opioid Remifentanil in humans. Mol Pain 2009;1(5):37.
106. Ray R, Ruparel K, Newberg A, et al. Human Mu Opioid Receptor (OPRM1 A118G) polymorphism is associated with brain mu-opioid receptor binding potential in smokers. Proc Natl Acad Sci U S A 2011;108(22):9268–73.
107. Szeto CY, Tang NL, Lee DT, et al. Association between mu opioid receptor gene polymorphisms and Chinese heroin addicts. Neuroreport 2001;12(6):1103–6.
108. Bart G, Kreek MJ, Ott J, et al. Increased attributable risk related to a functional mu-opioid receptor gene polymorphism in association with alcohol dependence in central Sweden. Neuropsychopharmacology 2005;30(2):417–22.

109. Hall FS, Sora I, Uhl GR. Ethanol consumption and reward are decreased in mu-opiate receptor knockout mice. Psychopharmacology (Berl) 2001; 154(1):43–9.

110. Namkoong K, Cheon KA, Kim JW, et al. Association study of dopamine D2, D4 receptor gene, GABAA receptor beta subunit gene, serotonin transporter gene polymorphism with children of alcoholics in Korea: a preliminary study. Alcohol 2008;42(2):77–81.

111. Mhatre M, Ticku MK. Chronic ethanol treatment upregulates the GABA receptor beta subunitexpression. Brain Res Mol Brain Res 1994;23(3):246–52.

112. Young RM, Lawford BR, Feeney GF, et al. Alcohol-related expectancies are associated with the D2 dopamine receptor and GABAA receptor beta3 subunit genes. Psychiatry Res 2004;127(3):171–83.

113. Feusner J, Ritchie T, Lawford B, et al. GABA(A) receptor beta 3 subunit gene and psychiatric morbidity in a post-traumatic stress disorder population. Psychiatry Res 2001;104(2):109–17.

114. Noble EP, Zhang X, Ritchie T, et al. D2 dopamine receptor and GABA(A) receptor beta3 subunitgenes and alcoholism. Psychiatry Res 1988;81(2):133–47.

115. Nikulina V, Widom CS, Brzustowicz LM. Child abuse and neglect, MAOA, and mental health outcomes: a prospective examination. Biol Psychiatry 2012; 71(4):350–7.

116. Nilsson KW, Comasco E, Åslund C, et al. MAOA genotype, family relations and sexual abuse in relation to adolescent alcohol consumption. Addict Biol 2011; 16(2):347–55.

117. Treister R, Pud D, Ebstein RP, et al. Associations between polymorphisms in dopamine neurotransmitter pathway genes and pain response in healthy humans. Pain 2009;147(1–3):187–93.

118. Tikkanen R, Auvinen-Lintunen L, Ducci F, et al. Psychopathy, PCL-R, and MAOA genotype as predictors of violent reconvictions. Psychiatry Res 2011;185(3): 382–6.

119. Gokturk C, Schultze S, Nilsson KW, et al. Serotonin transporter (5-HTTLPR) and monoamine oxidase (MAOA) promoter polymorphisms in women with severe alcoholism. Arch Womens Ment Health 2008;11(5–6):347–55.

120. Contini V, Marques FZ, Garcia CE, et al. MAOA-uVNTR polymorphism in a Brazilian sample: further support for the association with impulsive behaviors and alcohol dependence. Am J Med Genet B Neuropsychiatr Genet 2006; 141B(3):305–8.

121. Lee SY, Chen SL, Chen SH, et al. Interaction of the DRD3 and BDNF gene variants in subtyped bipolar disorder. Prog Neuropsychopharmacol Biol Psychiatry 2012;39(2):382–7.

122. Li T, Hou Y, Cao W, et al. Role of dopamine D3 receptors in basal nociception regulation and in morphine-induced tolerance and withdrawal. Brain Res 2012;1433:80–4.

123. Vengeliene V, Leonardi-Essmann F, Perreau-Lenz S, et al. The dopamine D3 receptor plays an essential role in alcohol-seeking and relapse. FASEB J 2006; 20(13):2223–33.

124. Mulert C, Juckel G, Giegling I, et al. A Ser9Gly polymorphism in the dopamine D3 receptor gene (DRD3) and event-related P300 potentials. Neuropsychopharmacology 2006;31(6):1335–44.

125. Limosin F, Romo L, Batel P, et al. Association between dopamine receptor D3 gene BalI polymorphism and cognitive impulsiveness in alcohol-dependent men. Eur Psychiatry 2005;20(3):304–6.

126. Duaux E, Gorwood P, Griffon N, et al. Homozygosity at the dopamine D3 receptor gene is associated with opiate dependence. Mol Psychiatry 1998;3(4): 333–6.
127. Spangler R, Wittkowski KM, Goddard NL, et al. Opiate-like effects of sugar on gene expression in reward areas of the rat brain. Brain Res Mol Brain Res 2004;124(2):134–42.
128. Comings DE, Gonzalez N, Wu S, et al. Homozygosity at the dopamine DRD3 receptor gene in cocaine dependence. Mol Psychiatry 1999;4(5):484–7.
129. Blum K, Han D, Giordano J, et al. Neurogenetics and nutrigenomics of Reward Deficiency Syndrome (RDS): stratification of addiction risk and meso-limbic nutrigenomic manipulation of hypodopaminergic function. In: Barh D, editor. Pharmacogenomics. London: Springer; 2015.
130. Do DN, Strathe AB, Ostersen T, et al. Genome-wide association study reveals genetic architecture of eating behavior in pigs and its implications for human obesity by comparative mapping. Obesity (Silver Spring) 2006;14:529–644.
131. Locke A, Kahali B, Berndt SI, et al. Genetic studies of body mass index yield new insights for obesity biology. Nature 2015;518:197–206.
132. Garfield AS, Li C, Madara JC, et al. A neural basis for melanocortin-4 receptor-regulated appetite. Nat Neurosci 2015. [Epub ahead of print].
133. Shah BP, Vong L, Olson DP, et al. MC4R-expressing glutamatergic neurons in the paraventricular hypothalamus regulate feeding and are synaptically connected to the parabrachial nucleus. Proc Natl Acad Sci U S A 2014;111: 13193–8.
134. Lim BK, Huang KW, Grueter BA, et al. Anhedonia requires MC4R-mediated synaptic adaptations in nucleus accumbens. Endocrinology 2014;155:1718–27.
135. Blum K, Oscar-Berman M, Gardner EL, et al. Chapter 10: neurogenetics and neurobiology of dopamine in anhedonia. In: Ritsner MS, editor. Anheonia: a comprehensive handbook, vol. 1. Dordrecht Heidelberg (NY); London: Springer; 2014. p. 209–44.
136. Baik JH. Dopamine signaling in food addiction: role of dopamine D2 receptors. BMB Rep 2013;46:519–26.
137. Begriche K, Girardet C, McDoald P, et al. Melanocortin-3 receptors and metabolic homeostasis. Prog Mol Biol Transl Sci 2013;114:109–46.
138. Lippert RN, Ellacott KL, Cone RD. Gender-specific roles for the melanocortin-3 receptor in the regulation of the mesolimbic dopamine system in mice. Nature 2012;487:183–9.
139. Żurawek D, Faron-Górecka A, Kuśmider M, et al. Mesolimbic dopamine D_2 receptor plasticity contributes to stress resilience in rats subjected to chronic mild stress. Psychopharmacology (Berl) 2013;227:583–93.
140. Kenny PJ. Reward mechanisms in obesity: new insights and future directions. Neuron 2011;69:664–79.
141. Blum K, Noble EP, Sheridan PJ, et al. Association of the A1 allele of the D2 dopamine receptor gene with severe alcoholism. Alcohol 1991;8:409–16.
142. Blum K, Sheridan PJ, Wood RC, et al. Dopamine D2 receptor gene variants: association and linkage studies in impulsive-addictive-compulsive behaviour. Pharmacogenetics 1995;5:121–41.
143. Gelernter J, Goldman D, Risch N. The A1 allele at the D2 dopamine receptor gene and alcoholism. A reappraisal. JAMA 1993;269:1673–7.
144. Yang BZ, Kranzler HR, Zhao H, et al. Haplotypic variants in DRD2, ANKK1, TTC12, and NCAM1 are associated with comorbid alcohol and drug dependence. Alcohol Clin Exp Res 2008;32:2117–27.

145. Comings DE, Blum K. Reward deficiency syndrome: genetic aspects of behavioral disorders. Prog Brain Res 2000;126:325–41.

146. Blum K, Oscar-Berman M, Badgaiyan RD, et al. Hypothesizing dopaminergic genetic antecedents in schizophrenia and substance seeking behavior. Med Hypotheses 2014;82:606–14.

147. Alguacil LF, González-Martín C. Target identification and validation in brain reward dysfunction. Drug Discov Today 2015;20:347–52.

148. Zhou Y, Leri F, Cummins E, et al. Individual differences in gene expression of vasopressin, D2 receptor, POMC and orexin: vulnerability to relapse to heroin-seeking in rats. Physiol Behav 2015;139:127–35.

149. Kobor MS, Weinberg J. Focus on: epigenetics and fetal alcohol spectrum disorders. Alcohol Res Health 2011;34:29–37.

150. Bonnin A, de Miguel R, Castro JG, et al. Effects of perinatal exposure to delta 9-tetrahydrocannabinol on the fetal and early postnatal development of tyrosine hydroxylase-containing neurons in rat brain. J Mol Neurosci 1996;7:291–308.

151. Dryden C, Young D, Hepburn M, et al. Maternal methadone use in pregnancy: factors associated with the development of neonatal abstinence syndrome and implications for healthcare resources. BJOG 2009;116:665–71.

152. Eiden RD, Godleski S, Schuetze P, et al. Prenatal substance exposure and child self-regulation: pathways to risk and protection. J Exp Child Psychol 2015;137: 12–29.

153. Narkowicz S, Płotka J, Polkowska Ż, et al. Prenatal exposure to substance of abuse: a worldwide problem. Environ Int 2013;54:141–63.

154. Novak G, Fan T, O'dowd BF, et al. Striatal development involves a switch in gene expression networks, followed by a myelination event: implications for neuropsychiatric disease. Synapse 2013;67:179–88.

155. Sikora M, Gese A, Czypicki R, et al. Correlations between polymorphisms in genes coding elements of dopaminergic pathways and body mass index in overweight and obese women. Endokrynol Pol 2013;64:101–7.

156. van der Zwaluw CS, Engels RC, Buitelaar J, et al. Polymorphisms in the dopamine transporter gene (SLC6A3/DAT1) and alcohol dependence in humans: a systematic review. Pharmacogenomics 2009;10:853–66.

157. Blum K, Chen TJ, Downs BW, et al. Neurogenetics of dopaminergic receptor supersensitivity in activation of brain reward circuitry and relapse: proposing "deprivation-amplification relapse therapy" (DART). Postgrad Med 2009;121: 176–96.

158. Blum K, Berman MO, Braverman ER, et al. Raising endogenous brain levels of kynurenic acid may produce anti-reward and enhance suicide ideation. J Alcohol Drug Depend 2014;2:151.

159. Sekine A, Okamoto M, Kanatani Y, et al. Amino acids inhibit kynurenic acid formation via suppression of kynurenine uptake or kynurenic acid synthesis in rat brain in vitro. Springerplus 2015;1(4):48.

160. Bruijnzeel AW, Repetto M, Gold MS. Neurobiological mechanisms in addictive and psychiatric disorders. Psychiatr Clin North Am 2004;4:661–74.

161. Gold MS, Dackis CA. New insights and treatments: narcotics and cocaine addiction. Clin Ther 1985;7:6–21.

162. Dackis CA, Gold MS. New concepts in cocaine addiction: the dopamine depletion hypothesis. Neurosci Biobehav Rev 1985;9:469–77.

163. Blum K, Febo M, Smith DE, et al. Neurogenetic and epigenetic correlates of adolescent predisposition to and risk for addictive behaviors as a function of

prefrontal cortex dysregulation. J Child Adolesc Psychopharmacol 2015;25(4): 286–92.

164. Daberkow DP, Brown HD, Bunner KD, et al. Amphetamine paradoxically augments exocytotic dopamine release and phasic dopamine signals. J Neurosci 2013;33:452–63.

165. Pelloux Y, Dilleen R, Economidou D, et al. Reduced forebrain serotonin transmission is causally involved in the development of compulsive cocaine seeking in rats. Neuropsychopharmacology 2012;37:2505–14.

166. Deng C, Li KY, Zhou C, et al. Ethanol enhances glutamate transmission by retrograde dopamine signaling in a postsynaptic neuron/synaptic bouton preparation from the ventral tegmental area. Neuropsychopharmacology 2009;34: 1233–44.

167. Yuan J, Cord BJ, McCann UD, et al. Effect of depleting vesicular and cytoplasmic dopamine on methylenedioxymethamphetamine neurotoxicity. J Neurochem 2002;80:960–9.

168. Edge PJ, Gold MS. Drug withdrawal and hyperphagia: lessons from tobacco and other drugs. Curr Pharm Des 2011;17:1173–9.

169. Zhang XL, Albers KM, Gold MS. Inflammation-induced increase in nicotinic acetylcholine receptor current in cutaneous nociceptive DRG neurons from the adult rat. Neuroscience 2015;284:483–99.

170. Koopmann A, Bez J, Lemenager T, et al. Effects of cigarette smoking on plasma concentration of the appetite-regulating peptide ghrelin. Ann Nutr Metab 2015; 66:155–61.

171. Gold MS, Avena NM. Animal models lead the way to further understanding food addiction as well as providing evidence that drugs used successfully in addictions can be successful in treating overeating. Biol Psychiatry 2013;74:e11.

172. Avena NM, Murray S, Gold MS. Comparing the effects of food restriction and overeating on brain reward systems. Exp Gerontol 2013;48:1062–7.

173. Avena NM, Murray S, Gold MS. The next generation of obesity treatments: beyond suppressing appetite. Front Psychol 2013;4:721.

174. Avena NM, Bocarsly ME, Hoebel BG, et al. Overlaps in the nosology of substance abuse and overeating: the translational implications of "food addiction". Curr Drug Abuse Rev 2011;4:133–9.

175. Blum K. Narcotic antagonism of seizures induced by a dopamine-derived tetrahydroisoquinoline alkaloid. Experientia 1988;44:751–3.

176. Blum K, DeLallo L, Briggs AH, et al. Opioid responses of isoquinoline alkaloids (TIQs). Prog Clin Biol Res 1982;90:387–98.

177. Blum K, Briggs AH, DeLallo L, et al. Naloxone antagonizes the action of low ethanol concentrations on mouse vas deferens. Subst Alcohol Actions Misuse 1980;1:327–34.

178. Verebey K, Blum K. Alcohol euphoria: possible mediation via endorphinergic mechanisms. J Psychedelic Drugs 1979;11:305–11.

179. Blum K, Hamilton MG, Hirst M, et al. Putative role of isoquinoline alkaloids in alcoholism: a link to opiates. Alcohol Clin Exp Res 1978;2:113–20.

180. Marshall A, Hirst M, Blum K. Analgesic effects of 3-carboxysalsolinol alone and in combination with morphine. Experientia 1977;33:754–5.

181. Blum K, Futterman S, Wallace JE, et al. Naloxone-induced inhibition of ethanol dependence in mice. Nature 1977;265:49–51.

182. Blum K, Eubanks JD, Wiggins B, et al. Morphine withdrawal reactions in male and female mice. Am J Drug Alcohol Abuse 1976;3:363–8.

183. Blum K, Hamilton MG, Meyer EK, et al. Isoquinoline alkaloids as possible regulators of alcohol addiction. Lancet 1977;1:799–800.
184. Blum K, Wallace JE, Schwerter HA, et al. Morphine suppression of ethanol withdrawal in mice. Experientia 1976;32:79–82.
185. Blum K, Elston SF, DeLallo L, et al. Ethanol acceptance as a function of genotype amounts of brain [Met]enkephalin. Proc Natl Acad Sci U S A 1983;80:6510–2.
186. Blum K, Briggs AH, Elston SF, et al. Reduced leucine-enkephalin–like immunoreactive substance in hamster basal ganglia after long-term ethanol exposure. Science 1982;216:1425–7.
187. Seevers MH, Davis VE, Walsh MJ. Morphine and ethanol physical dependence: a critique of a hypothesis. Science 1970;170:1113–5.
188. Warren MW, Gold MS. The relationship between obesity and drug use. Am J Psychiatry 2007;164:1268–9.
189. Newman MM, Gold MS. Preliminary findings of patterns of substance abuse in eating disorder patients. Am J Drug Alcohol Abuse 1992;18:207–11.
190. Jonas JM, Gold MS, Sweeney D, et al. Eating disorders and cocaine abuse: a survey of 259 cocaine abusers. J Clin Psychiatry 1987;48:47–50.
191. Gold MS, Pottash AL, Sweeney DR, et al. Further evidence of hypothalamic pituitary dysfunction in anorexia nervosa. Am J Psychiatry 1980;137:101–2.
192. Jonas JM, Gold MS. Naltrexone treatment of bulimia: clinical and theoretical findings linking eating disorders and substance abuse. Adv Alcohol Subst Abuse 1987;7:29–37.
193. Avena NM, Potenza MN, Gold MS. Why are we consuming so much sugar despite knowing too much can harm us? JAMA Intern Med 2015;175:145–6.
194. Murray S, Tulloch A, Gold MS, et al. Hormonal and neural mechanisms of food reward, eating behaviour and obesity. Nat Rev Endocrinol 2014;10:540–52.
195. Gold MS, Pottash AL, Martin DM, et al. 24 hour LH patterns test in the diagnosis and assessment of response to treatment of patients with anorexia nervosa. Int J Psychiatry Med 1981;11:245–50.
196. Orsini CA, Ginton G, Shimp KG, et al. Food consumption and weight gain after cessation of chronic amphetamine administration. Appetite 2014;78:76–80.
197. Davis C, Loxton NJ. A psycho-genetic study of hedonic responsiveness in relation to "food addiction". Nutrients 2014;6:4338–53.
198. Davis C. A narrative review of binge eating and addictive behaviors: shared associations with seasonality and personality factors. Front Psychiatry 2013;4:183.
199. Davis C, Loxton NJ, Levitan RD, et al. 'Food addiction' and its association with a dopaminergic multilocus genetic profile. Physiol Behav 2013;118:63–9.
200. Davis C, Levitan RD, Yilmaz Z, et al. Binge eating disorder and the dopamine D2 receptor: genotypes and sub-phenotypes. Prog Neuropsychopharmacol Biol Psychiatry 2012;38:328–35.
201. Levitan RD, Kaplan AS, Davis C, et al. A season-of-birth/DRD4 interaction predicts maximal body mass index in women with bulimia nervosa. Neuropsychopharmacology 2010;35:1729–33.
202. Gold MS, Blum K, Oscar-Berman M, et al. Low dopamine function in attention deficit/hyperactivity disorder: should genotyping signify early diagnosis in children? Postgrad Med 2014;126:153–77.
203. Archer T, Oscar-Berman M, Blum K. Epigenetics in developmental disorder: ADHD and endophenotypes. J Genet Syndr Gene Ther 2011;2 [pii:1000104].
204. Blum K, Chen AL, Braverman ER, et al. Attention-deficit-hyperactivity disorder and reward deficiency syndrome. Neuropsychiatr Dis Treat 2008;4:893–918.

205. Comings DE, Chen TJ, Blum K, et al. Neurogenetic interactions and aberrant behavioral co-morbidity of attention deficit hyperactivity disorder (ADHD): dispelling myths. Theor Biol Med Model 2005;2:50.
206. Reinblatt SP, Mahone EM, Tanofsky-Kraff M, et al. Pediatric loss of control eating syndrome: association with attention-deficit/hyperactivity disorder and impulsivity. Int J Eat Disord 2015. [Epub ahead of print].
207. Mantini D, Corbetta M, Romani GL, et al. Evolutionarily novel functional networks in the human brain? J Neurosci 2013;33:3259–75.
208. Zhai T, Shao Y, Chen G, et al. Nature of functional links in valuation networks differentiates impulsive behaviors between abstinent heroin-dependent subjects and nondrug-using subjects. Neuroimage 2015;115:76–84.
209. Smith MA, Lacy RT, Strickland JC. The effects of social learning on the acquisition of cocaine self-administration. Drug Alcohol Depend 2014;141:1–8.
210. Hu Y, Salmeron BJ, Gu H, et al. Impaired functional connectivity within and between frontostriatal circuits and its association with compulsive drug use and trait impulsivity in cocaine addiction. JAMA Psychiatry 2015. [Epub ahead of print].
211. Coveleskie K, Gupta A, Kilpatrick LA, et al. Altered functional connectivity within the central reward network in overweight and obese women. Nutr Diabetes 2015;5:e148.
212. Cheng H, Skosnik PD, Pruce BJ, et al. Resting state functional magnetic resonance imaging reveals distinct brain activity in heavy cannabis users - a multi-voxel pattern analysis. J Psychopharmacol 2014;28:1030–40.
213. Zhang JT, Yao YW, Li CS, et al. Altered resting-state functional connectivity of the insula in young adults with Internet gaming disorder. Addict Biol 2015. [Epub ahead of print].
214. Jung MH, Kim JH, Shin YC, et al. Decreased connectivity of the default mode network in pathological gambling: a resting state functional MRI study. Neurosci Lett 2014;583:120–5.
215. Lavagnino L, Amianto F, D'Agata F, et al. Reduced resting-state functional connectivity of the somatosensory cortex predicts psychopathological symptoms in women with bulimia nervosa. Front Behav Neurosci 2014;8:270.
216. Viswanath H, Velasquez KM, Thompson-Lake DG, et al. Alterations in interhemispheric functional and anatomical connectivity are associated with tobacco smoking in humans. Front Hum Neurosci 2015;9:116.
217. Blum K, Liu Y, Wang W, et al. rsfMRI effects of KB220Z™ on neural pathways in reward circuitry of abstinent genotyped heroin addicts. Postgrad Med 2015; 127:232–41.
218. Bruijnzeel AW, Alexander JC, Perez PD, et al. Acute nicotine administration increases BOLD fMRI signal in brain regions involved in reward signaling and compulsive drug intake in rats. Int J Neuropsychopharmacol 2014;18 [pii: pyu011].
219. Speca DJ, Rabbee N, Chihara D, et al. A genetic screen for behavioral mutations that perturb dopaminergic homeostasis in mice. Genes Brain Behav 2006;5:19–28.
220. Volkow ND, Wang GJ, Begleiter H, et al. High levels of dopamine D2 receptors in unaffected members of alcoholic families: possible protective factors. Arch Gen Psychiatry 2006;63:999–1008.
221. Bogomolova EV, Rauschenbach IY, Adonyeva NV, et al. Dopamine downregulates activity of alkaline phosphatase in Drosophila: the role of D2-like receptors. J Insect Physiol 2010;56:1155–9.

222. Boundy VA, Pacheco MA, Guan W, et al. Agonists and antagonists differentially regulate the high affinity state of the D2L receptor in human embryonic kidney 293 cells. Mol Pharmacol 1995;48:956–64.
223. Volkow ND, Baler RD. NOW vs LATER brain circuits: implications for obesity and addiction. Trends Neurosci 2015 [pii:S0166-2236(15) 00080-6].
224. Smith DE. The process addictions and the new ASAM definition of addiction. J Psychoactive Drugs 2012;44:1–4.
225. Grigson PS. Like drugs for chocolate: separate rewards modulated by common mechanisms? Physiol Behav 2000;76:389–95.
226. Kelley AE, Bakshi VP, Haber SN, et al. Opioid modulation of taste hedonics within the ventral striatum. Physiol Behav 2002;76:365–77.
227. Kalra SP, Kalra PS. Overlapping and interactive pathways regulating appetite and craving. J Addict Dis 2004;23:5–21.
228. Harrold JA, Williams G. The cannabinoid system: a role in both the homeostatic and hedonic control of eating? Br J Nutr 2003;90:729–34.
229. Cannon CM, Bseikri MR. Is dopamine required for natural reward? Physiol Behav 2004;81:741–8.
230. Carr KD. Augmentation of drug reward by chronic food restriction: behavioral evidence and underlying mechanisms. Physiol Behav 2002;76:353–64.
231. Wang GJ, Volkow ND, Logan J, et al. Brain dopamine and obesity. Lancet 2001; 357:354–7.
232. Volkow ND, O'Brien CP. Issues for DSM-V: should obesity be included as a brain disorder? Am J Psychiatry 2007;164:708–10.
233. Elmquist JK, Elias CF, Saper CB. From lesions to leptin: hypothalamic control of food intake and body weight. Neuron 1999;22:221–32.
234. Kleinridders A, Könner AC, Brüning JC. CNS-targets in control of energy and glucose homeostasis. Curr Opin Pharmacol 2009;9:794–804.
235. Hukshorn CJ, Van Dielen FM, Buurman WA, et al. The effect of pegylated recombinant human leptin (PEG-OB) on weight loss and inflammatory status in obese subjects. Int J Obes Relat Metab Disord 2002;26:504–9.
236. Neary NM, McGowan BM, Monteiro MP, et al. No evidence of an additive inhibitory feeding effect following PP and PYY 3-36 administration. Int J Obes (Lond) 2008;32:1438–40.
237. Kreier F. To be, or not to be obese - that's the challenge: a hypothesis on the cortical inhibition of the hypothalamus and its therapeutical consequences. Med Hypotheses 2010;75:214–7.
238. Zhang Y, Proenca R, Maffei M, et al. Positional cloning of the mouse obese gene and its human homologue. Nature 1994;372:425–32.
239. Rucker D, Padwal R, Li SK, et al. Long term pharmacotherapy for obesity and overweight: updated meta-analysis. BMJ 2007;335:1194–9.
240. Pollack A. Abbott Labs withdraws Meridia from the market. New York: New York Times; 2010.
241. Powell AG, Apovian CM, Aronne LJ. New drug targets for the treatment of obesity. Clin Pharmacol Ther 2011;90:40–51.
242. Yanovski SZ. Pharmacotherapy for obesity–promise and uncertainty. N Engl J Med 2005;353:2187–9.
243. Wadden TA, Berkowitz RI, Womble LG, et al. Randomized trial of lifestyle modification and pharmacotherapy for obesity. N Engl J Med 2005;353: 2111–20.
244. Oben JE, Ngondi JL, Blum K. Inhibition of Irvingia gabonensis seed extract (OB131) on adipogenesis as mediated via down regulation of the PPAR gamma

and leptin genes and up-regulation of the adiponectin gene. Lipids Health Dis 2008;7:44.

245. Yanovski SZ, Yanovski JA. Naltrexone extended-release plus bupropion extended-release for treatment of obesity. JAMA 2015;313:1213–4.

246. Bray GA. Medical treatment of obesity: the past, the present and the future. Best Pract Res Clin Gastroenterol 2014;28:665–84.

247. Trachtenberg MC, Blum K. Improvement of cocaine-induced neuromodulator deficits by the neuronutrient Tropamine. J Psychoactive Drugs 1988;20:315–31.

248. Brown RJ, Blum K, Trachtenberg MC. Neurodynamics of relapse prevention: a neuronutrient approach to outpatient DUI offenders. J Psychoactive Drugs 1990;22:173–87.

249. Chen TJ, Blum K, Payte JT, et al. Narcotic antagonists in drug dependence: pilot study showing enhancement of compliance with SYN-10, amino-acid precursors and enkephalinase inhibition therapy. Med Hypotheses 2004;63:538–48.

250. Blum K, Oscar-Berman M, Stuller E, et al. Neurogenetics and nutrigenomics of neuro-nutrient therapy for Reward Deficiency Syndrome (RDS): clinical ramifications as a function of molecular neurobiological mechanisms. J Addict Res Ther 2012;3:139.

251. Chen TJ, Blum K, Chen AL, et al. Neurogenetics and clinical evidence for the putative activation of the brain reward circuitry by a neuroadaptagen: proposing an addiction candidate gene panel map. J Psychoactive Drugs 2011;43: 108–27.

252. Blum K, Chen TJ, Morse S, et al. Overcoming qEEG abnormalities and reward gene deficits during protracted abstinence in male psychostimulant and poly-drug abusers utilizing putative dopamine D_2 agonist therapy: part 2. Postgrad 2010;122:214–26.

253. Miller DK, Bowirrat A, Manka M, et al. Acute intravenous synaptamine complex variant KB220™ "normalizes" neurological dysregulation in patients during protracted abstinence from alcohol and opiates as observed using quantitative electroencephalographic and genetic analysis for reward polymorphisms: part 1, pilot study with 2 case reports. Postgrad Med 2010;122:188–213.

254. Miller M, Chen AL, Stokes SD, et al. Early intervention of intravenous KB220IV–neuroadaptagen amino-acid therapy (NAAT) improves behavioral outcomes in a residential addiction treatment program: a pilot study. J Psychoactive Drugs 2012;44:398–409.

255. Blum K, Trachtenberg MC, Elliott CE, et al. Enkephalinase inhibition and precursor amino acid loading improves inpatient treatment of alcohol and polydrug abusers: double-blind placebo-controlled study of the nutritional adjunct SAAVE. Alcohol 1988;5:481–93.

256. Mclaughlin T, Blum K, Oscar-Berman M, et al. Putative dopamine agonist (KB20z) attenuates lucid dreams in PTSD: role of enhanced brain reward functional connectivity and homeostasis redeeming joy. J Behav Addict 2015. http://dx.doi.org/10.1556/2006.4. 2015.008.

257. McLaughlin T, Blum K, Oscar-Berman M, et al. Using the neuroadaptagen KB200z™ to ameliorate terrifying, lucid nightmares in RDS patients: the role of enhanced, brain-reward, functional connectivity, and dopaminergic homeostasis. J Reward Defic Syndr 2015;1:24–35.

258. Mclaughlin T, Oscar-Beramn M, Simpatico T, et al. Hypothesizing repetitive paraphilia behavior of a medication refractive Tourette's syndrome patient having rapid clinical attenuation with KB220Z-nutrigenomic amino-acid therapy (NAAT). J Behav Addict 2013;2:117–24.

259. Blum K, Chen ALC, Chen TLC, et al. Dopamine D2 receptor Taq A1 allele predicts treatment compliance of LG839 in a subset analysis of a pilot study in The Netherlands. Gene Ther Mol Biol 2008;12:129–40.

260. Downs BW, Chen AL, Chen TJ, et al. Nutrigenomic targeting of carbohydrate craving behavior: can we manage obesity and aberrant craving behaviors with neurochemical pathway manipulation by Immunological Compatible Substances (nutrients) using a Genetic Positioning System (GPS) Map? Med Hypotheses 2009;73:427–34.

261. Blum K, Chen TJH, Williams L, et al. A short term pilot open label study to evaluate efficacy and safety of LG839, a customized DNA directed nutraceutical in obesity: exploring nutrigenomics. Gene Ther Mol Biol 2008;12:371–82.

262. Blum K, Chen AL, Chen TJ, et al. LG839: anti-obesity effects and polymorphic gene correlates of reward deficiency syndrome. Adv Ther 2008;25:894–913.

263. Blum K, Chen TJ, Meshkin B, et al. Reward deficiency syndrome in obesity: a preliminary cross-sectional trial with a Genotrim variant. Adv Ther 2006;23: 1040–51.

264. Willuhn I, Burgeno LM, Groblewski PA, et al. Excessive cocaine use results from decreased phasic dopamine signaling in the striatum. Nat Neurosci 2014;17: 704–9.

265. Tomasi D, Wang GJ, Wang R, et al. Overlapping patterns of brain activation to food and cocaine cues in cocaine abusers: association to striatal D2/D3 receptors. Hum Brain Mapp 2015;36:120–36.

266. Dale LC, Schroeder DR, Wolter TD, et al. Weight change after smoking cessation using variable doses of transdermal nicotine replacement. J Gen Intern Med 1998;13:9–15.

267. Blum K, Febo M, Thanos PK, et al. Clinically combating reward deficiency syndrome (RDS) with dopamine agonist therapy as a paradigm shift: dopamine for dinner? Mol Neurobiol 2015. [Epub ahead of print].

268. Brownell KD, Gold MS. Food & addiction: a comprehensive handbook. Oxford (United kingdom): Oxford University Press; 2014.

269. Badgaiyan RD. Imaging dopamine neurotransmission in live human brain. Prog Brain Res 2014;211:165–82.

270. Blum K, Badgaiyan RD, Anges DH, et al. Should we embrace vaccines for treating substance-related disorder, a subset of reward deficiency syndrome (RDS)? J Reward Defic Syndr 2015;1:3–5.

271. Blum K, Thanos PK, Badgaiyan, et al. Neurogentics and gene therapy for Reward Deficiency Syndrome: are we going to the promised land? Expert Opin Biol Ther 2015;1–13.

272. State Department Study Finds Alarming Rates of Opium Products in Afghan Children. Available at: http://www.state.gov/j/inl/rls/fs/140668.htm. Accessed June 23, 2015.

273. Kandel DB, Kandel ER. A molecular basis for nicotine as a gateway drug. N Engl J Med 2014;371:2038–9.

274. Blum K, Febo M, McLaughlin T, et al. Hatching the behavioral addiction egg: Reward Deficiency Solution System (RDSS) as a function of dopaminergic neurogenetics and brain functional connectivity linking all addictions under a common rubric. J Behav Addict 2014;3:149–56.

275. Herman MA, Sidhu H, Stouffer DG, et al. GIRK3 gates activation of the mesolimbic dopaminergic pathway by ethanol. Proc Natl Acad Sci U S A 2015 [pii:201416146].

Integrated Care at the Interface of Psychiatry and Primary Care

Prevention of Cardiovascular Disease

Robert M. McCarron, DO[a,b,c],*

KEYWORDS

- Psychiatric education • Preventive care • Cardiovascular disease • Hypertension
- Diabetes and mental illness

KEY POINTS

- Persons with severe mental illness are at much higher risk for having diabetes, cardiovascular disease, and related early death.
- Psychiatrists can use psychotherapy to enhance patient education and motivation, while improving the preventive care for patients who have psychiatric disorders.
- Nonfasting total cholesterol, high-density lipoprotein, triglycerides, and hemoglobin A_{1c} are much more convenient for the patient and encompass all the blood work necessary to quantify the risk for cardiovascular disease.

MENTAL ILLNESS AND COMORBID GENERAL MEDICAL ILLNESS

In an historic study published in 2006 by the Centers for Disease Control and Prevention, Colton and Manderscheid[1] reported that persons with serious mental illness (SMI) have an average life expectancy 25 years less than that of the general population. The number of years of lost life is astonishing, and in part is related to a lack of primary and preventive medical care for those who have psychiatric illness. Persons with SMI not only face the stigma related to mental illness but also experience higher medical morbidity and mortality in comparison with the general population.

Fig. 1 provides estimates of standardized mortality ratios from different medical causes in persons with schizophrenia and bipolar disorder, based on systematic

[a] Department of Internal Medicine, University of California, Davis School of Medicine, Sacramento, CA, USA; [b] Department of Psychiatry and Behavioral Sciences, University of California, Davis School of Medicine, 2230 Stockton Boulevard, Sacramento, CA 95817, USA; [c] Division of Pain Medicine, Department of Anesthesiology, University of California, Davis School of Medicine, Sacramento, CA, USA
* 2230 Stockton Boulevard, Sacramento, CA 95817.
E-mail address: rmmccarron@ucdavis.edu

Psychiatr Clin N Am 38 (2015) 463–474
http://dx.doi.org/10.1016/j.psc.2015.05.005
0193-953X/15/$ – see front matter © 2015 Elsevier Inc. All rights reserved.
psych.theclinics.com

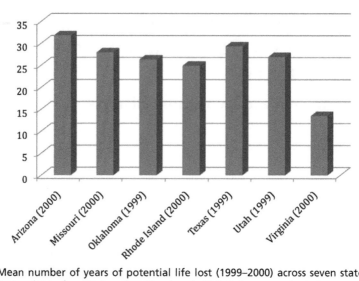

Fig. 1. Mean number of years of potential life lost (1999–2000) across seven states in the United States. (*Data from* Colton CW, Manderscheid RW. Congruencies in increased mortality rates, years of potential life lost, and causes of death among public mental health clients in eight states. Prev Chronic Dis 2006;2:A42.)

reviews and a population-based cohort study that provided data on more specific diseases for schizophrenia.[2,3] As shown in **Fig. 1**, individuals with SMI are more vulnerable and at higher risk of early death from chronic medical conditions in comparison with the general population. Conditions such as cardiovascular disease (CVD), diabetes, pulmonary disorders, and viral hepatitis are often not diagnosed or effectively managed in those with SMI.

In a report by the US National Association of State Mental Health Program Directors Medical Directors Council, the investigators estimated that whereas suicide and injury accounted for 40% of the excess mortality in schizophrenia, 60% of the excess mortality is attributed to CVD, diabetes (including kidney related deaths), respiratory infectious diseases, and other infections.[4] Persons with SMI have at least 2 to 3 times the risk of diabetes, dyslipidemia, hypertension, and obesity when compared with the general population.[5,6] Added to these medical conditions, 50% to 80% of those with SMI smoke cigarettes and consume more than one-third of available tobacco products.[7]

PREVENTING MEDICAL ILLNESS IN THE PSYCHIATRIC SETTING

CVD is the most common cause of mortality, which illustrates the urgency for physicians to more effectively and consistently provide cardiovascular-related primary preventive measures. Shorter life spans are not unique to those with schizophrenia. In one study, standardized mortality ratios in those with bipolar disorder were found to be 2.5 in men and 2.7 in women.[8] Patients with moderate to severe depression also have an elevated risk of myocardial dysfunction.[9] Patients with chronic mental illness, particularly severe mental illness, are inherently vulnerable and at increased risk of early death. What can be done to better implement preventive medical care for those with SMI?

Although this vulnerability in those who have SMI has been known for more than 2 decades, little has been done to change how we provide health care to this patient population; this is not surprising, as it is difficult to effectively change large systems of care without changing the way in which we train mental health providers. With the implementation of the Affordable Care Act and the call for evidence-based integrated mental health care, psychiatrists are well positioned to partner with primary care providers and help address common, preventable, and treatable disorders in those who have mental illness (eg, heart disease, infectious diseases, and cancers). This following sections aim to address what can be done to bridge these gaps in clinical knowledge and patient care, emphasizing the role of psychiatry in preventive care for those with mental illness. Risk assessment for CVD, in addition to an update on the diagnosis and prevention of hypertension, diabetes, and dyslipidemia, are discussed.

CLINICAL VIGNETTE

S.P. is a 38-year-old obese man with schizophrenia who presents for a follow-up visit. He has been inconsistently taking various antipsychotics for the past 9 years. He was prescribed olanzapine 11 months ago and says that he is "doing well." He denies current psychotic symptoms. His last psychiatric hospitalization was 1 year ago, which is when he moved in with his mother, who ensures that he takes his medication. He maintains a sedentary lifestyle and states that he has gradually gained weight over the past year (body mass index [BMI; weight in kilograms divided by height in meters squared, ie, kg/m^2] is 32.9 and waist circumference is 43 inches). He has a 12 pack-year history of smoking cigarettes and does not wish to stop smoking one half-pack per day. He denies alcohol and drug use. He has not seen a primary care physician since his hospitalization. S.P.'s father died of CVD at age 49 years. He has a paternal uncle with severe mental illness.

S.P.'s vitals are as follows: blood pressure, 164/90 mm Hg; pulse, 102 beats/min; respiratory rate, 14; temperature, 36.9°C (98.4°F); BMI, 32.9.

S.P.'s laboratory results are as follows: hemoglobin A_{1c} 8.2%, fasting blood glucose 205 mg/dL, total cholesterol 245 mg/dL, high-density lipoprotein (HDL) 32 mg/dL, low-density lipoprotein (LDL) 152 mg/dL, triglycerides 216 mg/dL, creatinine 0.8 mg/dL.

S.P. has numerous concerning metabolic derangements, which are likely linked to his schizophrenia and the treatment of this condition. He has the following medical concerns, which increase his risk for a heart attack or stroke:

- *Obesity*
- *Diabetes type 2*
- *Dyslipidemia*
- *Hypertension*
- *Schizophrenia*
- *Tobacco dependence*
- *Precontemplative stage of change or low motivation to make healthy lifestyle changes*
- *Family history of vascular disease*
- *Schizophrenia*
- *Greater than 20% atherosclerotic heart disease (Atherosclerotic Cardiovascular Disease [ASCVD] event 10-year risk)*

The following treatment considerations are discussed with S.P.

- *The reason(s) for suboptimal motivation to change is explored with S.P., and an action plan to improve his motivation level is developed. Part of this plan is assessing for depression and anxiety. S.P. should understand his actions are paramount when considering future medical complications and that his health care team will show ongoing support, independent of his choice or ability to initiate healthy lifestyle habits.*

- *Olanzapine may be cross-titrated to another atypical antipsychotic with relatively lower risk for metabolic derangements.*

- *S.P. is asked to consider participation in Weight Watchers, or any other program that supports assessment of daily caloric intake and exercise patterns.*

- *S.P should be started on both metformin for diabetes and an angiotensin-converting enzyme inhibitor (ACEI) for hypertension, in the context of diabetes. Both medications are renally protective and will decrease risk for a future vascular insult. The diagnosis of diabetes indicates that S.P. has existing vascular disease (risk equivalent) and is not merely at increased risk for vascular disease.*

- *Because S.P. likely has CVD and is at increased risk for a heart attack or stroke, he should be started on a high-potency statin, as tolerated.*

- *Use of cigarettes is the most preventable and reversible cardiac risk factor. S.P. should be encouraged to quit smoking.*

ASSESSING CARDIOVASCULAR RISK

Coronary vascular disease is the leading cause of death among men and women in the United States. CVD is the most common form of heart disease and was responsible for a reported 1 in 6 deaths in 2008 and a total of 385,000 deaths in in 2009. Risk-factor modification is an important strategy for decreasing morbidity and mortality from coronary artery disease (CAD) in the psychiatric patient population.[10]

Up to 60% of premature deaths in patients with schizophrenia are attributable to medical illnesses, and individuals with schizophrenia have a higher risk of coronary events than the general population.[11] Patients with bipolar affective disorder die 8 to 9 years earlier than controls, with CVD one of the leading causes of death.[12]

Box 1 provides a list of risk factors and risk equivalents for CVD, which can be used to approximate the risk of vascular-related morbidity.[13] Low (<10%), moderate (10%–20%), or high (>20%) 10-year risk of CAD can be quantified using the ASCVD risk

---

Box 1
Risk factors and risk equivalents for cardiovascular disease (CVD)

CVD risk equivalents (10-year risk of CVD ~20%, risk class high)

Diabetes mellitus

Abdominal aortic aneurysm

Peripheral arterial disease

Symptomatic carotid artery stenosis

Major risk factors

Family history of CVD in first-degree relative (male <55, female <65)

Cigarette smoking

Hypertension, treated or untreated

Age (male ≥45, female ≥55)

High-density lipoprotein <40 mg/dL

Adapted from Vanderlip ER, Fiedorowicz JG, Haynes WG. Screening, diagnosis, and treatment of dyslipidemia among persons with persistent mental illness: a literature review. Psychiatr Serv 2012;63:693–701.

assessment calculator, which was developed by the American College of Cardiology and the American Heart Association (http://tools.cardiosource.org/ASCVD-Risk-Estimator/). This online tool is easy to use and is now the standard of care when estimating risk for CVD-related morbidity. The preventive treatment plan, which often includes use of medications, will largely be based on this estimated risk. The United States Preventive Service Task Force (USPSTF) recommends against screening with either resting or exercise electrocardiogram (ECG) for individuals suspected of being at low risk for CAD because the information provided by the ECG testing does not add to the clinical risk assessment.[14] Lifestyle modification and attention to modifiable coronary risk factors are important primary prevention strategies. Dietary modifications, exercise, not smoking, and maintenance of normal BMI (<25) are associated with a lower risk of CAD.[15]

Situations warranting referral to a primary care provider and/or cardiologist include:

- New or worsening symptoms of possible cardiovascular event (eg, chest pain, dyspnea on exertion)
- New symptoms of left ventricular systolic dysfunction (eg, dyspnea, exercise intolerance, edema, paroxysmal nocturnal dyspnea, orthopnea)
- Any history of syncope, which could indicate arrhythmia or medication intolerance
- New diagnosis of diabetes mellitus
- Estimated CVD risk greater than 10%

HYPERTENSION
Diagnostic and Preventive Considerations

Hypertension is the most common diagnosis in the primary care setting and is a major risk factor for CVD, directly contributing to one-fourth of all heart attacks and one-third of all strokes.[16] Roughly 30% of Americans are diagnosed with hypertension each year, and only half of all Americans with hypertension have controlled blood pressure.[17] Hypertension has been associated with stress and poor social support, major depression, bipolar disorder, and generalized anxiety disorder.[18–21] Patients with schizophrenia have increased 10-year cardiac mortality when compared with controls in the CATIE (Clinical Trials of Antipsychotic Treatment Effectiveness) schizophrenia trial.[22] In a follow-up study, the rate of nontreatment of hypertension in patients with schizophrenia was 62.4%.[23] Psychiatrists are in a good position to monitor blood pressure in high-risk patients who have mental illness.

The Eighth Joint National Committee on the Prevention, Detection, Evaluation, and Treatment of High Blood Pressure (JNC 8) did not change the 2003 JNC 7 hypertension diagnostic criteria but instead focused more on specific targets for treatment (**Fig. 2**).[16,24] Normal blood pressure is defined as less than 120/80 mm Hg. Prehypertension is defined as a blood pressure between 120/80 and 139/89 mm Hg. Antihypertensive medication therapy is not indicated for prehypertension. Stage 1 hypertension is defined as blood pressure between 140/90 and 159/99 mm Hg, and stage 2 hypertension is >160/100 mm Hg. A diastolic blood pressure greater than 120 mm Hg with or without end organ damage (eg, retinal hemorrhage, hypertensive encephalopathy) is classified as hypertensive urgency and malignant hypertension, respectively (**Table 1**).

The USPSTF recommends screening for high blood pressure in adults aged 18 years or older. This recommendation is the evidence-based standard of care for the prevention of hypertension.[25] Patients with normal blood pressure should be screened at least every 2 years, whereas those with prehypertension should be screened annually.

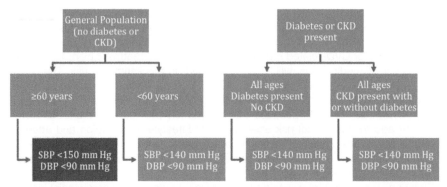

Fig. 2. Treatment goals for hypertension. CKD, chronic kidney disease; DBP, diastolic blood pressure; SBP, systolic blood pressure. (*Adapted from* James PA, Oparil S, Carter BL, et al. 2014 evidence-based guideline for the management of high blood pressure in adults—report from the panel members appointed to the Eighth Joint National Committee (JNC 8). JAMA 2014;311:507–20.)

The author suggests that blood pressure be measured at each mental health care visit, particularly if psychotropic medications are prescribed.

The medication-based treatment of hypertension consists of 4 main classes, all considered first line for the treatment of essential hypertension without other significant medical complications: thiazide-type diuretics, calcium channel blockers, ACEIs, and angiotensin receptor blockers. Of note, β-blockers are no longer a first-line treatment for hypertension. See **Fig. 3** for details on how best to use these classes of medications.

DIABETES
Diagnostic and Preventive Considerations

In the United States diabetes mellitus affects an estimated 8.3% of the population and is the seventh leading cause of death.[26] More than 7 million people live with diabetes and do not know it. If the prevalence of diabetes continues to grow at a steady rate, it is estimated that about 25% of Americans will have diabetes by 2030.[27] Diabetes is the leading cause of noncongenital blindness, kidney failure, and nontraumatic limb amputations. Patients with diabetes have a 2- to 4-fold increased risk of mortality, stroke, and CVD, this risk is even more pronounced in those who have SMI.

The diagnosis of diabetes requires one of the following:

- Fasting blood glucose greater than 126 mg/dL on 2 separate days
- Symptoms of hyperglycemia plus random plasma glucose of at least 200 mg/dL

Table 1
Joint National Committee diagnostic classification of blood pressure

Classification	Systolic (mm Hg)		Diastolic (mm Hg)
Normal	<120	And	<80
Prehypertension	120–129	Or	80–89
Stage 1 hypertension	140–159	Or	90–99
Stage 2 hypertension	≥160	Or	≥100

Adapted from U.S. Department of Health and Human Services (USDHHS). The seventh report of the Joint National Committee on prevention, detection, evaluation, and treatment of high blood pressure (JNC 7). Washington, DC: National Institutes of Health; 2003.

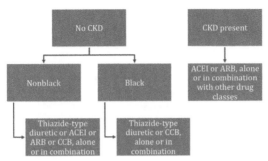

Fig. 3. Treatment of hypertension based on age, diabetes, and kidney function. ACEI, angiotensin-converting enzyme inhibitor; ARB, angiotensin receptor blocker; CCB, calcium channel blocker. (*Adapted from* James PA, Oparil S, Carter BL, et al. 2014 evidence-based guideline for the management of high blood pressure in adults—report from the panel members appointed to the Eighth Joint National Committee (JNC 8). JAMA 2014;311: 507–20.)

- Two-hour plasma glucose of at least 200 mg/dL during an oral glucose tolerance test (OGTT) with results duplicated on a separate day
- Hemoglobin A_{1c} greater than >6.5% (nonfasting test)

Prediabetes can be identified with the same tests used to diagnose diabetes, and is defined by:

- Fasting blood glucose of 100 to 125 mg/dL
- Two-hour plasma glucose of 140 to 199 mg/dL during an OGTT
- Hemoglobin A_{1c} of 5.7% to 6.4% (nonfasting test)

Identification of individuals at risk for type 2 diabetes and managing these risks can help in prevention. Patients with depression and schizophrenia should also be considered as being at particularly high risk, especially if they are also taking a medication associated with weight gain, hypertension, or metabolic syndrome.

Screening for diabetes should be considered in all adults who are older than 45 or those who are overweight (BMI ≥25) with 1 or more of the following risk factors:

- Physical inactivity
- First-degree relative with diabetes
- High-risk race/ethnicity (eg, African American, Latino, Native American, Asian American, Pacific Islander)
- Delivered a baby weighing more than 9 lb (4 kg) or were diagnosed with gestational diabetes mellitus
- Hypertension (≥140/90 mm Hg or on an antihypertensive)
- HDL-cholesterol level less than 35 mg/dL and/or a triglyceride level greater than 250 mg/dL
- Women with polycystic ovarian syndrome
- Hemoglobin A_{1c} at least 5.7%, impaired glucose tolerance, or impaired fasting glucose on previous testing
- History of established CVD

For patients with diabetes, prediabetes, or obesity, the provider may consider discussing secondary preventive measures with the patient. The following modifiable risk factors can be brought up in the context of psychotherapy and while assessing a patient's motivation to make significant lifestyle changes.

Modifiable risk factors for type 2 diabetes among patients with mental illness:

- Sedentary lifestyle
- Diet
- Obesity
- Medications that may contribute to weight gain
- Poor access to routine medical screening
- Poor adherence to medical regimen
- Depression, anxiety, and use of alcohol or illicit drugs

DYSLIPIDEMIA
Diagnostic and Preventive Considerations

Dyslipidemia is widely prevalent, often asymptomatic, and affects up to 25% of all adults in the United States.[28,29] As serum concentrations of non-HDL increase, and HDL decreases, there is a significantly higher likelihood of CVD-related morbidity.[21] Targeted lowering of total cholesterol and LDL levels in individuals with or without a prior history of myocardial infarction significantly reduces the likelihood of a CVD-related event.[28,30,31]

The prevalence of dyslipidemia among those with severe and persistent mental illness ranges from 25% to 70%, and is markedly higher than age-matched population controls.[6,32] This result is likely due to a confluence of multiple factors, which include at least sedentary lifestyle, high-fat/high-calorie diet, tobacco use, and treatment with antipsychotic or mood-stabilizing medications. Despite this growing recognition, up to 88% of patients with schizophrenia and diagnosed with dyslipidemia do not receive treatment, making it one of the most prevalent yet under-treated risk factors for CVD among those with SMI.[23]

Diagnosis and subsequent treatment of dyslipidemias is now based on CVD risk and no longer solely on an isolated LDL serum level (eg, previously <130 mg/dL, 100 mg/dL, or 70 mg/dL depending on cardiovascular risk). Individuals with established atherosclerotic CVD have a high (about 20%) risk of having another event in the subsequent 10 years. Unless otherwise contraindicated, they should be placed on high-potency statin therapy, as tolerated, without regard to their LDL-cholesterol values.

When considering primary prevention or treatment of those without evidence of diabetes or established CVD, individuals should be classified based on the estimated ASCVD 10-year risk of myocardial infarction or stroke. The use of "non-HDL" cholesterol is the primary criterion by which dyslipidemias may be defined and managed.[33] Non-HDL cholesterol can be calculated by subtracting HDL from the total cholesterol concentration, and varies less than 2% between fasting and nonfasting states, making nonfasting samples reliable, valid, and more convenient for the patient.

After cholesterol is measured and an individual's CVD risk is determined, he or she can be appropriately categorized according to treatment intensity. See **Table 2** for directions on when a statin should be considered as treatment.

PREVENTIVE GUIDELINES

The USPSTF recommends screening men at average risk for dyslipidemias at the age of 35, and women at the age of 45.[34] For those taking atypical antipsychotic medications, a consensus panel recommended obtaining cholesterol levels every 5 years in adults at average risk, although more recently experts have recommended yearly

Table 2
Four clinical classes of statin eligibility

Clinical Characteristic	Applicable Age Range (y)	Preferred Statin Intensity
Clinical presence of CVD	21–75	High
Serum LDL >190 mg/dL	21–75	High
Type 2 diabetes	40–75	Moderate to High
10-Year risk >7.5	40–75	Moderate

Abbreviation: LDL, low-density lipoprotein.
Adapted from Stone NJ, Robinson J, Lichtenstein AH, et al. 2013 ACC/AHA guideline on the treatment of blood cholesterol to reduce atherosclerotic cardiovascular risk in adults: a report of the American College of Cardiology/American Heart Association task force on practice guidelines. J Am Coll Cardiol 2014;63:2889–934; with permission.

screening with ongoing antipsychotic treatment, or in the presence of weight gain on treatment in excess of 7% from their baseline weight (**Table 3**).[32,35]

FINAL THOUGHTS

Patients with mental illness, particularly SMI, are more likely to suffer from common disorders without optimal treatment. The result is increased vulnerability, morbidity, and all-cause mortality in those with mental illness in comparison with the general population. Changes in preventive practice patters cannot be fully realized on a large scale until clinicians are trained on how to routinely provide this care.

Psychiatrists may consider using preventive care strategies in the area of cardiovascular health, as CVD is the most common cause of death and disproportionately affects patients with mental illness. At a minimum, psychiatrists are well positioned to work collaboratively with primary care providers to address psychopathology that may interfere with adherence to the treatment plan (eg, untreated mood disorders, lack of motivation, substance misuse, and anxiety related to general medical illness).

Table 3
Recommendations for metabolic monitoring of patients treated with second-generation antipsychotic medications

	Baseline	4 wk	8 wk	12 wk	Every 3 mo	Every 1 y
Personal/family history	X	—	—	—	—	X
Weight (BMI)	X	X	X	X	X	—
Waist circumference	X	—	—	—	—	X
Blood pressure	X	—	—	X	—	X
Fasting glucose	X	—	—	X	—	X
Fasting lipids	X	—	—	X	—	X

Abbreviation: BMI, body mass index.
Adapted from American Diabetes Association (ADA), American Psychiatric Association, American Association of Clinical Endocrinologists, North American Association for the Study of Obesity. Consensus development conference on antipsychotic drugs and obesity and diabetes. Diabetes Care 2004;27:596–601.

REFERENCES

1. Colton CW, Manderscheid RW. Congruencies in increased mortality rates, years of potential life lost, and causes of death among public mental health clients in eight states. Prev Chronic Dis 2006;2:A42.
2. Saha S, Chant D, McGrath J. A systematic review of mortality in schizophrenia. Arch Gen Psychiatry 2007;64:1123–31.
3. Roshanaei-Moghaddam B, Katon W. Premature mortality from general medical illnesses among persons with bipolar disorder: a review. Psychiatr Serv 2009;60: 147–56.
4. Parks J, Svendsen D, Singer P, et al. Morbidity and mortality in people with serious mental illness. Alexandria (VA): National Association of State Mental Health Program Directors (NASMHPD) Medical Directors Council; 2006.
5. Newcomer JW, Henneckens CH. Severe mental illness and risk of cardiovascular disease. JAMA 2007;298:1794–6.
6. McEvoy JP, Meyer JM, Goff DC, et al. Prevalence of the metabolic syndrome in patients with schizophrenia: baseline results from the Clinical Antipsychotic Trails of Intervention Effectiveness (CATIE) schizophrenia trial and comparison with national estimates from NHANES III. Schizophr Res 2005;80:19–32.
7. Compton MT, Daumit GL, Druss BG. Cigarette smoking and overweight/obesity among individuals with serious mental illnesses: a preventive perspective. Harv Rev Psychiatry 2006;14:212–22.
8. Osby U, Brandt L, Correi N, et al. Excess mortality in bipolar and unipolar disorder in Sweden. Arch Gen Psychiatry 2001;58:844–50.
9. Van der Kooy K, van Hout H, Marwijk H, et al. Depression and the risk for cardiovascular diseases: systematic review and meta analysis. Int J Geriatr Psychiatry 2007;22:613–26.
10. Bikdeli B, Ranasinghe I, Chen R, et al. Most important outcomes research papers on treatment of stable coronary artery disease. Circ Cardiovasc Qual Outcomes 2013;6:e17–25.
11. Darba J, Kaskens L, Aranda P, et al. A simulation model to estimate 10-year risk of coronary heart disease events in patients with schizophrenia spectrum disorders treated with second-generation antipsychotic drugs. Ann Clin Psychiatry 2013;25:17–26.
12. Crump C, Sundquist K, Winkleby MA, et al. Comorbidities and mortality in bipolar disorder: a Swedish national cohort study. JAMA Psychiatry 2013;70(9):931–9.
13. Vanderlip ER, Fiedorowicz JG, Haynes WG. Screening, diagnosis, and treatment of dyslipidemia among persons with persistent mental illness: a literature review. Psychiatr Serv 2012;63:693–701.
14. Moyer VA, U.S. Preventive Services Task Force (USPSTF). Screening for coronary heart disease with electrocardiography: U.S. Preventive Services Task Force recommendation statement. Ann Intern Med 2012;157:512–8.
15. Hartley L, Igbinedion E, Holmes J, et al. Increased consumption of fruit and vegetables for the primary prevention of cardiovascular diseases. Cochrane Database Syst Rev 2013;(6):CD009874.
16. U.S. Department of Health and Human Services (USDHHS). The seventh report of the Joint National Committee on prevention, detection, evaluation, and treatment of high blood pressure (JNC 7). Washington, DC: National Institutes of Health; 2003.
17. Egan BM, Zhao Y, Axon RN. US trends in prevalence, awareness, treatment, and control of hypertension, 1988-2008. JAMA 2010;303:2043–50.

18. Bosworth HB, Bartash RM, Olsen MK, et al. The association of psychosocial factors and depression with hypertension among older adults. Int J Geriatr Psychiatry 2003;18:1142–8.

19. Goldstein BI, Fagiolini A, Houck P, et al. Cardiovascular disease and hypertension among adults with bipolar I disorder in the United States. Bipolar Disord 2009;11:657–62.

20. Carroll D, Phillips AC, Gale CR, et al. Generalized anxiety and major depressive disorders, their comorbidity and hypertension in middle-aged men. Psychosom Med 2010;72:16–9.

21. Kannel WB, Castelli WP, Gordon T, et al. Serum cholesterol, lipoproteins, and the risk of coronary heart disease. Ann Intern Med 1971;74:1–12.

22. Goff DC, Sullivan LM, McEvoy JP, et al. A comparison of ten-year cardiac risk estimates in schizophrenia patients from the CATIE study and matched controls. Schizophr Res 2005;80:45–53.

23. Nasrallah HA, Meyer JM, Goff DC, et al. Low rates of treatment for hypertension, dyslipidemia and diabetes in schizophrenia: data from the CATIE schizophrenia trial sample at baseline. Schizophr Res 2006;86:15–22.

24. James PA, Oparil S, Carter BL, et al. 2014 evidence-based guideline for the management of high blood pressure in adults—report from the panel members appointed to the Eighth Joint National Committee (JNC 8). JAMA 2014;311:507–20.

25. Wolff T, Miller T. Evidence for the reaffirmation of the U.S. Preventive Services Task Force recommendation on screening for high blood pressure. Ann Intern Med 2007;147:787–91.

26. Centers for Disease Control and Prevention (CDC). Division of diabetes translation: long-term trends in diagnosed diabetes. 2011. Available at: http://www.cdc.gov/diabetes/statistics/slides/long_term_trends.pdf Accessed January 20, 2015.

27. Boyle JP, Thompson TJ, Gregg EW, et al. Projection of the year 2050 burden of diabetes in the US adult population: dynamic modeling of incidence, mortality, and prediabetes prevalence. Popul Health Metr 2010;8:1–12.

28. Expert Panel on Detection, Evaluation, and Treatment of High Blood Cholesterol in Adults. Executive summary of the third report of the National Cholesterol Education Program (NCEP) Expert Panel on Detection, Evaluation, And Treatment of High Blood Cholesterol In Adults (Adult Treatment Panel III). JAMA 2001;285:2486–97.

29. Ford ES, Mokdad AH, Giles WH, et al. Serum total cholesterol concentrations and awareness, treatment, and control of hypercholesterolemia among US adults: findings from the National Health and Nutrition Examination Survey, 1999 to 2000. Circulation 2013;107:2185–9.

30. Stone NJ, Robinson J, Lichtenstein AH, et al. 2013 ACC/AHA guideline on the treatment of blood cholesterol to reduce atherosclerotic cardiovascular risk in adults: a report of the American College of Cardiology/American Heart Association task force on practice guidelines. J Am Coll Cardiol 2014;63:2889–934.

31. Taylor F, Huffman MD, Macedo AF, et al. Statins for the primary prevention of cardiovascular disease. Cochrane Database Syst Rev 2013;(1):CD004816.

32. De Hert M, Correll CU, Bobes J, et al. Physical illness in patients with severe mental disorders. I. Prevalence, impact of medications and disparities in health care. World Psychiatry 2011;10:52–77.

33. Sniderman A, Kwiterovich PO. Update on the detection and treatment of atherogenic low-density lipoproteins. Curr Opin Endocrinol Diabetes Obes 2013;20:140–7.

34. US Preventive Services Task Force (USPSTF): Screening for lipid disorders in adults. 2008. Available at: http://www.uspreventiveservicestaskforce.org/uspstf/uspschol.htm. Accessed August 30, 2011.

35. American Diabetes Association (ADA), American Psychiatric Association, American Association of Clinical Endocrinologists, North American Association for the Study of Obesity. Consensus Development Conference on Antipsychotic Drugs and Obesity and Diabetes. Diabetes Care 2004;27:596–601.

The Next Big Thing in Child and Adolescent Psychiatry

Interventions to Prevent and Intervene Early in Psychiatric Illnesses

Erica Z. Shoemaker, MD, MPH[a],*, Laura M. Tully, PhD[b],
Tara A. Niendam, PhD[b], Bradley S. Peterson, MD[c]

KEYWORDS

- Prevention • Health promotion • Maternal depression • Familial depression
- Substance abuse • Adolescent depression • Ultra high risk for psychosis

KEY POINTS

- Psychiatrists have long spent much of their time working to reduce symptom burden in chronic conditions in their patients. However, an era is beginning in which psychiatrists can aim to prevent mental illness, reducing the number of people affected by mental illness in their lifetimes.
- Treating depression in mothers can have great benefit in treating and preventing mental illness in their children.
- Neuroimaging and psychological assessment may help clinicians to target preventive treatments to children who are at the highest risk of developing familial depression.
- Universal prevention programs delivered by teachers in schools can reduce the numbers of children who grow up to abuse alcohol and illicit drugs, and psychiatrists need to advocate strongly in their communities for the funding support and implementation of these programs.
- Interactive video games that teach cognitive behavioral techniques may provide a useful tool for early intervention in cases of mild to moderate depression in adolescents.
- Intensive psychosocial interventions reduce by more than one-third the number of youth who transition from the prodromal ultrahigh-risk state to first-episode psychosis.

[a] Department of Psychiatry and Behavioral Sciences, University of Southern California, 2250 Alcazar Street, Suite 2200, Los Angeles, CA 90033, USA; [b] Department of Psychiatry, UC Davis Imaging Research Center, University of California, Davis, 4701 X Street, Suite E, Sacramento, CA 95817, USA; [c] Institute for the Developing Mind, Children's Hospital Los Angeles, University of Southern California, 4650 Sunset Boulevard, MS# 135, Los Angeles, CA 90027, USA
* Corresponding author.
E-mail address: erica.shoemaker@med.usc.edu

Psychiatr Clin N Am 38 (2015) 475–494
http://dx.doi.org/10.1016/j.psc.2015.05.010
0193-953X/15/$ – see front matter © 2015 Elsevier Inc. All rights reserved.
psych.theclinics.com

INTRODUCTION

Patients who first seek treatment from a psychiatrist in adulthood frequently report that they manifested their first symptoms in childhood or adolescence. Many psychiatrists then wonder whether early intervention during their patient's childhood could have spared many years of suffering. However, many child psychiatrists treat disorders, such as childhood-onset schizophrenia and depression, that are typically more severe and more treatment resistant than adult-onset disorders. However, the allied fields of psychiatry, psychology, and social work, along with public health and prevention science, are making headway in the development and deployment of interventions that can prevent mental illness in some patients, and that offer the hope of reducing the incidence and prevalence of mental illness, and thereby of reducing the suffering and disability associated with psychiatric illness.

Childhood and adolescence are particularly propitious times in human development in which to intervene for the prevention of mental illness.[1] The architecture of the brains of children (the numbers and types of neurons; the circuits that they form; and the cognitive, behavioral, and emotional processes that those circuits support) are under dynamic construction, particularly in fetal life and infancy but also in later childhood and adolescence. Risk and protective factors exert their influences on the exceptionally dynamic formation of brain architecture during these sensitive periods in development, but they may not manifest their full effects until many years later. Therefore, early childhood and adolescence are opportune times to prevent mental illness not only in children but also in adults.

What is prevention? Gordon[2] defines preventive health interventions as "those which should be applied to persons not motivated by current suffering" and classifies preventive interventions as universal, selective, or indicated. Universal prevention interventions, such as counseling on good sleep hygiene, target everyone within a population. They are generally inexpensive to deliver, and even though effects may be weak at the level of each individual in the population, when amplified across the population their benefits can dramatically outweigh their costs in reducing population-based rates of illness. Selective interventions, such as educational programs designed to reduce child abuse in teen mothers, target populations of people at increased risk for adverse outcomes. Indicated preventions target specific persons who have conditions (usually early signs or symptoms) that warrant interventions designed to prevent or attenuate the development of further problems. Programs for youth at ultrahigh risk (UHR) of developing psychosis are in this category.

Prevention research has traditionally focused on reducing exposure to risk factors, such as poverty and child abuse. However, recent work has focused equally on health promotion: interventions that increase exposure to protective factors, such as good schools and healthy peer relationships. Prevention and health promotion both focus on changing common and important environmental influences on the development of children that will aid them in meeting maturational tasks and challenges and remaining free of cognitive, emotional, and behavioral problems.[1,3,4] Just as an individual patient's treatment plan highlights limitations and impairments to be remediated and assets and strengths on which to build, most effective prevention programs focus not only on reducing exposure to risk factors but also on enhancing exposure to protective factors. Health promotion approaches are especially important when risk factors (such as genetic risks) are not readily modifiable.

A comprehensive description of the available preventive interventions for children and adolescents is beyond the scope of this article. The interventions described in this article are instead selected as examples of the breadth and effectiveness of techniques that promise to reduce the incidence of mental illness and the progression to more severe disease from infancy to young adulthood. These program techniques range in their evidence base from being experimental (eg, the SPARX video game) to being grounded in many years of rigorous investigation (eg, the treatment of maternal depression).

Preventing the consequences of maternal depression in children

Susan is a 26-year-old woman who screens positive for depression on a questionnaire at her obstetrician's office. She is in her second trimester of pregnancy. After discussing the risks and benefits of antidepressant medication during pregnancy with her obstetrician, Susan declines medication and seeks no further mental health treatment.

Later, when her daughter is 6 months old, the pediatrician refers Susan to a psychiatrist. Susan reports that her depressive symptoms have only worsened since her daughter's birth. She denies suicidal ideation and psychotic symptoms, and denies any thoughts about harming her infant. On mental status examination she is tearful and poorly groomed. The psychiatrist refers Susan for a course of interpersonal psychotherapy, which relieves her symptoms somewhat. When her baby is 12 months old and Susan stops breastfeeding, the psychiatrist and Susan decide that she should try an antidepressant medication. She responds well to a selective serotonin reuptake inhibitor (SSRI), with complete remission of symptoms within 9 months of the initial referral. Susan continues with infrequent medication-management visits for another 2 years, and then is lost to follow-up.

Six years later, Susan contacts her former psychiatrist, asking to be evaluated for a recurrence of her depressive symptoms. Her daughter is having trouble with the transition to kindergarten, often refusing to separate from her mother. Susan is both worried about her daughter and concerned that her depression is making it hard to provide the consistency of parenting that her daughter requires.

Background

Perhaps one of the most powerful interventions an adult psychiatrist can undertake to foster the well-being of children is to treat depression in their mothers. The sequelae of maternal depression on children are diverse and profound. Depression in mothers has been linked to increased risk of numerous psychiatric illnesses in children, including anxiety disorders, depressive disorders, oppositional defiant disorder, and neurocognitive deficits.[5] Because depression is highly common in women, the Harvard Center for the Developing Child has stated that more children are disadvantaged by exposure to maternal depression than by exposure to child abuse.[6] Maternal depression also has wide-ranging impacts and costs; for example, reduced maternal earning power, increased child welfare costs, and even reduced earnings as the children enter adulthood. The Wilding Agency estimated that the 2-generational cost of untreated maternal depression is $22,647 each year a mother remains depressed.[7] The familial risk to children is likely mediated both by genetic influences and by the environmental influences of a child being reared by a depressed mother, who is likely to be less emotionally responsive to the need of her developing child.[8] Prioritizing psychiatric treatment of mothers with depression and addressing this environmental risk factor has the potential to prevent mental illness and adverse life consequences in their offspring, even when those children are not in psychiatric treatment themselves.

Treatment of Women with Depression During Pregnancy and Postpartum

Decisions concerning the treatment modality for maternal depression are affected by whether the mother is pregnant, breastfeeding, or just actively parenting. Pregnant women like Susan have justifiable worries about the effects of antidepressant medications on the developing fetus. SSRI medications cross the placental barrier, and maternal ingestion of an SSRI during pregnancy does, without question, alter central serotonergic signaling in her fetus.[9] Animal models have shown that serotonin acts as a trophic factor in fetal life, meaning that maternal SSRI ingestion affects cell division, cell migration, and synaptogenesis in the fetus.[9] SSRI exposure early in development in animals (at times corresponding with the third trimester of pregnancy in humans) produces anxiety and depression-related behaviors in adulthood.[10] These findings raise important questions about the long-term emotional and behavioral effects of prenatal exposure to antidepressant medications in humans. The neurodevelopmental effects of prenatal exposure to these medications have not been studied extensively in humans, and the existing studies thus far have been hampered by low numbers of participants, leading to poor statistical power to detect adverse effects. Nevertheless, studies in humans thus far suggest that SSRI exposure may be associated with premature birth and lower Apgar scores at birth and with poor fine motor and language abilities in early childhood.[11–13] Moreover, untreated depression in itself can contribute to poorer outcomes, with approximately 15% of emotional and behavioral problems in childhood estimated as attributable to the antenatal maternal stress and anxiety.[10] Thoughtful psychiatrists are still left to judge on a case-by-case basis the relative risks and benefits of medication and nonmedication therapies in pregnant women.

Use of antidepressants during breastfeeding can also be challenging. Women and their physicians may not want to risk exposing infants to the small amount of SSRIs that mothers secrete in their breast milk. Multiple case reports suggest that infants of mothers who began SSRIs while breastfeeding can quickly develop trouble with sleep and irritability in the short term, although the long-term effects of exposure via breast milk are unknown. Some women choose to continue the antidepressant but stop breastfeeding, whereas other women choose to discontinue the antidepressant and continue breastfeeding. For women who want to continue both, case reports suggest that sertraline and paroxetine may have fewer short-term effects than other SSRIs.[14]

These potential concerns with prenatal and early postnatal exposure to antidepressant medications make the use of psychological and behavioral therapies first-line treatments for depressed mothers with mild to moderate depression. However, growing evidence indicates that psychotherapy is an effective treatment of many women with perinatal depression. Interpersonal therapy for pregnant, depressed women has been found to be effective compared with wait-list controls, and both cognitive behavior therapy (CBT) and interpersonal therapy are reported to be effective for postpartum depression.[15] Women who respond to psychotherapy alone during the peripartum period benefit from reduced depressive symptoms and presumably can avoid the detrimental effects of their illness on their children's development. Patients like Susan may be willing to participate in psychotherapy even if they are too worried about adverse effects of taking antidepressants during pregnancy or when breastfeeding.

Treatment of Mothers Who have Older Children

The STAR*D (Sequenced Treatment Alternatives to Relieve Depression) Child study treated 151 women with major depression and then followed the women's children, aged 7 to 17 years, during the women's treatment. The first step in treatment was citalopram only. Those women who could not tolerate citalopram or for whom citalopram only was ineffective were offered a range of treatments, including alternative antidepressants, CBT, or a combination of treatments. The children of mothers who reached remission via any treatment modality had significantly fewer psychiatric symptoms and improved in their global functioning. Diagnoses of internalizing disorders (anxiety and depression) in particular decreased over time in the children of remitters. Temporally, the mothers' symptoms improved before their children's symptoms improved. These benefits to children were seen only in mothers who reached remission.[16] Psychiatrists can greatly benefit the children of their patients who are mothers by aggressively treating the mothers' depression.

The Potential for Preventing Depression in Asymptomatic Youth Who have a Family History of Major Depression

Until recently, biomarkers have not been useful in predicting which children or adults will go on to develop major depressive disorder (MDD). The best predictor of persons who will develop MDD has been family history. MDD is frequently transmitted across family generations.[3,17,18] Offspring of persons with MDD have a 2-fold to 5-fold increased lifetime risk for developing the illness, yielding heritability estimates of 40% to 70%.[19,20] Familial compared with nonfamilial MDD is more severe, more recurrent, and more treatment resistant,[21–25] and it tends to have an earlier age of onset, usually between 15 and 25 years of age. It is often heralded by an anxiety disorder in childhood.[26–28] A large, multisite preventive intervention study showed that CBT was more effective than treatment as usual in reducing the development of MDD symptoms in adolescents who have a family history of MDD.[29] Efficacy was sustained for at least 3 years following the intervention, with rates of MDD reduced by nearly 75% with the active intervention.[30] This study shows the feasibility of using family history as way of targeting a preventive intervention in this population.

Despite this important proof-of-concept demonstration that a targeted prevention of MDD is possible in the offspring of persons with this illness, only 30% to 60% of those offspring would be expected to develop MDD if left untreated, which means that many more youth at high familial risk for MDD need to receive preventive intervention under this model than would have MDD in their lifetimes without the intervention. Identifying additional risk factors for MDD in this population that could be used in conjunction with family history would aid in further refining the target population for the preventive intervention.

Our group has identified the structural features of the brain that seem to be passed between generations and that confer a biological vulnerability for development of MDD in high-risk families (**Fig. 1**).[31] This risk biomarker, or endophenotype, for familial MDD comprises thinning of the cortex along the entire lateral aspect of the right hemisphere and the mesial wall of the left hemisphere,[32] as well as bilaterally reduced volumes of frontal and parietal white matter.[33] This brain abnormality was enormous both in its spatial extent, extending from the front of the brain to the back of the brain, and in its magnitude at any single point on the surface of the brain, averaging 30% reduction in cortical thickness relative to values in low risk controls. This endophenotype was present at much higher rates in the offspring of persons with MDD than in the offspring of persons without MDD, even if the offspring did not have MDD. It was present in children and adults of the sample to the same degree. Those who had the endophenotype but who had never been ill with MDD nevertheless still had inattention and poor visual memory for social stimuli in direct proportion to the magnitude of cortical thinning and white matter hypoplasia within the brain regions that defined the endophenotype.[32,33] We then developed a computer algorithm that was able detect this pattern of structural brain abnormality within single individuals,[34] and on this basis we estimate that asymptomatic adolescents who have at least 1 depressed parent and this pattern of cortical thinning have a greater than 80% likelihood of becoming ill with MDD. The ability to predict with high likelihood which asymptomatic youth will develop MDD, if confirmed in future studies, affords the opportunity to use that predictive

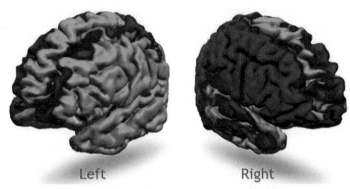

Left　　　　　　　　　　Right

Fig. 1. The endophenotype for brain structure that is transmitted between generations in families with major depression. The endophenotype consists of thinning of the cortical mantle (represented in purple) of the lateral surface of the right cerebral hemisphere, extending from the back of the brain to the front. The average reduction in cortical thickness in that large spatial expanse was 30%, which is a large biological effect. The thinning was present in the biological offspring of depressed people more than in the offspring of nondepressed people even if those offspring did not have any personal history of depressive illness, and it was present to the same degree regardless of age, confirming the status of the thinning as an endophenotype for trait vulnerability. The thinning did not affect the lateral surface of the left cerebral hemisphere (represented in green).

ability to identify youth who should be targeted for preventive interventions. The combined use of family history and identification of a brain-based marker of familial vulnerability for MDD is now being developed for that use in our laboratory and in others. Asymptomatic adolescents who have at least 1 depressed parent undergo brain imaging to determine whether they have the cortical thinning endophenotype. If they do, they enter a randomized clinical trial of CBT or an inactive control condition to determine whether the intervention is able to prevent the later onset of MDD. Brain imaging after the completion of the trial will allow clinicians to determine whether the intervention changes cortical thickness in any way. This kind of intervention is personalized for youth who have a specific biological abnormality that confers unique risk for onset of a specific illness.

Universal interventions for prevention of substance use

Carlos is a first-grade (6-year-old) boy in a school that serves mostly students from families with low income and low parental education. Carlos is bright, already reading above grade level and proud of his early arithmetical abilities, but he is defiant with his teacher and often disruptive to the degree that the teacher cannot attend to her other students. Carlos's teacher is concerned about him following the trajectory of his 13-year-old brother, Jessie, who was recently expelled from the local middle school for smoking marijuana on campus.

Background

Previous research has found that more than 90% of adults who have current substance abuse disorders started using substances before age 18 years, and half of those began before age 15 years.[35] Delivering services in schools, rather than trying to intervene through each child's family, can be an efficient way to ensure that large numbers of children receive an intervention designed to prevent substance use.[36] Interventions likely need to address skills both to delay the onset of experimentation with drugs in early adolescents and to reduce behavior problems (especially aggression and disruptive behavior) in early-school-aged children. These behaviors, even in early-school-aged children, have been shown repeatedly to be an important behavioral antecedent of adolescent and adult illicit drug use, conduct disorder, antisocial personality disorder, and school dropout.[37]

The PAX Good Behavior Game

What kind of preventive intervention might be helpful for Carlos and his peers in first grade? The PAX Good Behavior Game (GBG) is delivered by trained teachers, usually in the first and second grades. The game is played during regular school hours, occurring concurrently with regular school instruction. Teachers divide children into 2 to 5 teams per classroom, deliberately balancing teams as to numbers of high-achieving, shy, and disruptive students per team. The teacher counts the number of disruptive behaviors during game time, and rewards teams that have 3 or fewer of the designated behaviors per game period. Rewards vary from written notes praising an individual child to permission for the team to engage in activities not usually allowed during class time, such as tapping a pencil on a desk or throwing paper balls (http://nrepp.samhsa.gov/viewintervention.aspx?id=351).[38]

The developers of the GBG explain that all of these activities are designed to use behavioral reinforcement and peer pressure to socialize children to the role of student. The entire intervention uses positive and playful language. Disruptive behaviors are called spleems, notes praising a child are called tootles, and the rewards for good behavior (pencil tapping, ball throwing) are called Granny's wacky prizes. PAX language directed at teachers and parents is positive and aspirational; PAX materials refer to 4 miracles that happen when children go to school: learning to read, learning to write, learning mathematics, and "acquiring the mental ability to sustain attention, to self-regulate or self-manage, and to cooperate with others intentionally to create peace, productivity, health and happiness for self and others."[39] In mental wellness terminology, the goal of the GBG is to increase self-regulation of behavior and peer cooperation. Kellam and colleagues[37] emphasized that, when the GBG is effective, it not only reduces all students' exposure to risk factors for substance abuse (disruptive behaviors, poor academic achievement) but it also increases their exposure to protective elements (cooperative peers and more academic instruction).

The GBG's targeting of self-regulation in its interventions is a sensible choice, given that the development of the capacity for effective self-regulation in childhood leads to more adaptive interpersonal interactions, more positive health behaviors, improved cognitive flexibility, and better impulse control.[40,41] It predicts future academic and occupational achievement and reduces the severity or likelihood of manifesting psychiatric symptoms.[40] In contrast, poor self-regulation promotes risky and addictive behaviors,[42,43] and it undermines critical long-term pursuits such as educational attainment, social integration, and physical health.[40,44–46] Self-regulatory failures are implicated in many of the leading preventable causes of death, including tobacco use, alcohol use, other drug use, overeating, accidents, and violence, and account for up to 40% of all deaths in the United States.[47,48] Improving self-regulation relies on maturation of neural systems that comprise dorsal prefrontal, parietal, and anterior cingulate cortices, as well as on subcortical nuclei, including the basal ganglia and thalamus **Fig. 2**.[49–58]

Consistent with this broader research emphasizing the importance of self-regulatory capacities for long-term health, evaluation research of the GBG shows impressive long-term outcomes. Kellam and colleagues[37] initiated a trial of this intervention in Baltimore City public schools from 1985 to 1987. This study had a prospective design

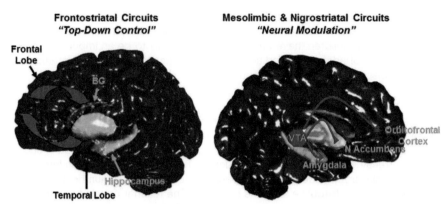

Fig. 2. Neural systems that support the capacity for self-regulation. (*Left*) The neural systems that support the capacity for self-regulation include cortical-subcortical circuits that project from all of the neocortex at the surface of the brain down to subcortical nuclei (*red arrows*) and then back to neocortex, particularly the frontal cortex. The frontal cortex exerts top-down control over activity in this circuit, particularly over activity in the subcortical nuclei, which include the basal ganglia (BG; *purple and green*) and thalamus. The hippocampus (*light blue*) within the temporal lobe supports the frontal cortex in the higher-order cognitive components of self-regulatory capacities. (Right) Neurochemical projections, particularly of dopamine, from the ventral tegmental area (VTA) and substantia nigra in the midbrain to the basal ganglia, nucleus accumbens, amygdala, and orbitofrontal cortex, modulate activity in these self-regulatory circuits. Early childhood interventions that strengthen the capacity for self-regulation likely affect activity within these various circuits. The neurochemical projections in the right panel are the target of stimulant medications that affect self-regulatory capacities in children with attention-deficit/hyperactivity disorder, which are affected by a wide range of drugs of abuse.

with complex procedures for randomization of both a large number of regionally representative schools and of classrooms within each school to receive either GBG, an enhanced educational intervention, or instruction as usual. Investigators worked with school staff to balance the composition of each class between disruptive and more cooperative students. For the preintervention measurement, students in all classrooms were rated by teachers as to their level of disruptive behaviors at the beginning of first grade. The postintervention measurement occurred when the grown-up students, now between 19 and 21 years old, were called by study personnel and given a semistructured diagnostic interview over the phone.

The effects of the GBG on adult psychopathology were statistically significant in male patients, and especially in male patients who had been highly disruptive in first grade.[37] In summary, based on the phone interview at 19 to 21 years old:

- For illicit drug use disorders:
  - Nineteen percent of GBG men had a drug abuse/dependence disorder compared with 38% of control men.
  - Of men who had been highly disruptive in first grade, 29% of GBG men had a drug use disorder compared with 83% of men in non-GBG classrooms.
- For alcohol use disorders: GBG men had a 50% reduction in risk for alcohol use disorder compared with non-GBG men,
- For antisocial personality disorder:
  - All men: GBG men had 17% lifetime incidence of antisocial personality disorder compared with 25% in non-GBG men.

o Men highly disruptive in first grade: 38% of GBG men compared with 80% in non-GBG classrooms.[37]

Findings such as these show that the GBG and interventions that target self-regulatory capacities have great potential for preventing substance abuse and antisocial behaviors in adults. It is difficult to overstate the societal and public health implications of these efforts.

Early intervention for mild to moderate depressive symptoms in adolescents:

A 14-year-old girl presents to her school guidance counselor. She tells her counselor that she has felt sad most of the time for the last 6 months, since the time that her grandmother passed away. She reports that her grades have deteriorated to Cs from As and Bs, and that she dropped out of the junior varsity soccer team, "because it just wasn't fun anymore." She continues to socialize with friends. She denies hopelessness and suicidal ideation. She continues to eat and sleep well. Her guidance counselor asks her to complete a depression-screening questionnaire (the PHQ9 [Patient Health Questionnaire 9]), in which she scores 10 (strong likelihood of mild clinical depression). The girl denies any new stressors, use of substances, history of abuse or trauma, and psychotic experiences.

Background

Rates of depressive disorders in adolescence are estimated to be 18% to 25%[4,59] (NIHCM) but only a small percentage of adolescents receive any sort of treatment.[59] Given that depression often has a slow and insidious onset, intervening early before the illness becomes full-blown or severe can reduce morbidity and mortality considerably. In this time window when adolescents do not meet criteria for a major depressive episode or for only a mild one, a nonintensive psychological intervention has the potential to be effective and acceptable to both the adolescents and their families. Treatment guidelines for minor to moderate major depressive episodes and other depressive disorders suggest a trial of psychotherapy before medications.[4] Despite these considerations and suggestions, finding and treating such a large number of adolescents could be prohibitive in terms of health care costs and the number of available clinicians to provide the care. Moreover, adolescents who are not yet experiencing the suffering and disability of a severe major depression may not be motivated to participate in treatment.

SPARX Video Game

One possible way to overcome barriers for these adolescents is the use of computerized psychotherapy. Video game play is nearly ubiquitous among American teenagers,[60] and therefore a particularly acceptable form of computerized psychotherapy may be psychotherapy delivered via an interactive video game. One such recently developed game is called SPARX, a fantasy-based platform that is both interactive and didactic. The appearance and shape of the game, in which players design their own avatar and move it through a three-dimensional, magical, and mythical world, are very much like commercial video fantasy games, such as World of Warcraft. However, in SPARX a mythical guide instructs players in basic CBT. The player is told that this mythical world has become bedeviled with gloomy negative automatic thoughts (GNATs). A total of 7 modules cover classic CBT content, such as psychoeducation about depression, behavioral activation, problem solving, and cognitive restructuring. Players are instructed to practice relaxation strategies with their real bodies and minds at certain points within the game. In-game activities (avatars can shoot GNATs with a gun) reinforce both the didactic and practical content.[61] Homework assignments appear at the end of game play, and safety checks are built into the game[62] (**Figs. 3–6**).

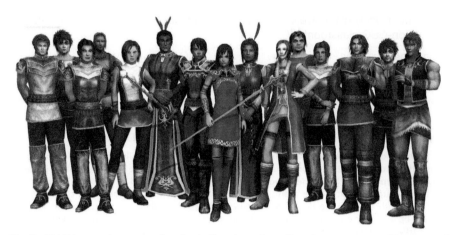

Fig. 3. SPARX uses characters that look like those in online fantasy games. (*Courtesy of* Auckland UniServices, LTD, Auckland, NZ; with permission.)

SPARX has been trialed in both New Zealand[61,62] and the Netherlands.[63] In all trials it has been used for adolescents whose depressive symptoms were mild to moderate in severity. This game can be thought of as either a treatment of illness or an indicated preventive intervention. The largest trial in New Zealand[61] tested its efficacy in reducing scores on the Children's Depression Rating Scale against treatment as usual by primary care physicians. The trial in the Netherlands tested it against a classroom-based program for depressed adolescents called Op Volle Kracht.[63]

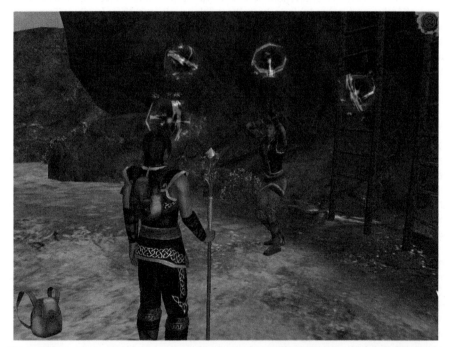

Fig. 4. Players in the game are encouraged to shoot GNATs. (*Courtesy of* Auckland UniServices, LTD, Auckland, NZ; with permission.)

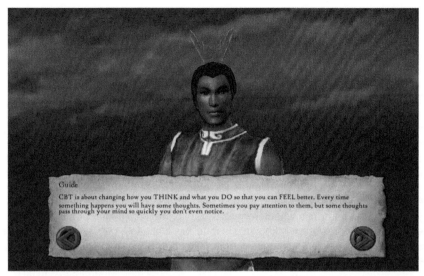

Fig. 5. A mythical guide educates players about CBT concepts. (*Courtesy of* Auckland UniServices, LTD, Auckland, NZ; with permission.)

Two aspects of SPARX may make it particularly useful with adolescents. First, it seems to be helpful in fostering autonomous motivation and in reducing guilt,[63] and in this respect in the Dutch trial it was better than the classroom, active-control intervention. Second, SPARX may have enhanced acceptability and cultural

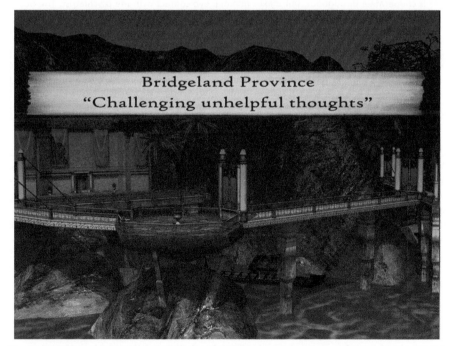

Fig. 6. SPARX integrates concepts from cognitive processing into a fantasy game world. (*Courtesy of* Auckland UniServices, LTD, Auckland, NZ; with permission.)

specificity. The company that developed the game consulted with adolescents in New Zealand and with Maori, Pacific Islander, and Asian cultural advisors[62]; the guides and characters in the game reflect culturally evocative content from those cultures. All characters speak in New Zealander accents. Investigators did not mention this cultural specificity as being an impediment when the game was used in the Netherlands.[63]

SPARX is only one of multiple games in development for the treatment of depression. Future games are likely to become more sophisticated and less clearly didactic in nature (Marientina Gotsis, personal communication, 2014). Moving these games to a mobile platform, such as a mobile phone application, may make them even more accessible and acceptable to adolescents.[64] In addition, games may be developed that can communicate in many languages and can even incorporate different cultural elements into the look of the guides and avatars.

As yet, no trials have followed participants in SPARX or similar games past the end of the use of the game, so whether it has a lasting preventive effect on recurrence or deepening of depression is unknown. Despite this limitation, gaming technology has great potential to deliver inexpensive, culturally compelling, and acceptable preventive interventions to children and adolescents.

Prevention of first-episode psychosis in adolescents at ultra high risk (UHR) of psychotic disorders

A 16-year-old boy is referred to a psychiatrist by his family doctor. This boy's paternal uncle has severely impairing schizophrenia and has had 10 hospitalizations in the past 5 years. The boy's mother is concerned because her son's grades have deteriorated from As to Cs over the past 6 months, and he has become increasingly socially withdrawn. At the psychiatric interview, the boy is clean, and is dressed in jeans and a black t-shirt. His hair is shaggy and he is unshaven. He is cooperative throughout, but makes minimal eye contact with the psychiatrist. The boy endorses symptoms of depression and reduced motivation to get his work done in the past month. Later in the interview, he reports that roughly twice per week he thinks that his teachers and classmates might be able to read his mind, which makes him anxious when he is near people at school. The boy reports that he is 50% convinced that it might be true that people can read his mind, and the associated distress has caused him to stay home from school twice in the past month. Further, he reports significant difficulty falling asleep because he sees shadows moving on the floor and walls at times, and he is so scared that he cannot close his eyes. A few weeks ago, he thought he heard one of the shadows giggling, keeping him awake all night.

Background

Over the last 20 years, considerable progress has been made in identifying and treating adolescents and young adults who are at UHR for developing psychotic disorders.[65,66] UHR individuals, like the boy described here, are familiar to psychiatrists. Although the onset of psychosis is associated with a variety of changes in brain structure and function, the utility of neuroimaging, genetics, and other biomarkers has not been established and they are not yet available for supporting psychotic disorder diagnoses.[67] Therefore, the identification of UHR individuals is based on a set of clinical risk markers, the presence of which are associated with a 20% to 36% risk for developing psychosis over 3 years.[68] The UHR state is defined clinically as:

1. Subthreshold psychotic symptoms (eg, seeing shadows out of the corner of the eye) that occur regularly (eg, once per week) and began within the past year.
2. Onset of psychotic symptoms within the past 3 months that only last for brief periods of time (eg, several minutes to a few hours per day but less than 1 day), and remit without treatment.

3. Familial risk factors (with the highest risk in the patient being associated with a first-degree relative who has psychosis) combined with significant functional decline in the past year.

Youth in the early stages of psychosis often present with depressed mood and anxiety as their chief complaint,[69] as in the case described earlier. Certain cultural factors can complicate the determination of whether a patient is psychotic. For example, some cultures speak about ancestors being with them as ghosts, and some religions believe that it is possible to speak to the dead. Symptoms therefore must be considered within the context of family and cultural settings before an experience is deemed psychotic. Using standardized screening instruments may help tease apart psychotic from cross-cultural phenomena.[65,66]

Psychotic disorders often present in adolescence or young adulthood,[70] making this developmental period an opportune time to prevent the progression to debilitating psychotic illness. Meta-analyses have shown that early intervention can reduce by 50% the risk of conversion from ultrahigh risk to first-episode psychosis over 12 months and by 37% over 24 to 36 months,[71] and it can reduce the long-term cost of care.[72] Most diagnostic and treatment programs for UHR individuals are located in academic medical centers that have established programs for early psychosis care and that employ highly trained and experienced staff, making extension and dissemination to nonacademic centers a priority for the future.

Description of Model Programs, Outcomes, and Treatment Elements

The standard of care for UHR individuals should encompass both the patient and family, and it should aim to prevent functional deterioration in work or school. The Family-aided Assertive Community Treatment (FACT) model represents an evidence-based coordinated specialty care (CSC) approach for UHR and first-episode psychosis.[73] Essential elements include community outreach and education to facilitate early identification, rapid referral to comprehensive assessment and care, and individual and family psychoeducation and treatment (including multifamily group, medical management, and supported education and employment) to reduce functional impairments and prevent deterioration in work or school. Many UHR individuals and families are most concerned about deterioration in work or school functioning, and the CSC model provides direct support in addressing these concerns, which are often key to engaging these individuals in care. Multifamily group treatment, in which multiple patients and their families receive psychoeducation and engage in collaborative problem solving,[74] has been shown to reduce symptoms and improve family well-being in first-episode psychosis[75] and UHR individuals.[76] A recent multisite trial of the FACT model within the United States reported greater improvements in functional outcomes for UHR individuals receiving FACT compared with standard community care.[77]

Similarly, family focused therapy (FFT), comprising 3 treatment stages that address knowledge of symptoms (psychoeducation), family communication, and problem solving,[78] has been shown to significantly reduce positive symptoms and improve role functioning in UHR individuals at 6-month follow-up compared with enhanced care (psychoeducation only).[79] Moreover, FFT decreases hostile and critical family communication styles,[80] which are the defining features of high expressed emotion, and are known to exacerbate symptoms and increase the risk for onset of psychosis.[81] Consequently, in the absence of access to a specialized early intervention program, family-based interventions that focus on psychoeducation, reduction in stigma, problem solving, communication skills training, and increasing family support are recommended as a primary line of treatment of UHR individuals.

Growing evidence also supports the use of CBT for psychosis (CBTp) with UHR individuals.[71] In CBTp, psychotic symptoms are conceptualized as distressing and stigmatizing interpretations of intrusions on normal awareness.[82] Thus, CBTp applies cognitive and behavioral techniques to evaluate objectively the content and accuracy of these interpretations and to generate alternative, more adaptive interpretations of psychotic experiences to reduce distress and improve functioning. These same techniques also are applied to treat the comorbid mood and anxiety symptoms that are common in UHR individuals. CBTp reduces positive symptoms[83,84] and the risk of transition to psychosis.[85]

Little evidence supports the prophylactic treatment of UHR individuals with antipsychotic medications. Early reports suggested that antipsychotic medication might be beneficial in UHR,[86] but a more recent trial of olanzapine 5 to 15 mg/d[87] did not produce significant benefit in preventing transition to first episode psychosis. Other studies suggest the presence of an increased risk to transition following antipsychotic treatment.[88,89] Consequently, clinical practice guidelines currently advise against the use of antipsychotic medications in UHR individuals,[90] and state that, if off-label prescription of antipsychotic medication is considered, very low doses should be used and should be prescribed by specialist psychiatric services as part of an early intervention treatment program.[91]

Other medications show early promise in treating UHR. One study reported that omega-3 polyunsaturated fatty acid supplements, when dosed at 1.2 g/d for 12 weeks and compared with placebo, produced statistically significant reductions in transition to psychosis at 12 months.[92] However, this finding has yet to be replicated. In addition, the use of antidepressants in combination with CBT to treat comorbid depression and anxiety seems to reduce significantly the rate of conversion to psychosis.[89]

The ideal intervention to prevent the transition to psychosis in UHR patients has not yet been identified. Nevertheless, early identification is important for connecting patients and their families to comprehensive, specialist services that simultaneously address multiple areas of need and can prevent further deterioration. Overall, sustained, long-term intervention seems important for success. Although the risk of transitioning to psychosis is highest in the first 2 years after identification of the UHR state, the risk can last 10 years or more.[93] Early studies that included a short duration of treatment (6 months) did not prevent the transition, but merely delayed it.[94] Therefore, many early intervention programs provide services for at least 2 to 3 years to monitor patients' symptoms and help support the patients and families to build the skills necessary to achieve wellness.

SUMMARY

Prevention of mental illness is possible. Interventions that are inexpensive and that have limited capacity to harm, such as the GBG and SPARX, can be implemented widely. Interventions that are more expensive and have some potential for harm, like treatment of psychiatric illness, should be applied more judiciously and in specific targeted populations. The development of biomarkers may one day help clinicians to determine which patients would benefit from interventions to prevent later illness.

One of the challenges of prevention work is funding. In many cases, the systems that fund interventions are not the systems that have the most to gain from reducing the incidence of disease. For example, the GBG is funded by school districts. School districts may see some benefits from reduced rates of substance use among their students (as well as reduced absenteeism, reduced dropout rates, and improved student achievement), but the greatest rewards may accrue to the future employers and family members of those students, as well as their medical insurance companies. In contrast, comprehensive psychiatric care for mothers with depression is funded by the mental health and medical systems, but the benefits of that intervention may accrue to their children's schools in terms of reduced absenteeism and better achievement. Their future employers may also benefit from reduced costs. If population-based, capitated medical care becomes a reality in the future, then health care providers in those systems may be motivated to support the costs of these preventive interventions, because the benefits of the interventions will accrue directly to the profit margin of the health care agency. Advocating for the funding of these powerful interventions is likely to devolve to child psychiatrists and other behavioral health care providers for children.

One of the limitations of prevention research is the short time to assessment following the interventions. With the exception of the GBG, knowledge of outcomes extends only to outcomes 1 to 2 years after the intervention. Clinicians need to –stay focused on the objective, which is prevention of psychiatric illnesses throughout the lifespan, and that will require much longer follow-up periods.

A point has now been reached at which psychiatrists can be optimistic about their power to prevent mental illness. As individual clinicians, they can all seek to aggressively treat mothers with depressive disorders, either with medication or psychotherapy. They can all seek to connect youth who present with prodromal symptoms to intensive psychosocial programs, usually at academic medical centers, that seek to prevent the development of serious psychotic illness in these youth. Encouraging the implementation of universal and selective preventive interventions (such as the GBG and SPARX) will require clinicians to exert their influence through advocacy at the level of state government and local school districts.

REFERENCES

1. O'Connell M, Boat T, Warner KE, editors. Committee on the Prevention of Mental Disorders and Substance Abuse Among Children, Youth and Young Adults: research advances and promising interventions; Institute of Medicine; National Research Council. Preventing mental, emotional, and behavioral disorders among young people: progress and possibilities. Washington, DC: National Academies Press; 2009.
2. Gordon R. An operational classification of disease prevention. Public Health Rep 1983;98:107–9.
3. Weissman MM, Wickramaratne P, Nomura Y, et al. Families at high and low risk for depression: a 3-generation study. Arch Gen Psychiatry 2005;62(1):29–36.
4. Boris Birmaher MD, David Brent MD, the AACAP Work Group on Quality Issues. Practice parameter for the assessment and treatment of children and adolescents with depressive disorders. J Am Acad Child Adolesc Psychiatry 2007; 46(11):1503–26.
5. Apter-Levy Y, Feldman M, Vakart A, et al. Impact of maternal depression across the first 6 years of life on the child's mental health, social engagement, and empathy: the moderating role of oxytocin. Am J Psychiatry 2013;170:1161–8.
6. Harvard Center for the Developing Child. Available at: http://developingchild. harvard.edu/index.php/resources/reports_and_working_papers/working_papers/ wp8/. Accessed January 10, 2015.
7. Diaz JY and Chase R Wilder Research. The cost of untreated maternal depression 2010. Available at: https://www.wilder.org/Wilder-Research/Publications/Studies/ Cost%20of%20Untreated%20Maternal%20Depression/The%20Cost%20of%20 Untreated%20Maternal%20Depression,%20Brief.pdf. Accessed January 10, 2015.

8. Cicchetti D, Toth SL, Rogosch FA. The efficacy of toddler-parent psychotherapy to increase attachment security in offspring of depressed mothers. Attach Hum Dev 1999;1(1):34–66.

9. Oberlander TF, Gingrich JA, Ansorge MS. Sustained neurobehavioral effects of exposure to SSRI antidepressants during development: molecular to clinical evidence. Clin Pharmacol Ther 2009;86(6):672–7.

10. Rebello TJ, Yu Q, Goodfellow NM, et al. Postnatal day 2 to 11 constitutes a 5-HT-sensitive period impacting adult mPFC function. J Neurosci 2014;34(37): 12379–93.

11. Wisner KL, Sit DK, Hanusa BH, et al. Major depression and antidepressant treatment: impact on pregnancy and neonatal outcomes. Am J Psychiatry 2009; 166(5):557–66.

12. Casper RC, Fleisher BE, Lee-Ancajas JC, et al. Follow-up of children of depressed mothers exposed or not exposed to antidepressant drugs during pregnancy. J Pediatr 2003;142(4):402–8.

13. Skurtveit S, Selmer R, Roth C, et al. Prenatal exposure to antidepressants and language competence at age three: results from a large population-based pregnancy cohort in Norway. BJOG 2014;121(13):1621–31.

14. Orsolini L, Bellantuono C. Serotonin reuptake inhibitors and breastfeeding: a systematic review. Hum Psychopharmacol Clin Exp 2015;30:4–20.

15. Stuart S, Koleva H. Psychological treatments for perinatal depression. Best Pract Res Clin Obstet Gynaecol 2014;28:61–70.

16. Pilowsky DJ, Wickramaratne P, Talati A, et al. Children of depressed mothers 1 year after the initiation of maternal treatment: findings from the STAR*D-Child Study. Am J Psychiatry 2008;165:1136–47.

17. Beardslee WR, Versage EM, Gladstone TR. Children of affectively ill parents: a review of the past 10 years. J Am Acad Child Adolesc Psychiatry 1998;37(11): 1134–41.

18. Kovacs M, Devlin B, Pollock M, et al. A controlled family history study of childhood-onset depressive disorder. Arch Gen Psychiatry 1997;54(7):613–23.

19. Bierut LJ, Heath AC, Bucholz KK, et al. Major depressive disorder in a community-based twin sample: are there different genetic and environmental contributions for men and women? Arch Gen Psychiatry 1999; 56(6):557–63.

20. Sullivan PF, Neale MC, Kendler KS. Genetic epidemiology of major depression: review and meta-analysis. Am J Psychiatry 2000;157(10):1552–62.

21. Lieb R, Isensee B, Hofler M, et al. Parental major depression and the risk of depression and other mental disorders in offspring: a prospective-longitudinal community study. Arch Gen Psychiatry 2002;59(4):365–74.

22. Keller MB, Beardslee WR, Dorer DJ, et al. Impact of severity and chronicity of parental affective illness on adaptive functioning and psychopathology in children. Arch Gen Psychiatry 1986;43(10):930–7.

23. Wickramaratne PJ, Greenwald S, Weissman MM. Psychiatric disorders in the relatives of probands with prepubertal-onset or adolescent-onset major depression. J Am Acad Child Adolesc Psychiatry 2000;39(11):1396–405.

24. Fava M, Uebelacker LA, Alpert JE, et al. Major depressive subtypes and treatment response. Biol Psychiatry 1997;42(7):568–76.

25. Kendler KS. Is seeking treatment for depression predicted by a history of depression in relatives? Implications for family studies of affective disorder. Psychol Med 1995;25(4):807–14.

26. Hammen C, Burge D, Burney E, et al. Longitudinal study of diagnoses in children of women with unipolar and bipolar affective disorder. Arch Gen Psychiatry 1990; 47(12):1112–7.
27. Pine DS, Cohen P, Gurley D, et al. The risk for early-adulthood anxiety and depressive disorders in adolescents with anxiety and depressive disorders. Arch Gen Psychiatry 1998;55:56–64.
28. Warner V, Wickramaratne P, Weissman MM. The role of fear and anxiety in the familial risk for major depression: a three-generation study. Psychol Med 2008; 38(11):1543–56.
29. Garber J, Clarke GN, Weersing VR, et al. Prevention of depression in at-risk adolescents: a randomized controlled trial. JAMA 2009;301(21):2215–24.
30. Beardslee WR, Brent DA, Weersing VR, et al. Prevention of depression in at-risk adolescents: longer-term effects. JAMA Psychiatry 2013;70(11):1161–70.
31. Peterson BS, Weissman MM. A brain-based endophenotype for major depressive disorder. Annu Rev Med 2011;62:461–74.
32. Peterson BS, Warner V, Bansal R, et al. Cortical thinning in persons at increased familial risk for major depression. Proc Natl Acad Sci U S A 2009;106(15):6273–8.
33. Dubin MJ, Weissman MM, Xu D, et al. Identification of a circuit-based endophenotype for familial depression. Psychiatry Res 2012;201(3):175–81.
34. Bansal R, Staib LH, Laine AF, et al. Anatomical brain images alone can accurately diagnose chronic neuropsychiatric illnesses. PLoS One 2012;7(12):e50698.
35. Holleran Steiker LK, Hopson LM, Goldback JT. Robinson C evidence for site-specific, systematic adaptation of substance prevention curriculum with high risk youth in community and alternative school settings. J Child Adolesc Subst Abuse 2014;23(5):307–17.
36. Furr-Holden Drug DM, Ialongo NS, Anthony JC, et al. Developmentally inspired drug prevention: middle school outcomes in a school-based randomized prevention trial. Drug Alcohol Depend 2004;73:149–58.
37. Kellam SG, Brown H, Poduska JM, et al. Wilcox effects of a universal classroom behavior management program in first and second grades on young adult behavioral, psychiatric, and social outcomes. Drug Alcohol Depend 2008;95:S5–28.
38. Available at: http://nrepp.samhsa.gov/viewintervention.aspx?id=351 PAX Good Behavior Game summary.
39. Available at: http://goodbehaviorgame.org/. GBG Web site.
40. Tangney JP, Baumeister RF, Boone AL. High self-control predicts good adjustment, less pathology, better grades, and interpersonal success. J Pers 2004; 72(2):271–324.
41. Mischel W, Shoda Y, Rodriguez MI. Delay of gratification in children. Science 1989;244(4907):933–8.
42. Kalivas PW. Addiction as a pathology in prefrontal cortical regulation of corticostriatal habit circuitry. Neurotox Res 2008;14(2–3):185–9.
43. Quinn PD, Fromme K. Self-regulation as a protective factor against risky drinking and sexual behavior. Psychol Addict Behav 2010;24(3):376–85.
44. Heatherton TF. Neuroscience of self and self-regulation. Annu Rev Psychol 2011; 62:363–90.
45. Ellis LK, Rothbart MK, Posner MI. Individual differences in executive attention predict self-regulation and adolescent psychosocial behaviors. Ann N Y Acad Sci 2004;1021:337–40.
46. Moffitt TE, Arseneault L, Belsky D, et al. A gradient of childhood self-control predicts health, wealth, and public safety. Proc Natl Acad Sci U S A 2011;108(7):2693–8.

47. Mokdad AH, Marks JS, Stroup DF, et al. Actual causes of death in the United States, 2000. JAMA 2004;291(10):1238–45.

48. Schroeder SA. Shattuck Lecture. We can do better–improving the health of the American people. N Engl J Med 2007;357(12):1221–8.

49. Leung HC, Skudlarski P, Gatenby JC, et al. An event-related functional MRI study of the Stroop color word interference task. Cereb Cortex 2000;10(6):552–60.

50. Peterson BS, Kane MJ, Alexander GE, et al. An event-related functional MRI study comparing interference effects in the Simon and Stroop tasks. Brain Res Cogn Brain Res 2002;13(3):427–40.

51. Peterson BS, Skudlarski P, Gatenby JC, et al. An fMRI Study of Stroop word-color interference: evidence for cingulate subregions subserving multiple distributed attentional systems. Biol Psychiatry 1999;45(10):1237–58.

52. Marsh R, Zhu H, Schultz RT, et al. A developmental fMRI study of self-regulatory control. Hum Brain Mapp 2006;27(11):848–63.

53. Adleman NE, Menon V, Blasey CM, et al. A developmental fMRI study of the Stroop color-word task. Neuroimage 2002;16(1):61–75.

54. Bunge SA, Dudukovic NM, Thomason ME, et al. Immature frontal lobe contributions to cognitive control in children: evidence from fMRI. Neuron 2002;33(2):301–11.

55. Casey BJ, Trainor RJ, Orendi JL, et al. A developmental functional MRI study of prefrontal activation during performance of a go-no-go task. J Cogn Neurosci 1997;9(6):835–47.

56. Rubia K, Overmeyer S, Taylor E, et al. Functional frontalisation with age: mapping neurodevelopmental trajectories with fMRI. Neurosci Biobehav Rev 2000;24(1):13–9.

57. Luna B, Thulborn KR, Munoz DP, et al. Maturation of widely distributed brain function subserves cognitive development. Neuroimage 2001;13(5):786–93.

58. Tamm L, Menon V, Reiss AL. Maturation of brain function associated with response inhibition. J Am Acad Child Adolesc Psychiatry 2002;41(10):1231–8.

59. NIHCM brief on adolescent depression. Available at: http://www.nihcm.org/pdf/Adol_MH_Issue_Brief_FINAL.pdf.

60. Granic I, Lobel A, Engels RC. The benefits of playing video games. Am Psychol 2014;69(1):66–78.

61. Merry SN, Stasiak K, Shepherd M, et al. The effectiveness of SPARX, a computerised self help intervention for adolescents seeking help for depression: randomised controlled non-inferiority trial. BMJ 2012;344:e2598.

62. Fleming T, Frampton C, Merry S. A pragmatic randomized controlled trial of computerized CBT (SPARX) for symptoms of depression among adolescents excluded from mainstream education. Behav Cogn Psychother 2012;40:529–41.

63. Poppelaars M, Tak YR, Lichtwarck-Aschoff A, et al. Autonomous and controlled motivation in a randomized controlled trial comparing school-based and computerized depression prevention programs. In: Schouten B, Fedtke S, Schijven M, et al, editors. Games for Health 2014: Proceedings of the 4th conference on gaming and playful interaction in healthcare. Berlin: Springer; 2014. p. 125–35.

64. Lee JS, Leong B. Having mentors and campus social networks moderates the impact of worries and video gaming on depressive symptoms: a moderated mediation analysis. BMC Public Health 2014;14:426.

65. Miller TJ, McGlashan TH, Rosen JL, et al. Prodromal assessment with the structured interview for prodromal syndromes and the scale of prodromal symptoms: predictive validity, interrater reliability, and training to reliability. Schizophr Bull 2003;29(4):703–15.

66. Yung AR, Yuen HP, McGorry PD, et al. Mapping the onset of psychosis: the comprehensive assessment of at-risk mental states. Aust N Z J Psychiatry 2005;39(11–12):964–71.
67. Fusar-Poli P, McGuire P, Borgwardt S. Mapping prodromal psychosis: a critical review of neuroimaging studies. Eur Psychiatry 2012;27(3):181–91.
68. Fusar-Poli P, Bonoldi I, Yung AR, et al. Predicting psychosis: meta-analysis of transition outcomes in individuals at high clinical risk. Arch Gen Psychiatry 2012;69(3):220–9.
69. Meyer SE, Bearden CE, Lux SR, et al. The psychosis prodrome in adolescent patients viewed through the lens of DSM-IV. J Child Adolesc Psychopharmacol 2005;15(3):434–51.
70. Liu P, Parker AG, Hetrick SE, et al. An evidence map of interventions across premorbid, ultra-high risk and first episode phases of psychosis. Schizophr Res 2010;123:37–44.
71. van der Gaag M, Smit F, Bechdolf A, et al. Preventing a first episode of psychosis: meta-analysis of randomized controlled prevention trials of 12 month and longer-term follow-ups. Schizophr Res 2013;149(1):56–62.
72. Valmaggia L, McCrone P, Knapp M, et al. Economic impact of early intervention in people at high risk of psychosis. Psychol Med 2009;39(10):1617–26.
73. McFarlane WR, Lukens E, Link B, et al. Multiple-family groups and psychoeducation in the treatment of schizophrenia. Arch Gen Psychiatry 1995;52(8): 679–87.
74. McFarlane WR. Multifamily groups in the treatment of severe psychiatric disorders. New York: Guilford Press; 2004.
75. McFarlane WR, Dixon L, Lukens E, et al. Family psychoeducation and schizophrenia: a review of the literature. J Marital Fam Ther 2003;29(2):223–45.
76. O'Brien MP, Zinberg JL, Bearden CE, et al. Psychoeducational multi-family group treatment with adolescents at high risk for developing psychosis. Early Interv Psychiatry 2007;1(4):325–32.
77. McFarlane WR, Levin B, Travis L, et al. Clinical and functional outcomes after 2 years in the early detection and intervention for the prevention of psychosis multisite effectiveness trial. Schizophr Bull 2015;41(1):30–43.
78. Schlosser DA, Miklowitz DJ, O'Brien MP, et al. A randomized trial of family focused treatment for adolescents and young adults at risk for psychosis: study rationale, design and methods. Early Interv Psychiatry 2012;6(3):283–91.
79. Miklowitz DJ, O'Brien MP, Schlosser DA, et al. Family-focused treatment for adolescents and young adults at high risk for psychosis: results of a randomized trial. J Am Acad Child Adolesc Psychiatry 2014;53(8):848–58.
80. O'Brien MP, Miklowitz DJ, Candan KA, et al. A randomized trial of family focused therapy with populations at clinical high risk for psychosis: effects on interactional behavior. J Consult Clin Psychol 2014;82(1):90–101.
81. Hooley JM. Expressed emotion and relapse of psychopathology. Annu Rev Clin Psychol 2007;3(1):329–52.
82. Morrison AP, Renton JC, Dunn H, et al. Cognitive therapy for psychosis: a formulation based approach. London: Routledge; 2004.
83. Morrison AP, French P, Walford L, et al. Cognitive therapy for the prevention of psychosis in people at ultra-high risk: randomised controlled trial. Br J Psychiatry 2004;185:291–7.
84. Phillips LJ, McGorry PD, Yuen HP, et al. Medium term follow-up of a randomized controlled trial of interventions for young people at ultra high risk of psychosis. Schizophr Res 2007;96(1):25–33.

85. Hutton P, Taylor PJ. Cognitive behavioural therapy for psychosis prevention: a systematic review and meta-analysis. Psychol Med 2014;44(03):449–68.
86. McGorry PD, Yung AR, Phillips LJ, et al. Randomized controlled trial of interventions designed to reduce the risk of progression to first-episode psychosis in a clinical sample with subthreshold symptoms. Arch Gen Psychiatry 2002;59(10): 921–8.
87. McGlashan TH, Zipursky RB, Perkins D, et al. Randomized, double-blind trial of olanzapine versus placebo in patients prodromally symptomatic for psychosis. Am J Psychiatry 2006;163(5):790–9.
88. Cannon TD, Cadenhead K, Cornblatt B, et al. Prediction of psychosis in youth at high clinical risk: a multisite longitudinal study in North America. Arch Gen Psychiatry 2008;65(1):28–37.
89. Fusar-Poli P, Frascarelli M, Valmaggia L, et al. Antidepressant, antipsychotic and psychological interventions in subjects at high clinical risk for psychosis: OASIS 6-year naturalistic study. Psychol Med 2015;45:1327–9.
90. International Early Psychosis Association Writing Group. International clinical practice guidelines for early psychosis. Br J Psychiatry 2005;187(48):s120–4.
91. Barnes TR, Schizophrenia Consensus Group of British Association for Psychopharmacology. Evidence-based guidelines for the pharmacological treatment of schizophrenia: recommendations from the British Association for Psychopharmacology. J Psychopharmacol 2011;25(5):567–620.
92. Amminger G, Schäfer MR, Papageorgiou K, et al. Long-chain ω-3 fatty acids for indicated prevention of psychotic disorders: a randomized, placebo-controlled trial. Arch Gen Psychiatry 2010;67(2):146–54.
93. Nelson B, Yuen HP, Wood SJ, et al. Long-term follow-up of a group at ultra high risk ("Prodromal") for psychosis: the PACE 400 study. JAMA Psychiatry 2013; 70(8):793–802.
94. Preti A, Cella M. Randomized-controlled trials in people at ultra high risk of psychosis: a review of treatment effectiveness,. Schizophr Res 2010;123:30–6.

Clinical Advances in Geriatric Psychiatry

A Focus on Prevention of Mood and Cognitive Disorders

Harris Eyre, MBBS[a,b], Bernhard Baune, MD, PhD[a],
Helen Lavretsky, MD, MS[c],*

KEYWORDS

- Late life • Psychiatry • Cognitive decline • Mood disorder • Depression
- Prevention • Treatment

KEY POINTS

- World population aging in the twenty-first century is unprecedented in human history, and will place substantial pressure on health systems across the world with concurrent rises in chronic diseases, particularly cognitive disorders and late-life affective disorders.
- Prevention of mood and cognitive disorders is of utmost importance to reduce morbidity and mortality and the high costs of health care for both patients and society.
- Recent data and innovative preventive interventions involving lifestyle, resilience building, and complementary, alternative, and integrative medicine for treatment and prevention of geriatric mood and cognitive disorders are discussed.
- Current clinical challenges and future directions for research are addressed.

INTRODUCTION

The world's population is aging in the twenty-first century at a rate unprecedented in human history, and this will place substantial pressure on health systems across the world along with concurrent rises in chronic diseases. In particular, rates of cognitive disorders and late-life affective disorders are expected to increase. A recent global report[1] suggests that the proportion of older people (aged ≥60 years) increased

[a] Discipline of Psychiatry, University of Adelaide, 55 Frome Road, Adelaide, South Australia 5005, Australia; [b] Semel Institute for Neuroscience, University of California, Los Angeles, 760 Westwood Boulevard, Los Angeles, CA 90095, USA; [c] Late Life Mood Stress and Wellness Research Program, Semel Institute for Neuroscience, University of California, Los Angeles, 760 Westwood Plaza, Room 37-465, Los Angeles, CA 90077, USA
* Corresponding author.
E-mail address: hlavretsky@mednet.ucla.edu

Psychiatr Clin N Am 38 (2015) 495–514
http://dx.doi.org/10.1016/j.psc.2015.05.002
0193-953X/15/$ – see front matter © 2015 Elsevier Inc. All rights reserved.

from 9.2% in 1990% to 11.7% in 2013, and will continue to grow as a proportion of the world population, reaching 21.1% by 2050. In tandem with aging, there are robust predictions suggesting that rates of age-related cognitive decline, dementia, and geriatric depression will increase, with serious consequences. As of 2013, there were an estimated 44.4 million people worldwide with dementia.[2] This number will increase to an estimated 75.6 million in 2030 and 135.5 million in 2050. The most recent data on geriatric depression[3] identified depressive disorders as a leading cause of burden internationally, and suggested major depressive disorder was also a contributor of burden allocated to suicide and ischemic heart disease. Depressive disorders were the second leading cause of years lived with disability in 2010.[3]

These large burdens of disease are met by modest efficacies of current therapies and poor access for many. Unfortunately for those with Alzheimer disease (AD), pharmacological agents temporarily treat symptoms without having an effect on the underlying pathophysiology of the disease.[4] In geriatric depression, a recent meta-analysis of clinical trials suggests a response rate of 48% and a remission rate of 33.7%, both very similar to response and remission rates found in adult patients.[5] Clearly innovative prevention and treatment strategies are needed.

Throughout health care, everything clinicians do should be aimed toward prevention. This approach ranges from preventing the onset of disease in those who are well, through preventing chronicity, disability, and other consequences of disease, to preventing relapses in those in recovery. When conceptualizing approaches in prevention science, the most commonly used models are those of the Institute of Medicine (IOM)[6] and the World Health Organization (WHO) framework of levels of prevention (ie, primary, secondary, and tertiary prevention).[7] A report from the IOM[6] suggests prevention may be directed toward the whole population (universal prevention), high-risk groups (selective prevention), or those with subsyndromal symptoms (indicated prevention). The WHO prevention framework[7] suggests primary prevention involves strategies aimed at preventing the development of disease; secondary prevention involves strategies to diagnose and treat existent disease in early stages before significant morbidity occurs; and tertiary prevention involves strategies to reduce the negative impact of existent disease by restoring function and reducing disease-related complications.

Fortunately, there are several innovative prevention and treatment strategies being developed. This article focuses on several key strategies that include preventive and treatment strategies coming from resilience-building interventions, and complementary, alternative and integrative therapies. Platforms such as telepsychiatry and Internet-based interventions are also promising mechanisms to enhance access to therapies. The latest clinical advances in geriatric psychiatry for the prevention and treatment of mood disorders and cognitive decline are outlined, followed by an exploration of clinically relevant scientific advances under way at present.

CLINICAL ADVANCES IN GERIATRIC DEPRESSION
Preventive Interventions for Geriatric Depression

This review focuses on the IOM framework of prevention comprising universal, selective, and indicated prevention.[6] A critique of prevention in geriatric psychiatry should focus on (1) feasibility, (2) effectiveness, and (3) ethical and economic considerations.[8] **Table 1** outlines these conceptual frameworks of preventive science, and gives clinical examples for the fields of geriatric psychiatry.

With respect to universal prevention, any universal preventive action for geriatric depression should be a "light" intervention in terms of cost, effort for patients, and

Table 1
Clinical implications of preventive science frameworks in geriatric psychiatry

Preventive Approach	Definition and Explanation	Clinical Examples for Geriatric Depression	Clinical Examples for Cognitive Decline
Universal	Strategies that involve the whole population. Provided without screening	Environmental design and modification (eg, green space development, walkway modification, food access, health communities); cross-governmental initiatives; Internet-based promotions; informational programs for the general public	
Selective	Strategies that involve targeted subpopulations whose risk of developing a disorder is above average. Involves identified exposure to specific risk factors	Risk factors: Preexisting disease: psychiatric illness (eg, anxiety disorder, age-related cognitive dysfunction, substance-related disorders); general medical conditions (eg, cardiovascular disease, obesity, diabetes) Health-related behaviors: eg, psychological stress; physical inactivity; alcohol, tobacco and other drugs; sleep disruption; dietary factors Biological factors	
Indicated	Strategies aimed at subjects who have early and subthreshold symptoms and signs of illness. Involves a screening process	Subthreshold; early intervention	
Primary	Strategies to avoid occurrence of disease	As per universal and selective approaches	
Secondary	Strategies to diagnose and treat existent disease in early stages before significant morbidity occurs	Relapse prevention; attenuation of episode duration and severity of episode; early intervention	Early intervention to prevent conversion to tertiary
Tertiary	Strategies to reduce negative impact of existent disease by restoring function and reducing disease-related complications	Prevention of cognitive decline; prevention of psychotropic drug use and therefore reduced side effects; prevention of catatonia; prevention of adverse effects of illness on social and occupational functioning	

Data from Refs.[4,6,7,72–75]

impact (reviewed extensively elsewhere[8]). An example is a public awareness campaign. Cuijpers[9] has described that, even in a disorder such as depression which has a relatively high incidence, studies testing universal prevention are not likely to be feasible. Such a study would require too many participants and be too costly to be run.[8] Cuijpers suggests "this does not imply that universal prevention may not be useful, but it does suggest that universal prevention is probably best seen as a 'primer'—a way to prepare the public that depression is a disorder that can be managed, to reduce stigma."[9] Fortunately, given technological advances and the widespread access to electronic media globally, electronic health preventive interventions for older people are in development.[8] These developments may drive down costs of programs, and increase opportunities for and scales of preventive interventions, hence shifting preventive action toward universal programs.

With respect to selective prevention, several tested interventions are available (for review see Ref.[8]). These interventions usually involve a way of identifying those at risk, and creating engagement with the intervention itself. Identification of older people at risk and engaging them effectively depends very much on local socioeconomic and cultural factors.[8] In high-resource settings with well-developed health services, the more prudent point of contact for selective prevention may be community health services. Encouragingly, epidemiological data show that most older people with risk factors for depression do contact their family physician regularly and that these doctors have reliable data about many known risk factors.[8] Engaging older people who are not clinically depressed in an intervention is not easy. Complicated factors include a lack of awareness of mental health; lack of trust in interventions; lack of time, trained personnel, and resources to engage in an intervention; and the societal stigma surrounding mental illness.[8] Beekman and colleagues[8] suggest "it is possible from an intrapersonal psychological perspective, humans tend to dislike doing things now to avoid harm later—ie, there is no immediate benefit." From the intervention perspective, the interventions that have been designed are mostly "light" versions of robust clinical interventions, such as cognitive therapy, interpersonal therapy, reminiscence, and problem solving.[8] Often these are modified to cater for persons exposed to specific risk factors and circumstances.[8] Other ingredients involve engaging in pleasant activities, physical activity, using nutritional supplements such as vitamin D and fish oils, and exposure to bright light (see for review Ref.[10]).

Indicated prevention engages older people who do have symptoms of depression but who have not developed a diagnosable major mood disorder. These individuals do have symptoms, and these symptoms interfere with their well-being and daily functioning. Indeed, older people with subthreshold depressive symptoms are at very high risk for developing diagnosable major mood disorders.[11] A drawback of indicated prevention is that participants need to be diagnosed with "symptoms but no disorder."[8] The trials that have been conducted in this area mostly recruited participants through screening.[11] A positive screen implies that some significant symptoms are present. In a next diagnostic step, the outcome may either (1) a diagnosable major mood disorder or (2) no such disorder. The patient is then referred for treatment or offered a preventive intervention, respectively. A study in the Netherlands by van't Veer-Tazleer and colleagues[12] tested a program that was organized along the lines of "stepped care." In this program all the older participants with "symptoms but major disorder" were offered a choice of educational and self-help interventions first, slowly stepping up the intensity of the intervention if the symptoms remained present. The intervention halved the 12-month incidence of depressive and anxiety disorders, from 0.24 in the usual care group to 0.12 in the stepped-care group (relative risk, 0.49; 95% confidence interval [CI], 0.24–0.98).

Resilience-Building Interventions

Advancing age is often associated with increased vulnerability to a unique set of stressors including retirement, medical comorbidity, loss of loved ones, and the threat of loss of independence. As such, there has been a surge of interest in exploring factors that contribute to older adults aging more successfully. One such aspect of successful aging is the concept of resilience.[13]

The critical role of resilience in successful aging has been well documented.[14–16] Positive constructs such as resilience may be thought of as being complements to traditional medicine in that they emphasize personal strength rather than disease or deficits.[17] The study of resilience coincides with the rising trend toward a strengths-based approach to aging, which is slowly starting to replace, or at least complement, the traditional negative deficits view of aging (see for review Ref.[18]). One of the goals of positive aging is for individuals to evolve, adapt, and find meaning and purpose in life events. One study found that older adults who were more resilient tended to report fewer adversities and were more likely to use adaptive, solution-driven coping rather than avoidant coping strategies in the face of challenge.[19] Additional individual characteristics that have been viewed as being important contributors to resilience include commitment, dynamism, humor in the face of adversity, optimism, faith, altruism, and perceiving adversity as an opportunity to learn and grow.[20]

To the authors' knowledge, there are no published interventions specifically targeting resilience in geriatric mood and cognitive disorders, but there are some data in adult populations. Padesky and Mooney[21] describe a 4-step strengths-based cognitive behavioral therapy model designed to enhance resilience. The 4 steps to resilience include: a search for strengths; construction of a personal model of resilience; applying the personal model of resilience to areas of life difficulties; and practicing resilience. In this treatment approach, individuals are supported to search for areas of competence such as good health, positive relationships with others, self-efficacy, emotion regulation skills, and the belief that one's life has meaning. The purpose of this search is based on the notion that all individuals possess resilience traits, however much they have been unaware of same. A personal model of resilience is created that may then be used by the individual in life situations.

When exploring resilience in older participants, a recent observational study by Jeste and colleagues[18] found significant associations between resilience and self-rated successful aging in a sample of more than 1000 community-dwelling older adults. The magnitude of these effects was reportedly comparable in size with that of physical health. This finding was supported by Manning and colleagues[22] who reported another observational study, finding high levels of resilience protect against the psychological impact of chronic new conditions in older adults. Some research has suggested that high levels of resilience significantly contribute to longevity and that this becomes even more significant at very advanced ages, centenarians being more resilient than any other age group.[23] In a cohort of middle- to older-aged women with breast cancer, Loprinzi and colleagues[24] demonstrated the possible efficacy of the Stress Management and Resiliency Training (SMART) program in increasing the quality of life. In this intervention, participants attended two 90-minute group sessions in which they were taught relaxation techniques, in addition to skills to delay judgment and attend to novel aspects of the environment rather than one's thoughts. Participants also learned to adopt a flexible disposition and practice gratitude, compassion, and acceptance. The investigators found that relative to the wait-list control group, women who received the SMART intervention reported improved resilience, quality of life, anxiety, stress, and fatigue. The evidence of the feasibility of such a brief intervention is promising in the context of adapting programs for older adults.

Complementary, Alternative, and Integrative Therapies for Geriatric Depression

Complementary and alternative medicine "is a group of diverse medical and health care systems, practices, and products that are not presently considered part of conventional medicine."[25] Some of these therapies provide promise as novel and effective therapies for treatment and prevention of geriatric psychiatric disorders with generally more modest side-effect profiles.[10] "Complementary" generally refers to using a nonmainstream approach together with conventional Western medicine. "Alternative" refers to using a nonmainstream approach in place of conventional Western medicine. "Integrative medicine" is another term often used when strategy combines alternative and complementary medicine with evidence-based Western medicine. In this article such therapies are referred to as complementary, alternative, and integrative medicine (CAIM). CAIM interventions have varying levels of efficacy and evidence; they can include mind-body practices, conventional physical activity, dietary interventions, and natural products, in addition to body-based practices and other medical system practices.

Mind-body practices refer to practices whereby there is both physical and mental activity that may be combined during training. These activities can be more exercise-focused (ie, yoga, tai chi, qigong) or more focused on practice and stress reduction (ie, mindfulness and relaxation). Physical activity refers to any bodily movement produced by skeletal muscles that requires energy expenditure, and may include aerobic, resistance, stretching and toning, or combination activities. Dietary interventions explore the effect of dietary patterns on health and illness, and may include, among others, Western, traditional, and Mediterranean dietary patterns, and caloric restriction. Natural products may include herbs, vitamins, minerals, natural supplements, and probiotics. Body-based practices may include spinal manipulation (eg, chiropractic, osteopathic medicine), aromatherapy, and massage therapy. Other medical systems include traditional Chinese medicine (including acupuncture), ayurvedic medicine, or homeopathy. These CAIM interventions are largely based on therapies that have been used in many civilizations and religions for hundreds and thousands of years. It is not since the past 50 to 100 years that empirical science has begun to explore the evidence behind these therapies.

Clinical importance

There are several major reasons why geriatric mental health providers need to recognize the importance of these interventions. (1) *CAIM therapy use is high and rising*. Research suggests 12-month prevalence of any CAIM usage (excluding prayer) in the United States is around 35% to 50%; Baby Boomers (adults born from 1946 to 1964) report significantly higher rates of use than the Silent Generation (born from 1925 to 1945) for chronic conditions.[26] (2) *The global population is aging*. See earlier discussion. (3) *CAIM therapies are increasingly cited in clinical guidelines*. It is now commonplace to note the use of therapies such as conventional exercise in the management of psychiatric conditions. (4) CAIM therapies are a source for innovative interventions and have a growing, quality empirical research basis. Empirical research into these therapies is exploring their clinical efficacy in trials and the neurobiological mechanism underlying their effects. (5) *CAIM therapies can help to lower utilization of conventional medicines*. CAIM therapies may be used in replacement of conventional medicines for the management of mild illnesses (eg, relaxation techniques for mild anxiety instead of benzodiazepines, which are known to have adverse effects in elderly populations).[10] (6) *CAIM therapies can have significant side effects and CAIM-drug interactions*. With the high use in geriatric populations, this is an important reason why clinicians need to better understand CAIM therapies.[10]

Conventional physical activity

Conventional physical exercise has received attention for its potential role in the treatment of geriatric depression. The effects of aerobic exercise on depressed adults ($\geq$50 years) was examined and compared with either monotherapy with sertraline as a standard antidepressant or a combination.[27] The study found that after 16 weeks, all groups demonstrated significant and equivalent reductions in depressive symptoms. Furthermore, a 10-month follow-up study showed that participants in the exercise group (who improved to the point of remission during the initial study) had lower rates of relapse with sertraline versus antidepressants. Another study of exercise in older adults found that 10 weeks of strength-training exercises classes, provided as an adjunctive treatment, lessened depressive symptoms in a group of older adults who failed antidepressant response alone when compared with a health education course.[28] A systematic review[29] examining the role of exercise in the treatment of depression in older adults was published in 2009. This study noted 11 randomized controlled trials (RCTs) with a total of 641 participants older than 60 years. The study noted short-term (0–3 months) positive outcomes in 9 studies, although there was variation in the type, intensity, and duration of exercise. The efficacy of exercise in the medium- and long-term (3–12 months and >12 months, respectively) was less clear. Methodological issues were noted, with only 5 studies showing appropriate allocation of concealment, 5 studies with intention-to-treat analysis, and 7 studies with blinding. From a more real-world perspective, the effectiveness of several lifestyle interventions promoting increases in conventional physical exercise were recently reviewed.[30] Interventions were relatively successful in initiating increased levels of physical activity in the short term; however, maintenance of these gains were diminished over time, and there was no convincing evidence that behavioral reinforcement strategies were beneficial; therefore, adherence is a major concern. Another review of exercise interventions found that although many older adults increase activity levels in response to a wide variety of interventions, the amount of increase is seldom enough to affect health outcomes in a positive manner.[30]

In conclusion, preliminary evidence points to exercise as having a significant potential to lessen symptoms in depressed older adults and, furthermore, to prevent relapse of depression and/or development of depressive symptoms in older adults experiencing acute stressors associated with aging. Therefore, the authors recommend physical exercise as a stand-alone therapy in the treatment of mild depression, and as an adjunct in moderate depression.

Currently, the American College of Sports Medicine[31] recommends that exercise programs for older adults include both aerobic and nonaerobic physical activities, such as resistance training, balance training, and stretching, for optimal general health. See **Box 1** for the latest clinical guidelines on physical activity for older adults.

Mind-body practices

Mindful exercise interventions have shown promise in addressing depressive symptoms in older adults. For example, a study of 82 older adult participants with depression randomized to either 16 weeks of qigong practice or newspaper reading groups found that qigong participants showed significantly greater improvements in mood, self-efficacy, and personal well-being.[32] Practice of yoga typically benefits from instruction by expert instructors, and requires the dedication by participants to multiple weekly sessions and continual use for maximal benefit. Prior review of published RCTs of yoga for depression in adults revealed that although all trials found benefit, trial methodologies have generally been weak with lack of blinding, short duration of the intervention, variable outcome measures, and limited information about subjects, randomization procedures, compliance, and dropout rates.[33] Comparative studies of yoga have likewise been limited, with one trial demonstrating that yoga was as effective as tricyclic antidepressants and another showing that yoga may provide benefit as an augmentation strategy for antidepressant treatment.[34] Yoga is commonly used in combination with other treatments for depression, anxiety, and stress-related disorders. Data on use of yoga for anxiety and depression in older adults are more limited; however, one significant study of 69 older adults in India did compare the impact of yoga with Ayurveda or a wait-list control condition on sleep and depressive symptoms.[35] Participants in the yoga group practiced physical postures, relaxation

---

Box 1
Clinical suggestions for geriatric populations

If 65 years or older, generally fit, and have no limiting health conditions.

- At least 150 minutes of moderate-intensity aerobic activity (ie, brisk walking) every week and muscle-strengthening activities on 2 or more days a week that work all major muscle groups (ie, legs, hips, back, abdomen, chest, shoulders, and arms) OR

- 75 minutes of vigorous-intensity aerobic activity (ie, jogging or running) every week and muscle-strengthening activities on 2 or more days a week that work all major muscle groups OR

- An equivalent mix of moderate- and vigorous-intensity aerobic activity and muscle-strengthening activities on 2 or more days a week that work all major muscle groups

Other comments:

- If there is a limiting condition, it is recommended that the health professional and patient consult a qualified exercise physiologist

- 10 minutes at a time is fine for physical activity

- The following activities count as muscle-strengthening activities: yoga, heavy gardening

Adapted from the Centers for Disease Control and Prevention Report 'Physical activity is essential to healthy aging'. How much physical activity do older adults need? 2014. Available at: http://www.cdc.gov/physicalactivity/everyone/guidelines/olderadults.html. Accessed October 28, 2014.

---

techniques, regulated breathing, and devotional songs, and attended lectures for more than 7 hours a week during the course of the 6-month trial. Practice of yoga significantly affected the quality of sleep and level of depressive symptoms when compared with the 2 control conditions, neither of which demonstrated significant effects. In particular, depressive symptoms, as measured by the short form of the Geriatric Depression Scale, decreased in the yoga group from a baseline average of 10.6 to 8.1 by 3 months and 6.7 by 6 months. The average time to fall asleep decreased in the yoga group by 10 minutes while the total number of hours slept increased by 60 minutes, and resulted in a greater feeling of being rested after 6 months. A recent study by Shahidi and colleagues[36] compared the effectiveness of laughter yoga, group exercise therapy, and a control arm in decreasing depression in older adult women (60–80 years). In this study, 70 depressed women were chosen if their Geriatric Depression Score was greater than 10. This study went for 10 sessions and found a significant improvement in depression score with both yoga and group exercise therapy in comparison with control activity. Although the evidence supporting the use of these therapies in the treatment of late-life mental illnesses is not strong, there are some interesting early results that require further high-quality research.[37]

The authors recommend the use of mind-body therapies as a stand-alone or adjunctive antidepressant treatment in the management of geriatric depression, based on individual preference and the severity of depression. Further high-quality data are needed to further inform these recommendations.

Dietary interventions

Dietary interventions are seen as a promising method to both treat and prevent geriatric depression. When considering the diet composition of older depressed adults, some concerning findings come from a recent cross-sectional study.[38] In this study of 278 older adults (144 with depression; 134 without depression), vitamin C, lutein, and cryptoxanthin intakes were significantly lower among depressed individuals than in controls. In addition, fruit and vegetable consumption, a primary determinant of antioxidant intake, was lower in depressed individuals. This type of dietary intake may indeed be a risk factor for depression. A recent systematic review[39] addressed associations between dietary patterns and depression in community-dwelling adult populations. A total of 21 studies were identified. Results from 13 observational studies were pooled, from cross-sectional to 15 years prospective. Two dietary patterns were identified. The healthy diet pattern was significantly associated with a reduced odds of depression (odds ratio [OR], 0.84; 95% CI, 0.76–0.92; $P<.001$). No statistically significant association was observed between the Western diet and depression (OR, 1.17; 95% CI, 0.97–1.68; $P = .094$); however, the studies were too few for a precise estimate of this effect. The results suggest that high intakes of fruit, vegetables, fish, and whole grains may be associated with a reduced risk of depression.

The authors are aware of only one RCT, currently under way in Australia, to explore the effect of dietary interventions on adult depression,[40] not specifically in an older-age population. This study is enrolling participants with a current major depressive episode who are randomized to a dietary intervention group or a social support group. The dietary intervention consists of 7 individual nutrition consulting sessions (60 minutes each) delivered by a dietician. Data will be explored across the 3-month trials and a 6-month follow-up. Data on the potential benefits of dietary coaching in the prevention of incident depression for older adults has recently been drawn from a larger randomized depression prevention trial that ran over 2 years.[41] Older adults (n = 122) receiving dietary coaching experienced a low incidence of major depressive episodes and exhibited a 40% to 50% decrease in depressive symptoms, and enhanced well-being, during the initial 6-week intervention; these gains were sustained over 2 years.[42] Clearly the role of dietary intervention is intriguing.

CLINICAL ADVANCES IN COGNITIVE DECLINE AND DEMENTIA
Prevention of Cognitive Decline and Dementia

The rising burden globally of mental, cognitive, and substance use disorders[2,43] supports the need for improved methods to aid prevention and early intervention.[44] Classic risk factor studies in dementia are hampered by the difficult phenotyping of the disease with large heterogeneity in severity and presentation, and by the fact that once symptomatic, irreversible brain damage is already present. The paradigm shift in medicine toward prevention calls for identification of potentially modifiable factors that affect disease at an earlier stage. The rising burden of cognitive disorders is occurring as our wider understanding of preventive lifestyle modifications and our understanding of the neurobiological underpinnings is rapidly evolving. For example, with AD, a recent study has highlighted the important role of risk factor reduction for reducing AD prevalence.[44] Barnes and Yaffe[44] explored the role of 7 potentially modifiable AD risk factors: diabetes, mid-life hypertension, mid-life obesity, smoking, depression, low educational attainment, and physical inactivity. The investigators determined that these factors contributed to up to half of AD cases globally (17.2 million), and that a 10% to 25% reduction in all risk factors could potentially prevent as many as 1.1 to 3.0 million cases. There is now an emerging body of literature exploring the effect of these risk factors on neurobiological factors. Other lifestyle factors that have been found to reduce the risk of AD include mind-body exercise (eg, yoga, tai chi, qi gong[45]), conventional physical activity (eg, aerobic, strength training[45]), supplements (eg, Ω3 fatty acids, flavanols[46]), stress-reduction techniques (eg, mindfulness-based stress reduction[47]), sleep modification strategies,[48] and dietary interventions (eg, fish consumption, Mediterranean diet).[49]

Conventional physical activity

Conventional physical activity is one of the most promising therapies for the treatment and prevention of cognitive decline and dementia.[4] There is a variety of subtypes of physical activity, from aerobic activity, to resistance, to stretching and toning.

A recent RCT[50] examined the efficacy of resistance and aerobic training in the improvement of cognitive functions in subjects with subjective mild cognitive impairment (MCI). The study occurred over 6 months and involved 86 community-dwelling women aged 70 to 80 years.

- Physical activity protocols included twice-weekly resistance training, twice-weekly aerobic training, or twice-weekly balance and toning (BAT) training (ie, control).
- Resistance training improved selective attention, conflict resolution, and associated memory compared with BAT.
- By contrast, aerobic physical activity improved general balance and mobility and cardiovascular capacity.
- The study also found that aerobic physical activity improved verbal memory, and both resistance and aerobic physical activity improved spatial memory.

A recent stringent meta-analysis[51] has examined the efficacy of exercise on cognition in older adults with MCI. MCI was diagnosed on documented criteria or via the Mini-Mental State Examination (MMSE). Fourteen RCTs with 1695 participants aged 65 to 95 years were analyzed, with a duration of 6 to 52 weeks. Overall, 42% of effect sizes (ESs) were potentially clinically relevant (ES >0.20) with only 8% of cognitive outcomes statistically significant. The meta-analysis revealed negligible but significant effects of exercise on verbal fluency (ES, 0.17; 95% CI, 0.04–0.30). No significant benefit was found for additional executive measures, memory, or information processing. The investigators critically appraised RCT methods and concluded on a moderate quality, with most trial samples being too small for sufficient power. There is clearly some effect for exercise at moderate to high levels of exertion. In addition, nowadays there is emerging evidence for the effect of low levels of physical activity or "sedentary behaviors" such as sitting. Physical inactivity may increase the risk of AD by 82%.[52] Approximately 13% of AD cases worldwide may be attributable to sedentary behaviors.[44] A 25% reduction in sedentary behavior could potentially prevent more than 1 million AD cases globally.[44] Sedentary behaviors may contribute to risk of AD and dementia by increased risk of cardiometabolic risk factors (diabetes, hypertension, obesity) associated with increased risk of dementia.[53]

Our clinical recommendation is that physical activity should be encouraged for all older adults. More work is required to discern whether physical activity recommendations or dementia prevention are the same as generic "healthy aging" recommendations (as in **Table 1**). Although shorter-term interventions are useful in the research setting, care must be taken to ensure a sustained engagement in physical activity. Care must also be taken to create an age-appropriate and physical function–appropriate prescription, given the risks of adverse health effects (eg, falls, cardiovascular events).

Mindful exercise

A recent meta-analysis[54] critically evaluated the effects of tai chi on individuals aged 60 and older with and without cognitive impairment. In this study, 20 eligible studies with a total of 2553 participants were identified who met inclusion criteria for the systematic review; 11 of the 20 eligible studies were RCTs, 1 was a prospective non-randomized controlled study, 4 were prospective noncontrolled observational studies, and 4 were cross-sectional studies. Overall quality of RCTs was modest, with 3 of 11 trials categorized as being at high risk of bias. Meta-analyses of outcomes related to executive function in RCTs of cognitively healthy adults indicated a large ES when tai chi participants were compared with nonintervention controls (Hedges g = 0.90; P = .04) and a moderate effect size when compared with exercise controls (g = 0.51; P = .003). Meta-analyses of outcomes related to global cognitive function in RCTs of cognitively impaired adults, ranging from MCI to dementia, showed smaller but statistically significant effects when tai chi was compared with nonintervention (g = 0.35; P = .004) and other active interventions (g = 0.30; P = .002).

There is a relative dearth of studies examining yoga and its effects on memory enhancement. One main study of which the authors are aware explores the effects of yoga and exercise in 135 healthy men and women aged 65 to 85 years.[55] In this study, subjects were exposed to 6 months of Hatha yoga classes, walking classes, or wait-list control; subjects were screened with a variety of mood and cognition tests (eg, Stroop test). After the intervention there were no effects from either of the active interventions on any of the cognitive and alertness outcome measures. The yoga intervention produced improvements in physical measures (eg, timed 1-legged standing, forward flexibility) and several quality-of-life measures related to sense of well-being, energy, and fatigue compared with control activity. This type of study needs to be replicated in populations with MCI to better understand the potential effects.

Mind-body practices and stress-reduction techniques

Relaxation techniques, such as breathing exercises, guided imagery, and progressive muscle relaxation, are designed to produce the body's natural relaxation response. These relaxation therapies are proved to lower stress levels in elderly subjects, and so are recommended for clinical use. A recent pilot randomized trial[47] with mindfulness-based stress reduction (MBSR) aimed to test the safety and feasibility of MBSR in older adults with MCI. The investigators found that adults with MCI can safely participate and adhere to an MBSR program. The qualitative interviews revealed that most enjoyed the program and described improved mindfulness skills, well-being, interpersonal skills, acceptance/awareness of MCI, and decreased stress reactivity. Most data suggest a trend toward improvement for measures of cognition and well-being. Nevertheless a more formal, large-scale RCT is needed.

Firm clinical recommendations for these activities are not possible given the paucity of sufficient evidence at this stage. However, the authors would recommend mind-body therapies as useful stand-alone or adjunctive therapies for the management of mild neuropsychiatric symptoms (eg, cognitive impairment and psychological distress) and physical health (eg, balance, strength, coordination). Care must be taken to create an age-appropriate, physically appropriate, and mental function–appropriate prescription.[56] The recommendations are based on clinical experience, emerging evidence, and the safe nature of these activities.

Dietary interventions

Examining the effect of nutrition on cognitive decline is a new area of research showing favorable results. Two significant studies are outlined here to illustrate the latest and most significant developments in this area. A recent analysis of the Australian Imaging, Biomarkers and Lifestyle Study of aging explores the association of 3 well-recognized dietary patterns with cognitive change over a 3-year follow-up period. In this study, 527 healthy older participants (age 69.3 ± 6.4 years) were enlisted and underwent dietary analysis using a food frequency question, in addition to neuropsychological analyses at baseline, 18 months, and 36 months. Three dietary patterns were delineated: the Australian-style Mediterranean diet (AusMeDi), the Western diet, and the prudent diet. The principal aspects of the AusMeDi diet include proportionally high consumption of olive oil, legumes, unrefined cereals, fruits, and vegetables, moderate to high consumption of fish, moderate consumption of dairy products (mostly as cheese and yogurt), moderate consumption of wine, and low consumption of meat and meat products. Western diets are characterized by high intakes of red meat, sugary desserts, high-fat foods, and refined grains. It also typically contains high-fat dairy products, high-sugar drinks, and higher intakes of processed meat. The prudent diet was characterized by high intakes of green leafy vegetables, fruits, nuts, grains, low-fat foods, and protein. Higher baseline adherence to the AusMeDi was associated with better performance in the executive function cognitive domain after 36 months in apolipoprotein E (APOE) ε4 allele carriers (P<.01). Higher baseline Western diet adherence was associated with greater cognitive decline after 36 months in the visuospatial cognitive domain in APOE ε4 allele noncarriers (P<.01). All other results were not significant. Systematic reviews of observation studies show similar results.[57]

The authors are aware of only one RCT exploring the role of diet in the prevention of cognitive impairment. This study was a multicenter, randomized, primary prevention trial named Prevención con Dieta Mediterránea (PREDIMED),[58] which assessed the effects of a nutritional intervention using the MeDi (supplemented with either extra-virgin olive oil [EVOO] or mixed nuts) in comparison with a low-fat control diet. This study assessed 522 participants at high vascular risk (age 74.6 ± 5.7) and examined cognitive performance (MMSE and Clock Drawing Test [CDT]) after 6.5 years of nutritional intervention. After full adjustment, the MeDi EVOO group showed higher mean MMSE and CDT scores versus control (adjusted differences: +0.62, 95% CI +0.18 to +1.05, P = .005 for MMSE; and +0.51, 95% CI +0.20 to +0.82, P = .001 for CDT). Similarly, the MeDi + nuts group showed higher mean MMSE and CDT scores (adjusted differences: +0.57, 95% CI +0.11 to +1.03, P = .015 for MMSE; and +0.33, 95% CI +0.003 to +0.67, P = .048 for CDT) versus control. Clearly, further RCTs are needed in this area of research to improve the quality.

From a clinical perspective, the authors recommend that the population in general adheres as closely as possible to the Mediterranean and healthy diets. Further clinical trials are needed to discover the best diet(s) for maintaining brain health.

Natural products
Natural products may include herbs, minerals, natural supplements, vitamins, and probiotics. A range of these products has been explored with regard to the treatment and prevention of cognitive impairment. There are too many of these products to thoroughly review here, so only the main products, with a larger body of research or epidemiological use, are reviewed, with further reading recommended.

Ω3 polyunsaturated fatty acid supplements One of the most widely used therapies is Ω3 polyunsaturated fatty acids (PUFAs). More than 37% of individuals who reported using a nonvitamin, nonmineral natural product in the 2007 National Health Interview Survey reported using Ω3 PUFAs.[59] Oily fish, such as salmon, mackerel, herring, and sardines, are a rich source of Ω3 PUFAs, which are essential for brain development. It is thought that Ω3 PUFAs may benefit neurodegenerative disorders owing to their antioxidant and anti-inflammatory effects.[60] Previous research from observational studies has suggested that increased consumption of fish oils rich in Ω3 PUFAs may reduce the chance of developing dementia. A recent Cochrane Database systematic review[60] explored the effects of Ω3 PUFAs on the prevention of dementia and cognitive decline in cognitively healthy older people. Information was available from 3 RCTs including 3536 participants in total. This meta-analysis found no evidence to support a preventive effect following 24 or 40 months of intervention. RCTs suggest that selected patients with an MMSE score greater than 27 were more likely to identify a positive effect of Ω3 PUFA supplementation. It would seem that studies of longer duration are required to further explore this area. The authors' clinical recommendation emphasizes clinician-patient discussions of evidence. Care must be taken with potential side effects of mild nausea, mild increased bleeding, and a fishy aftertaste.

Table 2 lists further details on other CAIM therapies for the treatment and prevention of cognitive decline.

Potential side effects and complementary, alternative, and integrative medicine-drug interactions

As alluded to earlier, when encountering natural products in a clinical environment, it is important to consider potential side effects and CAIM-drug interactions. **Table 3** outlines an array of clinical findings and potential pitfalls of natural products. Of importance is that CAIM use may exacerbate polypharmacy in the elderly, which is a risk factor for drug interactions, medication errors, and hospitalization. A survey of 271 British seniors found a mean of 5.91 (range 4–7) herbal and nutritional supplements and 2.26 prescription drugs.[61]

TELEPSYCHIATRY AND INTERNET-BASED APPROACHES FOR OLDER ADULTS

Because of the low rates of receiving adequate treatment among older adults, and the intrinsic and extrinsic barriers to mental health care, it is important to develop evidence-based treatments that are easily accessible to patients, and which keep time and costs low.[62] Telemedicine and Internet-based treatments have been proposed as interventions helpful for these issues.[63–65] Internet-guided and telepsychiatry interventions may save costs and time for patients and therapists, reach depressed older adults who are not reachable with traditional therapies, solve transportation problems, stimulate empowerment of patients, and reduce the stigma associated with mental illness.[62]

Internet-based therapies can be seen as a specific type of guided self-help intervention (for review see Ref.[62]). A self-help intervention can be defined as a psychological treatment whereby the patient or client takes home a standardized treatment and works through it more or less independently.[66,67] In the standardized psychological treatment, the patient can follow step-by-step instructions on what to do in applying a generally accepted psychological treatment. The standardized psychological treatment can be written down in hard-copy print, but can also be made available through other media such as a personal computer, television, video, or the Internet. Contact with therapists is not a necessity for the completion of the self-help therapy; if contact with a therapist takes place, it should only be for support or facilitation. Contact is not aimed at developing a traditional relationship between therapist and patient, and is only meant to support the carrying out of the psychological treatment. Interaction between patient and therapist can take place through face-to-face contact, telephone, email, or any other communication method.

Although a growing number of studies have examined the effects of Internet-based interventions and telephone-supported interventions, few have examined these in older adults.[67] However, research shows that these interventions are promising, and there is no reason to assume that they are not effective in older adults. Concerns may include lesser proficiency with information technology in old age and lesser visual acuity. More research is needed, especially as technological developments continue

Table 2
Other natural products and supplements suggested for the treatment of cognitive impairment

Herb/Supplement	Suggested Dose	Possible Mechanism of Action	Evidence Base	Side Effects
Bacopa monnieri	300 mg/d	An ayurvedic medicinal plant that acts as a free radical scavenger and in animal models reduces Aβ; may also boost cholinergic function	No convincing evidence: 9 RCTs; 518 subjects in meta-analysis. Limited evidence given poor study design	GI upset
Curcumin (yellow curry)	2000–8000 mg/d	Antioxidant, anti-inflammatory, induces heat-shock proteins; antiamyloid effects in animals	Mixed results; no convincing evidence: 2 studies find no effect; 1 study finds beneficial effect	GI upset
Dehydroepiandrosterone (DHEA)	100 mg/d	Adrenal steroid that declines with aging, is lower in AD patients, and is neurotrophic in animals	No convincing evidence of benefit. 3 RCTs	Acne, balding, insulin resistance, dyslipidemia, mood changes, hepatic dysfunction, possible effects on hormone-sensitive cancers
Hydergine	3 mg/d	Combination of 4 ergot derivatives with vasodilatory effects and possible effect on monoamine and cholinergic transmission	A 2000 Cochrane meta-analysis of 19 trials found some evidence of modest efficacy but many trials conducted before standardized criteria for diagnosing dementia	GI upset, psychosis, flushing, blood pressure changes
Lecithin	3600 mg/d	Acetylcholine precursor	Review of 11 randomized trials showed no consistent benefit	GI upset, rash, headache, dizziness
Resveratrol	Unknown (phase 1 trials 2500–5000 mg/d)	Polyphenol in the skin of red grapes and red wine with antioxidant and antiamyloid properties in animals	Clinical trial linking to increased cerebral blood flow. Needs further study on cognitive effects	Possible estrogen-like effects, as its chemical structure is similar to phytoestrogens
Vitamin E	800–2000 IU/d	Free radical scavenging	No convincing evidence. Cochrane review of 3 studies	High dose increases all-cause mortality

Abbreviations: AD, Alzheimer disease; GI, gastrointestinal; RCT, randomized controlled trial.
Data from Refs.[76–82]

Table 3
Potential CAIM-drug interactions between natural products and prescription medications

Herb/Supplement	Prescription Drug(s)	Possible Interaction
Chamomile	Sedatives (or alcohol)	Oversedation
Garlic extract	Protease inhibitors	Decreased efficacy against HIV

Ginkgo biloba	Anticoagulants
	Omeprazole (CYP2C19
	  substrates)
	Antipsychotic
		Excessive bleeding
		Decreased drug levels (2C19
		  induction)
		Priapism

Ginseng	Anticoagulants Monoamine oxidase inhibitors Sulfonylureas, insulin Stimulants	Excessive bleeding Mania, hypertension, headache Hypoglycemia Insomnia, anxiety, mania
Kava	Sedatives (or alcohol) Levodopa	Oversedation Increased parkinsonism
Omega-3 fatty acids	Warfarin	Excessive bleeding
St John's wort	Protease inhibitors cyclosporine Serotonergic antidepressants Oral contraceptives Tetracycline	Decreased efficacy against HIV Organ rejection Serotonin syndrome Ineffective contraception Photosensitivity
Valerian	Sedatives (or alcohol) CYP3A4 substrates	Oversedation Increased drug levels (3A4 inhibition)
Vitamin E	Anticoagulants	Excessive bleeding

Abbreviation: HIV, human immunodeficiency virus.

rapidly, and innovative types of intervention and new possibilities to reduce the disease burden are required.

PROMISING RESEARCH AGENDAS

In addition to these current clinical advances, there is a range of research advances that may pave the way for future clinical innovations.

Geroscience

Geroscience is an interdisciplinary field that aims to understand the relationship between aging and age-related diseases.[68] In geroscience, researchers in a variety of disciplines may work together, sharing data and ideas, with a common goal of explaining and intervening in age-related diseases. "Compression of morbidity," a major focus of geroscience research, is a concept whereby scientists discover ways to decrease the period of an individual's life in which there is poor health. With this aim, individuals hope to postpone and reduce disease onset, disability, dependency, and suffering. The exact mechanisms of aging are still under debate, although there are several mechanisms which are generally agreed on (see for discussion Ref.[69]). These mechanisms include genomic instability, telomere attrition, epigenetic alterations, loss of proteostasis, mitochondrial dysfunction, cellular senescence, and chronic inflammation.

Health Neuroscience

Health neuroscience was coined by Erickson and colleagues,[70] and is at the interface of health psychology and neuroscience. It is concerned with the interplay between the brain and physical health over the life span. A chief goal of health neuroscience is to characterize bidirectional and dynamic brain-behavior and brain-physiology relationships that are determinants, markers, and consequences of physical health states across the life span. The motivation behind this goal is that a better understanding of these relationships will provide mechanistic insights into how the brain links multilevel genetic, biological, psychological, behavioral, social, and environmental factors with physical health, especially vulnerability to and resilience against clinical illnesses.

Convergence Medicine

Convergence medicine is a novel derivative of convergence science, and refers to the discipline of how societal health can be optimized by the cross-pollination of clinical medical practice with nonclinical fields (eg, engineering, information technology, entrepreneurship, public health, business, finance, management, journalism, politics, law, and the arts).[71] The aim is for health innovation based on interdisciplinary team work and multidisciplinary mind-sets.

SUMMARY

Major problems are faced in geriatric psychiatry, and this article reviews the latest clinical advances that hold promise for assisting the prevention and treatment of depression, cognitive decline, and dementia. Several major factors coalesce to drive the need for innovation in geriatric psychiatry. First, the global population is aging. Second, age-related cognitive decline, dementia, and depression have a large burden. Third, the current treatment options for these conditions are modest. Finally, there is a relatively poor lack of access in low- and middle-income environments. Promising advances in geriatric psychiatry include preventive resilience-building interventions, complementary, alternative, and integrative therapies, and brain-stimulation techniques. Platforms such as telepsychiatry and Internet-based interventions are also promising mechanisms to enhance access to therapies.

REFERENCES

1. UN. World Population Ageing 2013. 2013. Available at: http://www.un.org/en/development/desa/population/publications/pdf/ageing/WorldPopulationAgeing2013.pdf. Accessed November 11, 2014.
2. Alzheimer's Disease International. World Alzheimer Report: journal of caring: an analysis of long-term care for dementia. London: Alzheimer's Disease International; 2013.
3. Ferrari AJ, Charlson FJ, Norman RE, et al. Burden of depressive disorders by country, sex, age, and year: findings from the global burden of disease study 2010. PLoS Med 2013;10(11):e1001547.
4. Selkoe DJ. Preventing Alzheimer's disease. Science 2012;337(6101):1488–92.
5. Kok RM, Nolen WA, Heeren TJ. Efficacy of treatment in older depressed patients: a systematic review and meta-analysis of double-blind randomized controlled trials with antidepressants. J Affect Disord 2012;141(2–3):103–15.
6. Institute of Medicine Committee on Prevention of Mental Disorders, Division of Biobehavioural Sciences and Mental Disorders. Reducing risks for mental disorders: frontiers for preventive intervention research. Washington, DC: National Academies Press; 1994. Available at: http://www.nap.edu/catalog/2139/reducing-risks-for-mental-disorders-frontiers-for-preventive-intervention-research.   Accessed November 11, 2014.

7. Beaglehole R, Bonita R, Kjellstrom T, et al. Basic epidemiology. Geneva: World Health Organization; 1993. Available at: http://apps.who.int/iris/handle/10665/36838. Accessed November 11, 2014.
8. Beekman AT, Cuijers P, Smit F. Prevention of depression in later life. In: Lavretsky H, Sajatovic M, Reynolds CF 3rd, editors. Late-life mood disorders. OUP; 2012.
9. Cuijpers P. Examining the effects of prevention programs on the incidence of new cases of mental disorders: the lack of statistical power. Am J Psychiatry 2003; 160(8):1385–91.
10. Lavretsky H. Complementary and alternative medicine use for treatment and prevention of late-life mood and cognitive disorders. Aging health 2009;5(1):61–78.
11. Beekman AT, Geerlings SW, Deeg DJ, et al. The natural history of late-life depression: a 6-year prospective study in the community. Arch Gen Psychiatry 2002; 59(7):605–11.
12. van't Veer-Tazelaar PJ, van Marwijk HW, van Oppen P, et al. Stepped-care prevention of anxiety and depression in late life: a randomized controlled trial. Arch Gen Psychiatry 2009;66(3):297–304.
13. Vaillant GE. Resilience and post-traumatic growth. In: Jeste DV, Palmer BW, editors. Positive psychiatry: a clinical handbook. Arlington (VA): American Psychiatric Press, Inc; 2015.
14. Lamond AJ, Depp CA, Allison M, et al. Measurement and predictors of resilience among community-dwelling older women. J Psychiatr Res 2008;43(2):148–54.
15. Montross LP, Depp C, Daly J, et al. Correlates of self-rated successful aging among community-dwelling older adults. Am J Geriatr Psychiatry 2006;14(1):43–51.
16. Moore RC, Martin AS, Kaup AR, et al. From suffering to caring: a model of differences among older adults in levels of compassion. Int J Geriatr Psychiatry 2015; 30(2):185–91.
17. Jeste DV, Palmer BW. Introduction. What is positive psychiatry?. In: Jeste DV, Palmer BW, editors. Positive psychiatry: a clinical handbook. Arlington (VA): American Psychiatric Press, Inc; 2015.
18. Jeste DV, Savla GN, Thompson WK, et al. Association between older age and more successful aging: critical role of resilience and depression. Am J Psychiatry 2013;170(2):188–96.
19. Hildon Z, Montgomery SM, Blane D, et al. Examining resilience of quality of life in the face of health-related and psychosocial adversity at older ages: what is "right" about the way we age? Gerontologist 2010;50(1):36–47.
20. Lavretsky H. Resilience and aging: research and practice. Baltimore (MD): Johns Hopkins University Press; 2014.
21. Padesky CA, Mooney KA. Strengths-based cognitive-behavioural therapy: a four-step model to build resilience. Clin Psychol Psychother 2012;19(4):283–90.
22. Manning LK, Carr DC, Kail BL. Do higher levels of resilience buffer the deleterious impact of chronic illness on disability in later life? Gerontologist 2014. [Epub ahead of print].
23. Zeng Y, Shen K. Resilience significantly contributes to exceptional longevity. Curr Gerontol Geriatr Res 2010;2010:525693.
24. Loprinzi CE, Prasad K, Schroeder DR, et al. Stress Management and Resilience Training (SMART) program to decrease stress and enhance resilience among breast cancer survivors: a pilot randomized clinical trial. Clin Breast Cancer 2011;11(6):364–8.
25. NCCAM. National Center for Complementary and Alternative Medicine. 2014. Available at: http://nccam.nih.gov/. Accessed October 28, 2014.

26. Ho TF, Rowland-Seymour A, Frankel ES, et al. Generational differences in complementary and alternative medicine (CAM) use in the context of chronic diseases and pain: baby boomers versus the silent generation. J Am Board Fam Med 2014;27(4):465–73.
27. Blumenthal JA, Babyak MA, Moore KA, et al. Effects of exercise training on older patients with major depression. Arch Intern Med 1999;159(19):2349–56.
28. Mather AS, Rodriguez C, Guthrie MF, et al. Effects of exercise on depressive symptoms in older adults with poorly responsive depressive disorder: randomised controlled trial. Br J Psychiatry 2002;180:411–5.
29. Blake H, Mo P, Malik S, et al. How effective are physical activity interventions for alleviating depressive symptoms in older people? A systematic review. Clin Rehabil 2009;23(10):873–87.
30. Spana TM, Rodrigues RC, Lourenco LB, et al. Integrative review: behavioral interventions for physical activity practice. Rev Lat Am Enfermagem 2009;17(6):1057–64.
31. American College of Sports Medicine, Chodzko-Zajko WJ, Proctor DN, et al. American College of Sports Medicine position stand. Exercise and physical activity for older adults. Med Sci Sports Exerc 2009;41(7):1510–30.
32. Tsang HW, Fung KM, Chan AS, et al. Effect of a qigong exercise programme on elderly with depression. Int J Geriatr Psychiatry 2006;21(9):890–7.
33. Pilkington K, Kirkwood G, Rampes H, et al. Yoga for depression: the research evidence. J Affect Disord 2005;89(1–3):13–24.
34. Janakiramaiah N, Gangadhar BN, Naga Venkatesha Murthy PJ, et al. Antidepressant efficacy of Sudarshan Kriya Yoga (SKY) in melancholia: a randomized comparison with electroconvulsive therapy (ECT) and imipramine. J Affect Disord 2000;57(1–3):255–9.
35. Krishnamurthy MN, Telles S. Assessing depression following two ancient Indian interventions: effects of yoga and ayurveda on older adults in a residential home. J Gerontol Nurs 2007;33(2):17–23.
36. Shahidi M, Mojtahed A, Modabbernia A, et al. Laughter yoga versus group exercise program in elderly depressed women: a randomized controlled trial. Int J Geriatr Psychiatry 2011;26(3):322–7.
37. Abbott R, Lavretsky H. Tai Chi and Qigong for the treatment and prevention of mental disorders. Psychiatr Clin North Am 2013;36(1):109–19.
38. Payne ME, Steck SE, George RR, et al. Fruit, vegetable, and antioxidant intakes are lower in older adults with depression. J Acad Nutr Diet 2012;112(12):2022–7.
39. Lai JS, Hiles S, Bisquera A, et al. A systematic review and meta-analysis of dietary patterns and depression in community-dwelling adults. Am J Clin Nutr 2014;99(1):181–97.
40. O'Neil A, Berk M, Itsiopoulos C, et al. A randomised, controlled trial of a dietary intervention for adults with major depression (the "SMILES" trial): study protocol. BMC Psychiatry 2013;13:114.
41. Reynolds CF 3rd, Thomas SB, Morse JQ, et al. Early intervention to preempt major depression among older black and white adults. Psychiatr Serv 2014;65(6):765–73.
42. Stahl ST, Albert SM, Dew MA, et al. Coaching in healthy dietary practices in at-risk older adults: a case of indicated depression prevention. Am J Psychiatry 2014;171(5):499–505.
43. Whiteford HA, Degenhardt L, Rehm J, et al. Global burden of disease attributable to mental and substance use disorders: findings from the Global Burden of Disease Study 2010. Lancet 2013;382(9904):1575–86.

44. Barnes DE, Yaffe K. The projected effect of risk factor reduction on Alzheimer's disease prevalence. Lancet Neurol 2011;10(9):819–28.
45. Eyre HA, Baune BT. Assessing for unique immunomodulatory and neuroplastic profiles of physical activity subtypes: a focus on psychiatric disorders. Brain Behav Immun 2014;39:42–55.
46. Varteresian T, Lavretsky H. Natural products and supplements for geriatric depression and cognitive disorders: an evaluation of the research. Curr Psychiatry Rep 2014;16(8):456.
47. Wells RE, Kerr CE, Wolkin J, et al. Meditation for adults with mild cognitive impairment: a pilot randomized trial. J Am Geriatr Soc 2013;61(4):642–5.
48. Coogan AN, Schutova B, Husung S, et al. The circadian system in Alzheimer's disease: disturbances, mechanisms, and opportunities. Biol Psychiatry 2013; 74(5):333–9.
49. Di Marco LY, Marzo A, Munoz-Ruiz M, et al. Modifiable lifestyle factors in dementia: a systematic review of longitudinal observational cohort studies. J Alzheimer's Dis 2014;42(1):119–35.
50. Nagamatsu LS, Handy TC, Hsu CL, et al. Resistance training promotes cognitive and functional brain plasticity in seniors with probable mild cognitive impairment. Arch Intern Med 2012;172(8):666–8.
51. Gates N, Fiatarone Singh MA, Sachdev PS, et al. The effect of exercise training on cognitive function in older adults with mild cognitive impairment: a meta-analysis of randomized controlled trials. Am J Geriatr Psychiatry 2013;21(11):1086–97.
52. Norton S, Matthews FE, Barnes DE, et al. Potential for primary prevention of Alzheimer's disease: an analysis of population-based data. Lancet Neurol 2014; 13(8):788–94.
53. de Rezende LF, Rey-Lopez JP, Matsudo VK, et al. Sedentary behavior and health outcomes among older adults: a systematic review. BMC Public Health 2014;14:333.
54. Wayne PM, Walsh JN, Taylor-Piliae RE, et al. Effect of tai chi on cognitive performance in older adults: systematic review and meta-analysis. J Am Geriatr Soc 2014;62(1):25–39.
55. Oken BS, Zajdel D, Kishiyama S, et al. Randomized, controlled, six-month trial of yoga in healthy seniors: effects on cognition and quality of life. Altern Ther Health Med 2006;12(1):40–7.
56. Sarris J, Moylan S, Camfield DA, et al. Complementary medicine, exercise, meditation, diet, and lifestyle modification for anxiety disorders: a review of current evidence. Evid Based Complement Altern Med 2012;2012:809653.
57. Panza F, Solfrizzi V, Tortelli R, et al. Prevention of late-life cognitive disorders: diet-related factors, dietary patterns, and frailty models. Curr Nutr Rep 2014;3(2): 119–29.
58. Martinez-Lapiscina EH, Clavero P, Toledo E, et al. Mediterranean diet improves cognition: the PREDIMED-NAVARRA randomised trial. J Neurol Neurosurg Psychiatry 2013;84(12):1318–25.
59. Barnes PM, Bloom B, Nahin RL. Complementary and alternative medicine use among adults and children: United States, 2007. Natl Health Stat Rep 2008;12: 1–23.
60. Sydenham E, Dangour AD, Lim WS. Omega 3 fatty acid for the prevention of cognitive decline and dementia. Cochrane Database Syst Rev 2012;(6):CD005379.
61. Canter PH, Ernst E. Herbal supplement use by persons aged over 50 years in Britain: frequently used herbs, concomitant use of herbs, nutritional supplements and prescription drugs, rate of informing doctors and potential for negative interactions. Drugs Aging 2004;21(9):597–605.

62. Cuijpers P, Riper H, Beelman AT. Novel platforms for care delivery: internet-based interventions and telepsychiatry. In: Lavretsky H, Sajatovic M, Reynolds C III, editors. Late-life mood disorders. New York: Oxford University Press; 2012.
63. Leach LS, Christensen H. A systematic review of telephone-based interventions for mental disorders. J Telemed Telecare 2006;12(3):122–9.
64. Andrews G, Cuijpers P, Craske MG, et al. Computer therapy for the anxiety and depressive disorders is effective, acceptable and practical health care: a meta-analysis. PloS One 2010;5(10):e13196.
65. Andersson G, Cuijpers P, Carlbring P, et al. Guided Internet-based vs. face-to-face cognitive behavior therapy for psychiatric and somatic disorders: a systematic review and meta-analysis. World Psychiatry 2014;13(3):288–95.
66. Cuijpers P, Schuurmans J. Self-help interventions for anxiety disorders: an overview. Curr Psychiatry Rep 2007;9(4):284–90.
67. Marrs RW. A meta-analysis of bibliotherapy studies. Am J Community Psychol 1995;23(6):843–70.
68. Burch JB, Augustine AD, Frieden LA, et al. Advances in geroscience: impact on healthspan and chronic disease. J Gerontol A, Biol Sci Med Sci 2014;69(Suppl 1):S1–3.
69. Lopez-Otin C, Blasco MA, Partridge L, et al. The hallmarks of aging. Cell 2013; 153(6):1194–217.
70. Erickson KI, Creswell JD, Verstynen TD, et al. Health neuroscience: defining a new field. Curr Dir Psychol Sci 2014;23(6):446–53.
71. NRC. Convergence: facilitating transdisciplinary integration of life sciences, physical sciences, engineering, and beyond. 2014. Available at: http://www.nap.edu/catalog/18722/convergence-facilitating-transdisciplinary-integration-of-life-sciences-physical-sciences-engineering. Accessed November 11, 2014.
72. Dobson KS, Dozois DJA. Risk factors in depression. New York: Academic Press; 2008.
73. Berk M, Jacka F. Preventive strategies in depression: gathering evidence for risk factors and potential interventions. Br J Psychiatry 2012;201(5):339–41.
74. Miller AH, Haroon E, Raison CL, et al. Cytokine targets in the brain: impact on neurotransmitters and neurocircuits. Depress Anxiety 2013;30(4):297–306.
75. CDCP. How much physical activity do older adults need? 2014. Available at: http://www.cdc.gov/physicalactivity/everyone/guidelines/olderadults.html. Accessed October 28, 2014.
76. Kongkeaw C, Dilokthornsakul P, Thanarangsarit P, et al. Meta-analysis of randomized controlled trials on cognitive effects of *Bacopa monnieri* extract. J Ethnopharmacol 2014;151(1):528–35.
77. Cox KH, Pipingas A, Scholey AB. Investigation of the effects of solid lipid curcumin on cognition and mood in a healthy older population. J Psychopharmacol 2014;29(5):642–51.
78. Naqvi R, Liberman D, Rosenberg J, et al. Preventing cognitive decline in healthy older adults. CMAJ 2013;185(10):881–5.
79. Olin J, Schneider L, Novit A, et al. Hydergine for dementia. Cochrane Database Syst Rev 2000;(2):CD000359.
80. Higgins JP, Flicker L. Lecithin for dementia and cognitive impairment. Cochrane Database Syst Rev 2003;(3):CD001015.
81. Kennedy DO, Wightman EL, Reay JL, et al. Effects of resveratrol on cerebral blood flow variables and cognitive performance in humans: a double-blind, placebo-controlled, crossover investigation. Am J Clin Nutr 2010;91(6):1590–7.
82. Farina N, Isaac MG, Clark AR, et al. Vitamin E for Alzheimer's dementia and mild cognitive impairment. Cochrane Database Syst Rev 2012;(11):CD002854.

Complex Trauma in Adolescents and Adults

Effects and Treatment

John Briere, PhD*, Catherine Scott, MD

KEYWORDS

- Complex trauma • Trauma • PTSD • Complex PTSD • Treatment of complex trauma

KEY POINTS

- Exposure to multiple interpersonal traumas over the life span can have significant later psychological effects, both on the likelihood of posttraumatic stress disorder (PTSD) in response to a given stressor and in terms of a wide range of other symptoms and problems.
- Complex trauma can sometimes result in what has been referred to as complex PTSD, developmental trauma disorder, or enduring personality change after catastrophic events, often involving some combination of relational dysfunction, affect dysregulation, identity disturbance, and dysfunctional behavior.
- There are several empirically validated psychological and pharmacologic treatments relevant to complex trauma, most of which target individual symptom clusters.
- Psychological treatments for complex trauma effects tend to focus on processing trauma memories and cognitions and developing affect regulation skills and coping responses.
- Although selective serotonin reuptake inhibitors and related drugs can be helpful for the posttraumatic stress that sometimes follows complex trauma exposure, there are less data to suggest that the other, more personality-level difficulties associated with complex trauma respond well to pharmacologic interventions.

Recent research indicates that the number and variety of interpersonal traumas an individual has experienced over his or her lifespan significantly predicts the extent and composition of his or her subsequent psychological symptoms and disorders. At high levels, this phenomenon is referred to as *complex trauma*, defined as exposure to

Neither Dr J. Briere nor Dr C. Scott has commercial or financial conflicts of interest to declare. Preparation of this review was supported by grant No. 1U79SM061262-01 from the Substance Abuse and Mental Health Administration, U.S. Department of Health and Human Services.
Department of Psychiatry and Behavioral Sciences, Keck School of Medicine, University of Southern California, Los Angeles, CA 90089, USA
* Corresponding author. USC Psychiatry, Clinical Sciences Center, 2250 Alcazar Street, Suite 2200, Los Angeles, CA 90089.
E-mail address: jbriere@usc.edu

Psychiatr Clin N Am 38 (2015) 515–527
http://dx.doi.org/10.1016/j.psc.2015.05.004
0193-953X/15/$ – see front matter
psych.theclinics.com

multiple, often prolonged or extended traumas over time, potentially including events such as rape, physical assault, sex trafficking, torture, and combat and frequently in the context of previous childhood abuse and/or neglect.[1,2] As described in this article, complex trauma exposure not only increases the likelihood of posttraumatic stress in response to a given event but it also can result in several simultaneously presenting but phenomenologically discrete psychological difficulties, described in the empirical literature as *symptom complexity*.[3–5]

Research on the effects of complex trauma has had significant impacts on empirical and clinical models of posttraumatic distress and disorder. Most importantly, it reinforces the notion of multidimensional symptoms arising from multiple traumatic events and challenges traditional assumptions regarding the single-event cause of posttraumatic stress disorder (PTSD).

RISK OF POSTTRAUMATIC STRESS DISORDER

PTSD, as defined by the *Diagnostic and Statistical Manual of Mental Disorders* (Fifth Edition) (*DSM-5*), consists of 4 clusters or symptom dimensions: re-experiencing of the traumatic event; avoidance of trauma-relevant stimuli; numbing, negative cognitions, and mood; and hyperarousal and hyperreactivity.[6] Historically, *DSM-III* through *DSM-IV* linked all the symptoms of PTSD to a single traumatic event, such as an instance of sexual or physical assault or a natural disaster. As a result, by definition, PTSD could not be diagnosed if some of its symptoms, for example, flashbacks or numbing, arose from one trauma and others, for example, hyperarousal or effortful avoidance, were related to one or more other traumatic events.

Despite this narrow trauma requirement, a study of more than 2000 nonclinical individuals indicated that previous exposure to multiple traumatic events was associated with a greater risk of PTSD in response to a current (index) trauma and that multiple previous traumas had a stronger effect than did a single event.[7] Similarly, data from the World Health Organization's World Mental Health Survey Initiative (combined $N = 51,295$) found that approximately 20% of people with PTSD, if asked, attributed their disorder to the effects more than a single traumatic event. This study also indicated a risk threshold of 4 traumatic events, at or greater than which PTSD tended to involve greater functional impairment, more chronic symptoms, earlier onset, greater hyperarousal, and higher comorbidity with mood and anxiety disorders.[8] Other studies also have found that previous traumas increase the likelihood of PTSD in response to a later trauma as well as indicate that multiple trauma exposures are the norm in the general population rather than the exception.[9,10]

These findings suggest that although an index traumatic event may be immediately associated with the development of PTSD, this trauma may best be understood in some cases as the tipping point for the cumulative impacts of prior, more complex traumas. Apropos of this, *DSM-5* criterion A for PTSD specifies traumatic "*event(s)*",[6(pp271, 272)] in contrast to previous *DSM's* requirement of a single traumatic event. This *DSM* transition from a single-trauma to a potentially multi-trauma criterion highlights the notion that PTSD can arise from complex trauma, perhaps especially when it is accompanied by other symptoms and difficulties.[9]

RISK OF COMPLEX OUTCOMES

Because complex trauma typically involves exposure to multiple types of events, it is logical to assume that their combined effects might also be complex. For example, sexual assaults are often associated with different outcomes than physical assaults; the effects of disaster can differ from those of interpersonal trauma; and childhood maltreatment often has different impacts than adolescent or adult victimization,[11] such that an accumulation of different traumas generally leads to a wider range of symptom types. Further, trauma is, itself, a risk factor for revictimization at later points in time[12] and, thus, even more complex outcomes.

Other variables further complicate this clinical picture. Multiple trauma exposures are frequently associated with reduced affect regulation capacity,[13] premorbid or comorbid anxiety, depressive or personality-level disorders,[8,14] impulsivity,[15] dissociation,[16] drugs or alcohol abuse,[17] and a history of insecure parent-child attachment.[2] These phenomena not only represent complex posttraumatic outcomes, they can intensify or mediate the effects of trauma exposure.[7,16] Finally, posttraumatic symptoms may motivate subsequent maladaptive coping responses, such as suicidality related to sustained posttraumatic stress[18] and avoidance activities, such as dissociation and substance abuse in response to trauma-related dysphoria.[17,19]

Given these findings, it is not surprising that a history of complex trauma exposures is associated with multiple symptoms or symptom clusters experienced simultaneously by the same individual. Although the literature describes an extensive list of these outcomes,[1–3,20–23] clinical researchers have repeatedly identified a more specific group of psychological symptoms and problems, generally involving self-related difficulties,[1] such as affect dysregulation, relational disturbance (including abandonment concerns and interpersonal sensitivity), identity problems, cognitive distortions, somatization, and avoidance responses such as dissociation, substance abuse, and self-injurious behavior.[1,20,22,23] Despite the overlap of many of these symptoms and problems with diagnostic features of borderline personality disorder,[24] their relationship to multiple childhood and adult traumas, and the frequent copresence of posttraumatic stress symptoms, have led them to be characterized as *complex PTSD*,[22] *disorders of extreme stress not otherwise specified*,[23] *developmental trauma disorder*,[25] *self-capacity disturbance*,[11] and *enduring personality change after catastrophic events* (EPCACE).[26] Most recently, the proposed *International Classification of Diseases, 11th Revision*, is slated to replace EPCACE with a diagnosis of *complex PTSD*. There is controversy, however, regarding whether such disturbance reflects a specific syndrome, as opposed to dimensions of symptoms that vary according to characteristics and developmental timing of the traumas involved.[1,23]

TREATMENT OF COMPLEX TRAUMA-RELATED DISTURBANCE

Because complex posttraumatic outcomes are, by definition, wide ranging, there are several psychological and psychopharmacological interventions relevant to their treatment. In both psychological and biological domains, these can be divided into single- and multi-target treatments. Most single-target interventions address one aspect of complex trauma outcomes, although they may have additional effects. For example, exposure therapy is targeted at symptoms of PTSD but also impacts trauma-related cognitive distortions[27]; the selective serotonin reuptake inhibitors (SSRIs) have effects not only on PTSD but also on depression and anxiety.[28] Multi-target interventions, on the other hand, often consist of several different components and have been developed explicitly to address a wider range of trauma symptoms.

Psychological Interventions

Treatments for complex posttraumatic outcomes generally consist of (1) cognitive-behavioral therapy (CBT), (2) affect regulation and coping skills training, (3) relational/psychodynamic approaches, and (4) multi-target intervention models. These methodologies are briefly presented later, primarily for clinically referred older adolescents and adults.

Cognitive-behavioral

CBT is described in the trauma literature as the most commonly applied empirically based treatment of PTSD and, to a lesser extent, acute stress disorder (ASD).[29,30] The most efficacious aspects of CBT for trauma symptoms seem to be *therapeutic exposure*, involving the activation and habituation and/or extinction of trauma-related memories within the context of a safe therapeutic environment,[27] and *cognitive processing*, during which negative thoughts and schemas, such as self-blame, helplessness, and overgeneralized danger appraisals, are explored, challenged, and ideally replaced with more accurate information.[31] Also potentially included in this domain is *eye movement desensitization and reprocessing*,[32] during which the client recalls a traumatic event, focuses on his or her internal responses, and then, typically, tracks the therapist's finger as it moves across his or her visual field. Each of these methodologies has been shown in outcome studies to reduce symptoms associated with PTSD.[29]

Affect regulation training

A second form of psychological treatment attends less to the direct processing of traumatic memories and cognitions and more to the development of affect tolerance and regulation as well as emotional coping skills. This distinction is often important in the treatment of complex trauma effects because affect dysregulation is associated with affective instability, difficulties in tolerating and processing potentially overwhelming traumatic memories, and the use of maladaptive coping strategies, such as substance abuse, excessive dissociation, self-injury, dysfunctional sexual behavior, and binge-purge eating.[33] Empirically based interventions in this area teach several skills, including emotion identification, increased self-awareness, relaxation, mindfulness, de-escalation of catastrophic cognitions, and the development of coping strategies to deal with triggered trauma-related thoughts and feelings.[34–39]

Psychodynamic

A third class of interventions in complex trauma effects includes those calling on psychodynamic and relational principles and therapies. Although less studied in the empirical literature, a limited number of studies suggest that relational/dynamic treatments can be helpful in the treatment of the self-related aspects of complex trauma, including interpersonal dysfunction, attachment-related problems, and identity disturbance.[30,40] It is likely that, among other components, these treatments call on the most powerful common factors identified in psychotherapy outcome research: a positive therapeutic relationship, empathy, warmth, attunement, and positive regard.[41]

Multi-target therapies

Although the 3 approaches described here have demonstrated efficacy for trauma-related symptoms and problems, the breadth and range of complex posttraumatic symptoms often require more than one interventional modality. For example, although CBT might be helpful resolving a client's trauma-related flashbacks and hyperarousal, he or she might additionally require affect regulation interventions to address his or her impulsive or self-injurious behavior, both of which might be most helpful in the context of a caring and attuned therapeutic relationship.

For this reason, there are currently several empirically based, multi-target interventions available for the treatment of complex trauma effects. Among these are dialectical behavior therapy (DBT)[38] and skill training in affect regulation (STAIR),[36] along with several programs developed specifically for adolescents, including Attachment, Self-Regulation, and Competency[37]; Integrative Treatment of Complex Trauma for Adolescents[35]; and Structured Psychotherapy for Adolescents Responding to Chronic Stress.[42] Two of the best known of these approaches for adults, DBT and STAIR, have especially encouraging treatment outcome data for the treatment of complex trauma symptoms,[38,43] although DBT originally identified borderline personality disorder (BPD) as its focus. Almost all these hybrid interventions stress some combination of the following:

- A positive therapeutic relationship, characterized by caring, attunement, compassion, and boundary awareness
- When appropriate, affect regulation training before major emotional processing of trauma is initiated
- Titrated therapeutic exposure, in which the client is only asked to recall and process traumatic memories that do not exceed his or her affect regulation capacity and, thus, do not overwhelm or retraumatize
- Cognitive and relational processing of negative attachment and relational schema
- Strategies for the management of posttraumatic triggers and activated emotional states

Pharmacotherapeutic Interventions

There is a dearth of literature on the pharmacotherapy of complex posttraumatic stress. The multidimensional nature of complex trauma presentations makes outcome research into this area particularly challenging: comorbidities, such as medical problems, ongoing domestic violence and other maltreatment, substance use, suicidal ideation, and dissociation, are typically excluded from treatment outcome studies.[44] MEDLINE searches for pharmacotherapy of *complex trauma*, *disorders of extreme stress not otherwise specified*, *self-capacities disturbance*, and *affect regulation/affect tolerance* yield virtually no results. Thus, treatment of complex trauma presentations must be adapted from the literature on PTSD, borderline personality disorder, and dissociation and most often involves targeting the various symptom clusters rather than specific diagnostic categories.[33]

Pharmacotherapy of Posttraumatic Stress Disorder

It must be noted that pharmacotherapy for PTSD is typically not curative and that generally the amount of symptom reduction obtained with psychotherapy is larger than that associated with pharmacology.[45,46] On the other hand, several medications have been found to be useful in the treatment of PTSD and other potential complex trauma effects.[33] Because there is less research available on the biological treatment of trauma symptoms in adolescents, this review is limited to pharmacotherapy with adults.

Antidepressants

The SSRIs are generally considered first-line pharmacotherapy for PTSD.[28] At this time, the only medications approved by the Food and Drug Administration for the treatment of PTSD are SSRIs: sertraline and paroxetine. Randomized placebo-controlled trials (RCTs) of SSRIs including sertraline, paroxetine, and fluoxetine[47–49] have demonstrated efficacy across all 3 *DSM-IV* PTSD symptom clusters (re-experiencing, hyperarousal, and avoidance) and are now widely prescribed for posttraumatic stress. As SSRIs are also the first-line treatment of other anxiety and depressive disorders, SSRIs may be used to address this broader spectrum of comorbidity in complex trauma.

Other antidepressants also have been investigated, with mixed results. Venlafaxine[50] and mirtazapine[51] seem promising, whereas bupropion shows less potential efficacy.[52] Monoamine oxidase inhibitors and tricyclic antidepressants seem to be similarly equivocal[53,54]; given their high number of side effects, as well as lethality in overdose, these medications are not currently recommended for PTSD.

Benzodiazepines

Benzodiazepines are generally contraindicated for traumatized individuals, except when they are necessary for downregulation of severe acute anxiety or panic.[55] Research with benzodiazepines has overwhelmingly indicated that they are specifically unhelpful in ameliorating the symptoms of PTSD[56] and may in fact increase the risk for later PTSD.[57,58] In complex trauma presentations, particular caution is warranted when prescribing benzodiazepines, given their tolerance effects and addictive potential.[33]

Mood stabilizers

Data on mood stabilizers in PTSD are sparse; most studies involve small sample sizes, are not randomized, and results are equivocal. Researchers have investigated lamotrigine,[59] divalproex sodium,[60] carbamazepine,[61] and tiagabine.[62] Mood stabilizers are not considered a primary treatment of PTSD.

Adrenergic agents

Both alpha- and beta-adrenergic blocking agents have been investigated in the treatment of PTSD. Although some open trials indicate promise,[63,64] data from larger studies suggest that beta-blockers are not effective in either preventing PTSD or ameliorating symptoms.[65,66] However, several open trials of clonidine[67,68] and RCTs of prazosin[69,70] indicate that alpha-blockade is useful for improving sleep and reducing nightmares and trauma-related dream content in PTSD.

Antipsychotics

There has been much interest in antipsychotics for PTSD; despite the limited evidence of effectiveness, they are used with some frequency in clinical practice. Of the second-generation antipsychotics, risperidone and olanzapine have been evaluated in RCTs. Initial studies of risperidone were promising[71,72]; however, in a recent 6-month multicenter RCT with more than 300 subjects, risperidone was not associated with a reduction in symptoms of anxiety, depression, or PTSD.[73] Similarly, although an initial RCT of olanzapine as an adjunctive treatment indicated moderate response in symptoms,[74] a second found no benefit over placebo.[75] The single RCT of olanzapine monotherapy[76] did show a robust response in 70% of the treated individuals but has not been replicated.

The aforementioned results are interpreted variously, with some reviewers suggesting that antipsychotics show promise for the treatment of PTSD,[77] whereas others conclude that there is not a role for antipsychotics as a first-line treatment.[28] According to the American Psychiatric Association's (APA) guidelines,[55] antipsychotics should be reserved for individuals with comorbid psychosis or overwhelming agitation and aggression.

Pharmacotherapy of Dissociation

The literature on pharmacotherapy of dissociative symptoms is extremely sparse. Symptoms such as derealization, depersonalization, and time loss are generally considered to be nonresponsive to medications. Although this is largely correct, there are some limited data on pharmacotherapy for dissociative symptoms. Several open trials[78] and one RCT[79] have suggested that naltrexone may help to reduce dissociative symptoms and posttraumatic flashbacks in borderline patients. Others have described its effectiveness in reducing self-injurious behavior in dissociative identity disorder.[80]

Initial open trials suggested that SSRIs might be effective for treating dissociation[81]: however, an RCT of fluoxetine did not support this practice.[82] Similarly, although open trials suggested the antiepileptic lamotrigine might be helpful for dissociative symptoms,[83] an RCT[84] did not indicate efficacy. In the lone study of an antipsychotic in dissociation, aripiprazole was found to be helpful in 3 cases of depersonalization disorder.[85]

Pharmacotherapy for Self-capacity Disturbance

There is virtually no literature on pharmacologic treatment of those complex posttraumatic outcomes characterized earlier as self-capacity disturbance. The only data available in the larger literature involves the pharmacotherapy of BPD, which also involves altered self-capacities. BPD is one of the most difficult psychiatric conditions to treat, and almost every medication in the psychopharmacotherapy armamentarium has been investigated.

Guidelines for the treatment of BPD vary: the APA recommends mood stabilizers and antipsychotics to treat aggression and transient paranoid ideation,[86] whereas the National Institute for Clinical Excellence recommends that pharmacotherapy of specific borderline symptoms, in the absence of comorbidities, be avoided.[87] Two extensive reviews of pharmacotherapy for BPD indicate, respectively, the following: "Notably, no evidence was found for several borderline personality disorder symptoms – avoidance of abandonment, chronic feelings of emptiness, identity disturbance and dissociation"[88] and "In particular, no drugs were found efficacious to treat core domains of BPD."[89]

Despite the aforementioned information, there are a handful of RCTs indicating that there might be a role for medications in the treatment of 2 domains relevant to complex trauma: rejection sensitivity and interpersonal relatedness. The mood stabilizer divalproex sodium was found in 2 studies to be helpful for social functioning in BPD[90] and for interpersonal sensitivity,[91] respectively. Similarly, the antiepileptic topiramate decreased levels of both somatization and interpersonal sensitivity[92] and the antipsychotic olanzapine was superior to placebo in improving measures of interpersonal sensitivity.[93]

SUMMARY

Exposure to complex trauma is both relatively common and potentially associated with a range of psychological outcomes, including a decreased threshold for PTSD and a cluster of symptoms especially characterized by identity disturbance, affect dysregulation, relational difficulties, and dysfunctional behaviors. Empirical studies indicate that both psychological and pharmacologic interventions can be helpful, although psychotherapy seems to be markedly more effective for self-related symptoms.

CLINICAL VIGNETTE: YOUNG WOMAN WITH COMPLEX POSTTRAUMATIC SYMPTOMS

M.K. is a 24-year-old single Caucasian woman brought to a university-based emergency department (ED) by police following an overdose with twenty 0.5-mg tablets of lorazepam (Ativan). ED records indicate 4 previous ED admissions for suicidal behavior, generally precipitated by relational strife with romantic partners. She was hospitalized following 2 of these incidents and in both cases was discharged after 72 hours. Discharge diagnoses were, variously, borderline personality disorder, posttraumatic stress disorder, mood disorder not otherwise specified, and substance use disorder. On interview, M.K. reports a childhood history of sexual abuse by her stepfather and oldest stepbrother, from 7 to 16 years of age, and psychological neglect combined with an episode of physical abuse by her mother. She describes herself as always in trouble from her early teens until the present, reporting chronic methamphetamine abuse, truancy, running away from home, physical fights with other girls, and relatively indiscriminant sexual behavior since 16 years of age, soon after being gang-raped by her ex-boyfriend and 2 of his friends. Her last methamphetamine use was reportedly 1 week before her ED admission. On mental status examination, she appeared alert and oriented but somewhat dissociated, with depressed mood and constricted/numb affect. She reported a history of chronic self-cutting, bulimia, hypervigilance around men, and flashbacks of the gang rape and an especially violent sexual assault by her stepbrother.

M.K. was referred to a trauma-specialized female psychologist and a psychiatrist who started her on sertraline hydrochloride (Zoloft), with limited supplies of medication because of her recent history of suicide attempts. After a relatively rocky beginning, characterized by rejection sensitivity and distrust of her therapist, she seems to be gaining from the affect regulation training component of therapy, which has reduced her self-injurious and dysfunctional behaviors, and has experienced some lifting of her depression. After 3 months of therapy, however, she is still unable to engage in significant therapeutic exposure or cognitive processing of her trauma history.

REFERENCES

1. Briere J, Spinazzola J. Phenomenology and psychological assessment of complex posttraumatic states. J Trauma Stress 2005;18:401–12.
2. Cook A, Spinazzola J, Ford J, et al. Complex trauma in children and adolescents. Psychiatr Ann 2005;35:390–8.
3. Briere J, Kaltman S, Green BL. Accumulated childhood trauma and symptom complexity. J Trauma Stress 2008;21:223–6.
4. Cloitre M, Stolbach BC, Herman JL, et al. A developmental approach to complex PTSD. Childhood and adult cumulative trauma as predictors of symptom complexity. J Trauma Stress 2009;22:399–408.
5. Hodges M, Godbout N, Briere J, et al. Cumulative trauma and symptom complexity in children: a path analysis. Child Abuse Negl 2013;37:891–8.
6. American Psychiatric Association. Diagnostic and statistical manual of mental disorders. 5th edition. Washington, DC: American Psychiatric Publishing; 2013.
7. Breslau N, Chilcoat HD, Kessler RC, et al. Previous exposure to trauma and PTSD effects of subsequent trauma: results from the Detroit area survey of trauma. Am J Psychiatry 1999;156:902–7.
8. Karam EG, Friedman MJ, Hill ED, et al. Cumulative traumas and risk thresholds: 12-month PTSD in the World Mental Health (WMH) surveys. Depress Anxiety 2014;31:130–42.
9. Kilpatrick DG, Resnick HS, Milanak ME, et al. National estimates of exposure to traumatic events and PTSD prevalence using DSM-IV and DSM-5 criteria. J Trauma Stress 2013;26:537–47.

10. Walsh K, Danielson CK, McCauley JL, et al. National prevalence of posttraumatic stress disorder among sexually revictimized adolescent, college, and adult household-residing women. Arch Gen Psychiatry 2012;69:935–42.

11. Briere J. Psychological assessment of adult posttraumatic states: phenomenology, diagnosis, and measurement. 2nd edition. Washington, DC: American Psychological Association; 2004.

12. Classen CC, Palesh OG, Aggarwal R. Sexual revictimization: a review of the empirical literature. Trauma Violence Abuse 2005;6:103–29.

13. Ford JD. Treatment implications of altered affect regulation and information processing following child maltreatment. Psychiatr Ann 2005;35:410–9.

14. Breslau N, Davis GC, Andreski P, et al. Traumatic events and posttraumatic stress disorder in an urban population of young adults. Arch Gen Psychiatry 1991;48: 216–22.

15. Nickerson A, Aderka IM, Bryant RA, et al. The relationship between childhood exposure to trauma and intermittent explosive disorder. Psychiatry Res 2012; 197:128–34.

16. Briere J, Hodges M, Godbout N. Traumatic stress, affect dysregulation, and dysfunctional avoidance: a structural equation model. J Trauma Stress 2010; 23:767–74.

17. Ouimette P, Brown PJ. Trauma and substance abuse: causes, consequences, and treatment of comorbid disorders. Washington, DC: American Psychological Association; 2003.

18. Briere J, Godbout N, Dias C. Trauma, hyperarousal, and suicidality: a path analysis. J Trauma Dissociation 2015;16(2):153–69.

19. Briere J, Scott C, Weathers FW. Peritraumatic and persistent dissociation in the presumed etiology of PTSD. Am J Psychiatry 2005;162:2295–301.

20. Complex Trauma Taskforce. The ISTSS Expert Consensus treatment guidelines for complex PTSD in adults. 2012. Available at: http://www.istss.org/ISTSS_Main/media/Documents/ISTSS-Expert-Concesnsus-Guidelines-for-Complex-PTSD-Updated-060315.pdf. Accessed June 11, 2015.

21. Follette VM, Polusny MA, Bechtle AE, et al. Cumulative trauma: the impact of child sexual abuse, adult sexual assault, and spouse abuse. J Trauma Stress 1996;9: 25–35.

22. Herman JL. Complex PTSD: a syndrome in survivors of prolonged and repeated trauma. J Trauma Stress 1992;5:377–92.

23. van der Kolk BA, Roth S, Pelcovitz D, et al. Disorders of extreme stress: the empirical foundation of a complex adaptation to trauma. J Trauma Stress 2005;18: 389–99.

24. Gunderson J. Borderline personality disorder. N Engl J Med 2011;364:2037–42.

25. van der Kolk BA. Developmental trauma disorder: towards a rational diagnosis for chronically traumatized children. Psychiatr Ann 2005;35:401–8.

26. World Health Organization. International statistical classification of diseases and related health problems (10th revision). Geneva (Switzerland): World Health Organization; 1992.

27. Foa EB, Hembree EA, Rothbaum BO. Prolonged exposure therapy for PTSD: emotional processing of traumatic experiences: therapist guide. New York: Oxford University Press; 2007.

28. Friedman MJ, Davidson JR, Stein DJ. Psychopharmacotherapy for adults. In: Foa EB, Keane TM, Friedman MJ, et al, editors. Effective treatments for PTSD: practice guidelines from the International Society for Traumatic Stress Studies. New York: Guilford; 2009. p. 245–68.

29. Foa EB, Keane TM, Friedman MJ, et al, editors. Effective treatments for PTSD: practice guidelines from the International Society for Traumatic Stress Studies. 2nd edition. New York: The Guilford Press; 2008.

30. Roberts NP, Kitchiner NJ, Kenardy J, et al. Early psychological interventions to treat acute traumatic stress symptoms. Cochrane Database Syst Rev 2010;(3):CD007944.

31. Resick PA, Schnicke MK. Cognitive processing therapy for rape victims: a treatment manual. Newbury Park (CA): Sage; 1993.

32. Shapiro F. Eye movement desensitization and reprocessing: basic principles, protocols, and procedures. New York: Guilford; 1995.

33. Briere J, Scott C. Principles of trauma therapy: a guide to symptoms, evaluation, and treatment. DSM-5 update. 2nd edition. Thousand Oaks (CA): Sage; 2014.

34. Blaustein ME, Kinniburgh KM. Treating traumatic stress in children and adolescents: how to foster resilience through attachment, self-regulation, and competency. New York: Guilford Publications; 2010.

35. Briere J, Lanktree CB. Treating complex trauma in adolescents and young adults. Thousand Oaks (CA): Sage; 2011.

36. Cloitre M, Stovall-McClough KC, Nooner K, et al. Treatment for PTSD related to childhood abuse: a randomized controlled trial. Am J Psychiatry 2010;167: 915–24.

37. Ford JD, Russo E. A trauma-focused, present-centered, emotion self-regulation approach to integrated treatment for PTSD and addiction. Am J Psychother 2006;60:335–55.

38. Linehan MM. Cognitive-behavioral treatment of borderline personality disorder. New York: Guilford; 1993.

39. Lampe A, Mitmansgruber H, Gast U, et al. [Treatment outcome of psychodynamic trauma therapy in an inpatient setting]. [Therapieevaluation der Psychodynamisch Imaginativen Traumatherapie (PITT) im stationären Setting]. Neuropsychiatr 2008;22:189–97 [in German].

40. Schottenbauer MA, Glass CR, Arnkoff DB, et al. Contributions of psychodynamic approaches to treatment of PTSD and trauma: a review of the empirical treatment and psychopathology literature. Psychiatry 2008;71:13–34.

41. Lambert MJ, Barley DE. Research summary on the therapeutic relationship and psychotherapy outcome. Psychother Theor Res Pract Train 2001;38:357–61.

42. Habib M, Labruna V, Newman J. Complex histories and complex presentations: implementation of a manually-guided group treatment for traumatized adolescents. J Fam Violence 2013;28:717–28.

43. Linehan MM, Comtois KA, Murray AM. Two-year randomized controlled trial and follow-up of dialectical behavior therapy vs therapy by experts for suicidal behaviors and borderline personality disorder. Arch Gen Psychiatry 2006;63: 757–66.

44. Spinazzola J, Blaustein M, van der Kolk BA. Posttraumatic stress disorder treatment outcome research: the study of unrepresentative samples? J Trauma Stress 2005;18(5):425–36.

45. Cahill SP, Rothbaum BO, Resick PA, et al. Cognitive behavioral therapy for adults. In: Foa EB, Keane TM, Friedman MJ, et al, editors. Effective treatments for PTSD: practice guidelines from the International Society for Traumatic Stress Studies. New York: Guilford; 2009. p. 139–222.

46. Cukor J, Difede J. Review: psychotherapy, somatic therapy and pharmacotherapy are all more effective than control for the treatment of PTSD. Evid Based Ment Health 2014;17(1):7. Accessed January 21, 2015.

47. Davidson JRT, Rothbaum BO, van der Kolk BA, et al. Multi-center, double-blind comparison of sertraline and placebo in the treatment of posttraumatic stress disorder. Arch Gen Psychiatry 2001;58:485–92.
48. Stein DJ, Davidson J, Seedat S, et al. Paroxetine in the treatment of posttraumatic stress disorder: pooled analysis of placebo-controlled studies. Expert Opin Pharmacother 2003;4:1829–38.
49. Martenyi F, Soldatenkova V. Fluoxetine in the acute treatment and relapse prevention of combat-related post-traumatic stress disorder: analysis of the veteran group of a placebo-controlled, randomized clinical trial. Eur Neuropsychopharmacol 2006;16:340–9.
50. Pae CU, Lim HK, Ajwani N, et al. Extended-release formulation of venlafaxine in the treatment of post-traumatic stress disorder. Expert Rev Neurother 2007;7(6): 603–15.
51. Davidson JRT, Weisler RH, Butterfield MI, et al. Mirtazapine vs placebo in posttraumatic stress disorder: a pilot trial. Biol Psychiatry 2003;53:188–91.
52. Becker ME, Hertzberg MA, Moore SD, et al. A placebo-controlled trial of bupropion SR in the treatment of chronic posttraumatic stress disorder. J Clin Psychopharmacol 2007;27:193–7.
53. Frank JB, Kosten TR, Giller EL, et al. A randomized clinical trial of phenelzine and imipramine for posttraumatic stress disorder. Am J Psychiatry 1988;145: 1289–2291.
54. Reist C, Kauffmann CD, Haier RJ, et al. A controlled trial of desipramine in 18 men with posttraumatic stress disorder. Am J Psychiatry 1989;146:513–6.
55. American Psychiatric Association (APA). Practice guideline for the treatment of patients with acute stress disorder and posttraumatic stress disorder. Psychiatry Online. 2004. Available at: http://psychiatryonline.org/pb/assets/raw/sitewide/practice_guidelines/guidelines/acutestressdisorderptsd.pdf. Accessed June 11, 2015.
56. Braun P, Greenberg D, Dasberg H, et al. Core symptoms of posttraumatic stress disorder unimproved by alprazolam treatment. J Clin Psychiatry 1990;51:236–8.
57. Gelpin E, Bonne O, Peri T, et al. Treatment of recent trauma survivors with benzodiazepines: a prospective study. J Clin Psychiatry 1996;57:390–4.
58. Girard TD, Shintani AK, Jackson JC, et al. Risk factors for post-traumatic stress disorder symptoms following critical illness requiring mechanical ventilation: a prospective cohort study. Crit Care 2007;11:28.
59. Hertzberg MA, Butterfield MI, Feldman ME, et al. A preliminary study of lamotrigine for the treatment of posttraumatic stress disorder. Biol Psychiatry 1999;45: 1226–9.
60. Hamner MB, Faldowski RA, Robert S, et al. A preliminary controlled trial of divalproex in posttraumatic stress disorder. Ann Clin Psychiatry 2009;21:89–94.
61. Keck P, McElroy S, Friedman L. Valproate and carbamazepine in the treatment of panic and posttraumatic stress disorders, withdrawal states, and behavioral dyscontrol syndromes. J Clin Psychopharmacol 1992;12:368–418.
62. Connor KM, Davidson JR, Weisler RH, et al. Tiagabine for posttraumatic stress disorder: effects of open-label and double-blind discontinuation treatment. Psychopharmacology (Berl) 2006;184:21–5.
63. Jiménez JP, Romero CC, Diéguez NG, et al. Pharmacological treatment of acute stress disorder with propranolol and hypnotics. Actas Esp Psyquiatr 2007;35(6): 351–8.
64. Vaiva G, Ducrocq F, Jezequel K, et al. Immediate treatment with propranolol decreases posttraumatic stress disorder two months after trauma. Biol Psychiatry 2003;52:947–9.

65. Pitman RK, Sanders KM, Zusman RM. Pilot study of secondary prevention of posttraumatic stress disorder with propranolol. Biol Psychiatry 2002;51:189–92.

66. Stein MB, Kerridge C, Dimsdale JE, et al. Pharmacotherapy to prevent PTSD: results from a randomized controlled proof-of-concept trial in physically injured patients. J Trauma Stress 2007;20(6):923–32.

67. Kolb LC, Burris BC, Griffiths S. Propranolol and clonidine in the treatment of the chronic post-traumatic stress disorders of war. In: van der Kolk BA, editor. Posttraumatic stress disorder: psychological and biological sequelae. Washington, DC: American Psychiatric Press; 1984. p. 98–108.

68. Kinzie JD, Leung P. Clonidine in Cambodian patients with posttraumatic stress disorder. J Nerv Ment Dis 1989;177:546–50.

69. Taylor FB, Martin P, Thompson C, et al. Prazosin effects on objective sleep measures and clinical symptoms in civilian trauma posttraumatic stress disorder: a placebo-controlled study. Biol Psychiatry 2008;63:629–32.

70. Raskind MA, Peskind ER, Kanter ED, et al. Reduction of nightmares and other PTSD symptoms in combat veterans by prazosin: a placebo-controlled study. Am J Psychiatry 2003;160:371–3.

71. Monnelly EP, Ciraulo DA. Risperidone effects on irritable aggression in posttraumatic stress disorder. J Clin Psychopharmacol 1999;19:377–8.

72. Rothbaum BO, Killeen TK, Davidson JR, et al. Placebo-controlled trial of risperidone augmentation for selective serotonin reuptake inhibitor-resistant civilian posttraumatic stress disorder. J Clin Psychiatry 2008;69:520–5.

73. Krystal JH, Rosenheck RA, Cramer JA. Adjunctive risperidone treatment for antidepressant-resistant symptoms of chronic military service-related PTSD: a randomized trial. JAMA 2011;306:493–502.

74. Stein MB, Kline NA, Matloff JL. Adjunctive olanzapine for SSRI-resistant combat-related PTSD: a double-blind, placebo-controlled study. Am J Psychiatry 2002; 159:1777–9.

75. Butterfield MI, Becker ME, Connor KM, et al. Olanzapine in the treatment of posttraumatic stress disorder: a pilot study. Int Clin Psychopharmacol 2001;16: 197–203.

76. Carey P, Suliman S, Ganesan K, et al. Olanzapine monotherapy in posttraumatic stress disorder: efficacy in a randomized, double-blind, placebo-controlled study. Hum Psychopharmacol 2012;27(4):386–91.

77. Wang HR, Woo YS, Bahk WM. Atypical antipsychotics in the treatment of posttraumatic stress disorder. Clin Neuropharmacol 2013;36(6):216–22.

78. Bohus MJ, Landwehrmeyer GB, Stiglmayr CE, et al. Naltrexone in the treatment of dissociative symptoms in patients with borderline personality disorder: an open-label trial. J Clin Psychiatry 1999;60:598–603.

79. Schmahl C, Kleindienst N, Limberger M, et al. Evaluation of naltrexone for dissociative symptoms in borderline personality disorder. Int Clin Psychopharmacol 2012;27(1):61–8.

80. Simeon D, Knutelska M. An open trial of naltrexone in the treatment of depersonalization disorder. J Clin Psychopharmacol 2005;25(3):267–70.

81. Preve M, Mula M, Cassano G, et al. Venlafaxine in somatopsychic and autopsychic depersonalization. Prog Neuropsychopharmacol Biol Psychiatry 2011;35(8): 1808–9.

82. Simeon D, Guralnik O, Schmeidler J, et al. Fluoxetine therapy in depersonalisation disorder: randomised controlled trial. Br J Psychiatry 2004;185:31–6.

83. Sierra M, Phillips ML, Lambert MV, et al. Lamotrigine in the treatment of depersonalization disorder. J Clin Psychiatry 2001;62(10):826–7.

84. Sierra M, Phillips ML, Ivin G, et al. A placebo-controlled, cross-over trial of lamotrigine in depersonalization disorder. J Psychopharmacol 2003;17(1):103–5.
85. Uguz F, Sahingoz M. Aripiprazole in depersonalization disorder comorbid with major depression and obsessive-compulsive disorder: 3 cases. Clin Neuropharmacol 2014;37(4):125–7.
86. American Psychiatric Association. Practice guideline for the treatment of patients with borderline personality disorder. Washington, DC: Author; 2001.
87. National Institute for Clinical Excellence (NICE). Borderline personality disorder: treatment and management. 2009. Available at: https://www.nice.org.uk/guidance/cg78/resources/guidance-borderline-personality-disorder-pdf. Accessed January 21, 2015.
88. Lieb K, Völlm B, Rücker G, et al. Pharmacotherapy for borderline personality disorder: Cochrane systematic review of randomised trials. Br J Psychiatry 2010; 196(1):4–12.
89. Bellino S, Rinaldi C, Bozzatello P, et al. Pharmacotherapy of borderline personality disorder: a systematic review for publication purpose. Curr Med Chem 2011; 18(22):3322–9.
90. Hollander E, Allen A, Lopez RP, et al. A preliminary double-blind, placebo-controlled trial of divalproex sodium in borderline personality disorder. J Clin Psychiatry 2001;62(3):199–203.
91. Frankenburg FR, Zanarini MC. Divalproex sodium treatment of women with borderline personality disorder and bipolar II disorder: a double-blind placebo-controlled pilot study. J Clin Psychiatry 2002;63(5):442–6.
92. Loew TH, Nickel MK, Muehlbacher M, et al. Topiramate treatment for women with borderline personality disorder: a double-blind, placebo-controlled study. J Clin Psychopharmacol 2006;26(1):61–6.
93. Zanarini MC, Frankenberg FR. Olanzapine treatment of female borderline personality disorder patients: a double blind, placebo-controlled pilot study. J Clin Psychiatry 2001;62(11):849–54.

Facing Violence – A Global Challenge

Thomas Wenzel, Dr med[a],*, Hanna Kienzler, PhD[b], Andreas Wollmann, Mag[c]

KEYWORDS

- Violence • Trauma • Refugees • Transcultural differences • Posttraumatic stress
- Idioms of distress • Prevention

KEY POINTS

- Sequels to violence can, due to their high prevalence and potentially severe long-term impact, be seen globally as the potentially largest mental health challenge.
- Displacement can add additional challenges for victims and health care systems.
- An interdisciplinary approach integrating medical and psychological, but also legal and sociological, aspects is required to address understanding, treating, and preventing violence.
- A stronger focus on subjective, culture-based, and dimensional factors, as partly reflected in the new DSM-5 models, needs to be part of any intervention.

INTRODUCTION

Violence has been shown to lead to a global challenge resulting in long-lasting social, medical, and mental health sequelae. In this article, we focus on massive social violence affecting groups, although it should be noted that especially sexual and domestic violence can have an equally severe impact on the life of individuals.[1,2] As Williams Nester[3] has observed, the problem is substantial, as "269 wars involving 591 states broke out between 1945 and 1988 alone," with an additional tendency of civil wars to be seen as a key challenge as "more than 85% of all wars between 1945 and 1976 were civil wars," and numbers appear to be growing since then. Although regions such as Syria or Iraq currently receive great public attention, with traumatic stress and suffering present in large parts of the populations, similar conditions apply for at least parts of many other countries, either on a long-term basis or during often-reoccurring outbreaks of unrest, civil war, and war.

No conflict of interests.
a Division of Social Psychiatry, Department of Psychiatry and Psychotherapy, Medical University of Vienna, Waehringer Guertel 18, Vienna A-1090, Austria; b Department of Social Science, Health and Medicine, King's College London, Strand, London WC2R 2LS, UK; c Sigmund Freud University, Schnirchgasse 3A, Vienna A-1030, Austria
* Corresponding author.
E-mail address: drthomaswenzel@web.de

> **Box 1**
> **Violence: relevance for mental health, key points**
>
> Violence is highly prevalent in most countries or regions; risk of exposure is high, especially if a longer observation period is used.
>
> Violence can, and frequently has, a long-term impact on mental health, including indirect trauma affecting the second-generation, third-generation and helpers.
>
> The impact of violence usually affects multiple levels, including the individual, group, and society.
>
> The long-term sequelae of violence can be severe and partly treatment resistant.
>
> Violence is seen as a possible predictor of future violence.
>
> *Data from* Refs.[3,7–14]

Models developed in Western Europe and North America for understanding trauma-related health problems and developing interventions cannot be sufficient to address this global health challenge. Culture is an important aspect of this challenge. Revisions of the American Psychiatric Association's *Diagnostic and Statistical Manual* in DSM-5,[4] the discussion of dimensional approaches,[5] new approaches in public mental and community health,[6] and closer interdisciplinary collaboration indicate a paradigm shift that reflects the complexity of issues. For instance, in displaced populations, the benefit of flight might be unbalanced by further problems due to forced migration and experiences of exclusion and discrimination in the host country. To simplify the complex issue, we summarize key challenges and models for solutions by two main areas of concern.

VIOLENCE

An increasing host of data demonstrate long-term impact not only on the individual, but also on social networks, economy, and society[15] that must be seen as interfacing (**Box 1**). Interconnections shape and are shaped by the kinds of violence encountered, physical and psychological injuries, increase in general morbidity, economic crises, and the breakdown of societal structures, frequently accompanied by the brain drain of health care experts. These complexities in combination with the persistent threat to personal and communal security create particular situations that cannot be compared with peace-time conditions even in developing countries.[15–17] Additionally, there is usually a lack of resources, which can be expected to further reduce support for patients with preconflict health and social problems, severe mental disorders, and disabilities,[18] and a general reconstruction of services besides development of specific services for trauma-related disorders might be a major challenge.[19]

Because of the often cumulative exposure to violence in contexts of conflict, particularly in settings of so-called "low"-intensity warfare areas, it is difficult to measure, generalize, or quantify stressors that might lead to or increase mental health problems, although it might be helpful to distinguish between isolated and repeated events or catastrophic environments (**Box 2**).

Diagnostic Considerations

Besides specific disorders that usually result only from extreme life events, especially posttraumatic stress disorder (PTSD), depression, and other mood and anxiety disorders are also equally or even more common in populations exposed to violence.[20–22] Secondary complications, like substance abuse or suicidal ideation, in a prevalence

| Box 2 |
| Types of severe life events by time |

Type I event (exposure): One-time event

Type II events (exposure): Repeated exposure or multiple events

Type III events (exposure): Continuous or intermittent exposure over longer time period

Type IV events (exposure): Longer exposure in childhood during psychological development

Data from Wenzel T. Challenges in implementing the Istanbul protocol. Göttingen, Germany: VR Unipress; 2015.

rate that depends also on social and cultural factors,[23,24] are common. PTSD is the trauma-specific disorder that is best explored and has been demonstrated to have severe impact on the survivor's life. And it has been shown to be highly prevalent in most affected regions even years after hostilities have ended, although patterns of expression and coping might differ.[25] Less or nearly no data are available on adjustment disorders, and the category describing the results of especially catastrophic events are included only in the *International Classification of Diseases, 10th Revision* ("Enduring *personality change* after catastrophic experience," F 62.0), This is partly related to a lack of translated and validated instruments for the last two disorders. Specific problems like trauma-related and culture-related psychosis[26] or brain trauma[27–29] might constitute additional and underrated problems besides more common stress-related disorders. Limitations of the PTSD concept on the background of culture have been the focus of continuous debate.[30] The recent changes in DSM-5 do not address all controversial aspects raised,[4] but can be seen as helpful as they integrate complex sociopsychological symptoms. They will require substantial adaptation of diagnostic and research tools, including culture-sensitive translation and revalidation also in regions with already limited resources.

Ethnographic research has highlighted that medicalizing the experiences of trauma, and thereby treating survivors of violence as patients, precludes our understanding of how individuals, families, and other social groups actually respond to violence, what their particular complex health and social care needs are, and through what capacities they contribute to the wider communities they belong to.[31] This can be best achieved by conducting comparative qualitative or mixed method research. Particularly through participant observation, important insights may be gained into people's everyday lives and routine practices, their social relations, and behaviors, whereas qualitative interviews allow researchers to elicit complex narratives of symptom and illness experiences, explanatory models, and local idioms of distress,[32] as well as information related to health-seeking behaviors and treatment experiences and possible resources to be mobilized for healing.[33] These considerations have been taken up by DSM-5 through its "Cultural Formation Interview," which, instead of providing a "list" of idioms of distress or syndromes of suffering, provides a semi-structured qualitative interview to elicit these aspects. DSM-5 includes culture-based "idioms of distress" and "cultural explanation or perceived illness (**Fig. 1**)."[34] Examples for such idioms are the West African "Kiyang-yang," as outlined by de Jong and Resi,[35] or llaki and nakary, as described by Pedersen and colleagues.[31] Idioms and illness behavior can be expected to be of substantial clinical relevance, as they would influence factors such as help-seeking and compliance.[36]

Although it is largely acknowledged that suffering itself is a universal human experience, the ways in which suffering is experienced and expressed differs depending on

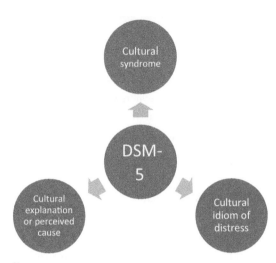

Fig. 1. DSM and culture.

social and cultural determinants, such as gender, age, ethnicity, and religion, as well as on economic situations and wider global processes that impact on local worlds and people's lives. Moreover, different forms of suffering can be distinguished. For instance, research in cultural anthropology has shown that the cultural meaning of suffering differs greatly between "routinized forms of suffering" that can be considered shared aspects of human conditions (eg, chronic illness or death) or experiences of deprivation and exploitation and "suffering resulting from extreme conditions," such as survivorship of genocide.[37] The complexity of these reactions is illustrated by, for example, Coker,[38] who found that southern Sudanese refugees in Cairo told stories of physical and social suffering that could be considered mourning for a lost cultural and physical normalcy as well as moral rage at their present circumstances. The investigator concludes that "illnesses were historicized and given meaning through the constant juxtaposition of time, place, and movement in narrative" (p. 27). Zarowsky[39] contributes to the understating of emotion, suffering, and trauma in different cultural and sociopolitical contexts by focusing on Ethiopian Somali returnees' narratives of emotion and suffering and comparing those with the literature on emotion in relation to trauma and the "refugee experience." According to her, emotional distress was about social rupture and injuries and not simply about private suffering. In fact, making a living under such harsh circumstances was a "recognition of the destruction of much of the fabric of the community at the same time as a refusal to vanish, a collective mourning of both private and collective losses at the same time as a deliberate creation of both history and the possibility of a future through the rhetorical (…) telling of the story of dispossession to each other, to their children, and to any outsiders who might be made to listen" (p. 202).

Interventions

Culturally and socially sensitive prevention strategies are of crucial importance due to the high prevalence and impact of sequels faced by individuals and groups exposed to armed conflict.

Primary prevention

Primary prevention strategies usually focus on social, psychological, and legal strategies. In contexts of mass violence during ethnic and political conflicts in countries like Rwanda or Syria, etiology tends to reflect social and political factors. Safety and political stability might at first have to be supported by military action, if not caused by the same military, but cannot be achieved by the same means, and a stable civil society is required to offer real safety as precondition for prevention and healing. As Worthington summarizes, "troops might effectively suppress military activities and reduce (but not usually eliminate) violence. Rarely can troops heal trauma, promote a re-establishment of the emotional bond between conflicting parties, and promote forgiveness and reconciliation, including the reduction or elimination of prejudices."[40]

Investigators, such as the psychiatrist and psychoanalyst Vamik Volkan, have drawn attention to psychological factors that permit manipulation of large groups as prerequisite to such violence and have demonstrated that interventions based on group analytical models can contribute to early prevention. Volkan[41] described "chosen" traumata, a symbolic representation of long-distant earlier historical loss, like the catastrophe of the "Kosovo Polje" in Serb history, as a key instrument used in manipulation of group regression and preparation for violence. Other investigators have followed similar approaches to explain the genesis and possible interventions.[42]

The development of human rights standards and treaty systems, such as the Geneva Conventions and the United Nations (UN) Convention against Torture, can be seen as socio-legal contributions to primary prevention. The obligatory Istanbul protocol (IP) (*Manual on Effective Investigation and Documentation of Torture and Other Cruel, Inhuman, or Degrading Treatment or Punishment*[43]), an interdisciplinary medico-legal document supported by the UN and the World Medical Association, assists medical doctors in the documentation of torture and inhuman and degrading treatment, contributing to prevention of torture practices, supporting criteria for protection in asylum and other procedures, and as secondary and tertiary prevention strategy in helping victims to receive justice and redress.[44] Ethical standards, including the IP, demand a clear position and underline both the importance of health professionals and a close collaboration with legal professionals.

Secondary prevention
Although critical incidence stress debriefing and critical incidence management have over the past decade been established especially in the United States as interventions that can in some cases prevent the development of stress-related disorders,[45] data must still be seen as ambivalent, controversial, or lacking, especially in developing and postconflict countries (see also the new World Health Organization [WHO] guidelines for management of acute stress, PTSD, and bereavement[46]). Because of the complex interaction between concrete event-related challenges and religious and cultural background, an uncritical transfer of models to local conditions should be seen as a dubious strategy. Existing cultural resources and strategies should be identified, evaluated, and supported in place or as part of intervention packages.[47]

Treatment and tertiary prevention
Present treatment models are most commonly developed in Western Europe and North America reflecting at least in principle availability of necessary experts (ie, especially psychiatrists and psychotherapists). The independent UK-based National Institute for Clinical Excellence treatment guidelines on, for example, PTSD, recommend seroxate and especially cognitive behavior therapy as standards in evidence-based treatment (https://www.nice.org.uk/guidance/cg26, in review March 2015). It is

---

Box 3
Five essential elements of immediate and midterm mass trauma intervention

1. A sense of safety,

2. Calming,

3. A sense of self- and community efficacy,

4. Connectedness,

5. Hope.

Data from Hobfoll SE, Watson P, Bell CC, et al. Five essential elements of immediate and mid-term mass trauma intervention: empirical evidence. Psychiatry 2007;70:283–315; [discussion: 316–69].

---

good to keep in mind that trained psychotherapists or even psychiatrists are not available in most regions of the world, might not be accepted as care providers by clients because of mental health stigma and local health belief models, or are unaffordable if available at all. In case of massive and far-spread violence, existing resources might not at all suffice even to cover the most urgent needs. Any intervention must be embedded in a more complex framework. The loss of local experts due to brain drain,[48] displacement, and death cannot sustainably be balanced by third-country humanitarian aid and treatment by foreign experts.

An expert consortium headed by Hobfoll and colleagues[49] proposed 5 simple key needs, listed in **Box 3**.

The new WHO guidelines provide a comprehensive framework that needs future exploration.[46]

Specific forms of psychotherapy focusing on trauma as the most common mental health problem that do not cover the complete range of clinical disorders or are based on a short-time intervention model have been successfully tested in crisis regions as components for interventions. Basoglu and colleagues[50,51] developed a focused approach of ultra-short treatment based on cognitive behavior therapy (CBT), tested first in earthquake survivors. A recent study reported positive results in a pilot study with former child soldiers using a culture-adapted CBT approach.[52] Murray and colleagues[53] developed and tested a "Common Elements Treatment Approach" (CETA) targeting mood or anxiety problems developed for use with lay counselors in low-income and middle-income countries. Testimony therapy, an approach developed originally to face widespread torture in Latin American dictatorships, has influenced specialized approaches developed over the past decade, but also has been proposed if embedded in local culture.[47,54,55] Narrative Exposure Therapy can be seen as a method well established in conflict zones[56] and as in principle open to local culture. The application of EMDR (Eye Movement Desensitization and Reprocessing) has been well established as an evidence-based intervention, and first studies have been performed with refugee populations,[57] but most data are based on application by trained psychotherapists.[58] The recent Cochrane review for interventions of torture survivors is skeptical as to this subgroup, summarizing data for intervention as existing but still weak and limited mainly to narrative therapy and CBT.[59] Criteria for medical evidence-based interventions as in this model might be difficult to realize in postconflict situations and might have to be adapted to complex interdisciplinary settings and outcome criteria (**Box 4**).[60]

Box 4
Proposed general criteria for interventions in postconflict areas and refugee populations

Limited training required

Training of available professionals or lay helpers

Low barrier

Culture sensitive

Resource oriented

Sustainable

Evidence-based, monitoring, and outcome evaluation

Data from Wenzel T. Challenges in Implementing the Istanbul Protocol. Göttingen, Germany: VR Unipress; 2015.

An increasing number of investigators have underlined the importance of existing resilience and healing models,[61] and community-based solutions are seen by most investigators working in developing countries and postconflict zones to be highly relevant, as suffering is seen as a social rather than purely individual experience.[62] Examples include the family support project in Kosovo,[63] whereas many centers in regions such as Gaza have been pioneers in community-oriented models, although again, most publications are descriptive and outcome studies are mostly missing. A general community orientation in this context should be differentiated from specific trauma-related intervention community projects.

The concepts of curative or transitional justice can be seen as characteristic examples of community-based approaches especially addressing the injustice gap perceived by the victims that might interfere also with psychological recovery. The use of "truth and reconciliation" committees like the South African Truth and Reconciliation Commission or of a modified version of traditional court systems in Rwanda can be seen as important and culture-sensitive models that might need further considerations and adaptation to achieve lasting positive results.[64]

Decisions of international courts, such as the European Court on Human Rights, (http://hudoc.echr.coe.int/sites/eng/pages/search.aspx?i=001-144151#{%22itemid %22:[%22001-144151%22]}) and the Inter-American Court (www.corteidh.or.cr/docs/casos/articulos/seriec_160_ing.pdf), complement these local culture-based models and confirm the importance of psychological suffering in family members and indirect victims caused by complex factors like the impact of uncertain fate and lack of closure and urge rapid and complete action by authorities to avoid such suffering. Reparations and the right to rehabilitation include not only provision of treatment but also symbolic interventions like the recognition and social respect for victims.

DISPLACEMENT AS AN ADDITIONAL CHALLENGE

Both internal and external displacement and refugee status are common results of violence, and the UN High Commissioner for Refugees estimates an overall number of 51,200,000, including those internally displaced, a high point since World War II, with approximately half younger than 18.[65]

In spite of a tendency to treat refugees as homogeneous population groups, data and especially qualitative results also indicate that the individual situation and stressors, and even biological factors relevant for treatment, might greatly differ.[66] In a global context and for many groups, all steps starting from flight through survival in often far from safe refugee camps, to return or forced return where feasible, raise multiple challenges. Although internal displacement that affects a large part of the populations might not always add transcultural factors, this becomes a key factor in external displacement. The diverse situations encountered and heterogeneous population structures often add to challenges, such as asylum procedures; separation from family members who might be in an unclear situation, lost, or at risk; cultural differences; or discrimination.[67] The loss of frameworks for individuals or small groups creates a situation different from that of larger populations who might create their own local networks, whereas role changes, especially in second-generation refugees, lead to new forms of coping or distress.[68,69] Treatment recommendations would require a longer review to address the diverse complex challenges mentioned, but will be summarized shortly.

The mutual culture "shock" between host and refugee culture, take out and transcultural aspects of public health,[70] and biological aspects such as cytochromes and competition or interaction between traditional and "Western" medicines are additional factors,[71,72] as outlined before. Rehabilitation, especially in severe PTSD, can be a major challenge as (re)integration might be inhibited.[73] Cultural idioms of distress not recognized and understood in the host country are part of the communication problems that can be expected to interfere with treatment. In spite of the better public health resources, for example in the United States, many traumatized victims in need of support and treatment arriving as refugees are therefore not recognized and consequently are not sufficiently supported,[74,75] and the available models might not be effective in cases of severe trauma, like torture,[13,76] pain being an adverse predictor.[77,78] A recent comprehensive project has led to similarly critical assessment with a larger refugee population regarding psychopharmacological treatment and psychotherapy of PTSD,[66] whereas a review by Palic and Elklit[79] found a stronger effect of CBT. New and community-based approaches are therefore explored through a number of projects. Drozdek and colleagues,[80] for example, reported improvement with a new group treatment approach. Community-based basic interventions have been demonstrated to be effective by Bolton and colleagues,[81] again using CETA. Palic and Carlsson[82] have drawn attention to the special care required if planning interventions with refugee groups.

Children,[73] and especially child soldiers,[83–86] who require special culture-sensitive (re)integration programs but also family systems as a whole,[87,88] have been described as a group of special concern that, because of the limited frame of this article, will be illustrated only in an example later in this article. The joint impact on parents and children neutralizes needed family support parallel to the lack of local social and medical resources or in case of "unaccompanied minors" loss of even core stuctures.[87] Economic stress and social isolation are common aggravating problems encountered in postconflict zones before flight and on return, but also in host countries.[89] Simple, although per se evidence-based interventions, can again not address the complexity of rehabilitation and treatment needs,[90,91] and specific intervention packages will be required for special groups.[76,92,93]

In a recent study for UNICEF of children returned to Kosovo after longer stays in European host countries, using a mixed method approach integrating qualitative and quantitative data, we followed parents and their children after repatriation, and found high rates of untreated PTSD and depression in both parents and children who lost most network contacts acquired before forced return ("repatriation").[89]

CASE VIGNETTE

A 16-year-old girl had witnessed the war in an eastern European country. Living conditions were difficult even before the war, as the region and its ethnic groups were discriminated against, and the village was mostly destroyed by overwhelming military forces. The girl's family tried to survive for some time, but intermittent raids, when several family members were killed, forced the girl and her mother and small sister to flee the country and ask for asylum in a neighboring country. For some time, the family feared that the father, who had been separated from the rest of the family, had been killed, but they could neither mourn nor do anything to help. The family received a temporary permit to stay. When the father finally could escape and join the family, he was withdrawn and irritable, and fights erupted with his wife at minor occasions. He started to drink alcohol in the evening, as he claimed he needed it to be able to sleep. The girl's mother consulted a "wise person," who claimed that her husband's behavior was "bewitched" through a spell of a jealous neighbor and gave her a charm to use, but the problem did not greatly improve. The girl's father refused to go to treatment, as "he was not crazy" and also "did not trust doctors here." The girl felt guilty, as she felt she was responsible for having caused dissatisfaction and she attributed his behavior to her shortcomings. Feelings of unhappiness and anxiety were partly balanced when she found new friends in school and a teacher who praised her quick wit and intelligence. Her teacher had also observed her distress, but interpreted it as being caused by the new cultural environment. With time, the girl developed a large group of friends, was invited to their families, and planned for a higher education and felt completely happy in her new home country, with only rare thoughts about her "old" country and the atrocities she had witnessed as a child. After 12 years, in the early morning hours, a group of police with a dog broke into their home, stating that the family's permit to stay had been revoked as the war "was over," and put the family on a plane to the country of origin for "repatriation."

She had no time to contact her friends. In her town of birth, the girl did not have any friends or relatives. At school, which was hard to reach, she was mocked and could not understand the language properly. Her earlier achievements were useless, and when returning home, her father had started drinking again as memories of the war had become stronger, and there was no work available. The family was shunned, because the other villagers thought they had had "a good time" abroad, being jealous and critical of their "Western" behavior. She became depressed, developed flashbacks of childhood war experiences, thought about suicide, and started seeing a ghost of a friend who had been killed during the war. No psychotherapy was available, and the nearest psychiatrist was in the capital, too far away to afford the costs for regular visits. No resolution has been found so far.

SUMMARY

Social suffering and mental health problems related to violence as a global public health problem can only be tackled with a holistic approach that takes cultural, social, legal, and economic determinants into account, and might also need a strong focus on human rights. Research that can give a reliable assessment of complex long-term outcomes is still largely missing, and can be seen as a major and complex challenge for future study.

REFERENCES

1. Garcia-Moreno C, Zimmerman C, Morris-Gehring A, et al. Addressing violence against women: a call to action. Lancet 2015;385(9978):1685–95.
2. Decker MR, Peitzmeier S, Olumide A, et al. Prevalence and health impact of intimate partner violence and non-partner sexual violence among female adolescents aged 15-19 years in vulnerable urban environments: a multi-country study. J Adolesc Health 2014;55:S58–67.

3. Nester WR. Globalization, war, and peace in the twenty-first century. 1st edition. New York: Palgrave Macmillan; 2010.

4. Levin AP, Kleinman SB, Adler JS. DSM-5 and posttraumatic stress disorder. J Am Acad Psychiatry Law 2014;42:146–58.

5. Braca M, Berardi D, Mencacci E, et al. Understanding psychopathology in migrants: a mixed categorical-dimensional approach. Int J Soc Psychiatry 2014; 60:243–53.

6. Dirscherl H, McConnell SC, Yoder JA, et al. The MHC class I genes of zebrafish. Dev Comp Immunol 2014;46:11–23.

7. Slone M, Shoshani A. Psychiatric effects of protracted conflict and political life events exposure among adolescents in Israel: 1998-2011. J Trauma Stress 2014;27:353–60.

8. Muhtz C, Wittekind C, Godemann K, et al. Mental health in offspring of traumatized refugees with and without post-traumatic stress disorder. Stress Health 2015. [Epub ahead of print].

9. Zerach G, Aloni R. Secondary traumatization among former prisoners of wars' adult children: the mediating role of parental bonding. Anxiety Stress Coping 2015;28:162–78.

10. Scharf M. Long-term effects of trauma: psychosocial functioning of the second and third generation of Holocaust survivors. Dev Psychopathol 2007;19:603–22.

11. O'Neill LK. Mental health support in northern communities: reviewing issues on isolated practice and secondary trauma. Rural Remote Health 2010;10:1369.

12. Symonds M. The "second injury" to victims of violent acts. 1980. Am J Psychoanal 2010;70:34–41.

13. Carlsson JM, Mortensen EL, Kastrup M. A follow-up study of mental health and health-related quality of life in tortured refugees in multidisciplinary treatment. J Nerv Ment Dis 2005;193:651–7.

14. Marie-Alsana W, Haj-Yahia MM, Greenbaum CW. Violence among Arab elementary school pupils in Israel. J Interpersonal Violence 2006;21:58–88.

15. Halileh SO, Daoud AR, Khatib RA, et al. The impact of the intifada on the health of a nation. Med Confl Surviv 2002;18:239–48.

16. Haar RJ, Footer KH, Singh S, et al. Measurement of attacks and interferences with health care in conflict: validation of an incident reporting tool for attacks on and interferences with health care in eastern Burma. Confl Health 2014;8:23.

17. de Jong JT. Challenges of creating synergy between global mental health and cultural psychiatry. Transcult Psychiatry 2014;51:806–28.

18. Hadary A, Schecter W, Embon OM, et al. Impact of military conflict on a civilian receiving hospital in a war zone. Ann Surg 2009;249:502–9.

19. De Vries AK, Klazinga NS. Mental health reform in post-conflict areas: a policy analysis based on experiences in Bosnia Herzegovina and Kosovo. Eur J Public Health 2006;16:247–52.

20. Priebe S, Bogic M, Ashcroft R, et al. Experience of human rights violations and subsequent mental disorders—a study following the war in the Balkans. Soc Sci Med 2010;71:2170–7.

21. de Jong JT, Komproe IH, Van Ommeren M. Common mental disorders in post-conflict settings. Lancet 2003;361:2128–30.

22. de Jong JT, Komproe IH, Van Ommeren M, et al. Lifetime events and posttraumatic stress disorder in 4 postconflict settings. JAMA 2001;286:555–62.

23. Panagioti M, Gooding P, Taylor PJ, et al. Negative self-appraisals and suicidal behavior among trauma victims experiencing PTSD symptoms: the mediating role of defeat and entrapment. Depress Anxiety 2012;29:187–94.

24. Wenzel T, Rushiti F, Aghani F, et al. Suicidal ideation, post-traumatic stress and suicide statistics in Kosovo. An analysis five years after the war. Suicidal ideation in Kosovo. Torture 2009;19:238–47.

25. Eytan A, Munyandamutsa N, Mahoro Nkubamugisha P, et al. Long-term mental health outcome in post-conflict settings: similarities and differences between Kosovo and Rwanda. Int J Soc Psychiatry 2015;61(4):363–72.

26. Soosay I, Silove D, Bateman-Steel C, et al. Trauma exposure, PTSD and psychotic-like symptoms in post-conflict timor leste: an epidemiological survey. BMC Psychiatry 2012;12:229.

27. Keatley E, d'Alfonso A, Abeare C, et al. Health outcomes of traumatic brain injury among refugee survivors of torture. J Head Trauma Rehabil 2013;28(6): E8–13.

28. Keatley E, Ashman T, Im B, et al. Self-reported head injury among refugee survivors of torture. J Head Trauma Rehabil 2013;28:E8–13.

29. Mollica RF, Chernoff MC, Megan Berthold S, et al. The mental health sequelae of traumatic head injury in South Vietnamese ex-political detainees who survived torture. Compr Psychiatry 2014;55:1626–38.

30. Summerfield D, Hume F. War and posttraumatic stress disorder: the question of social context. J Nerv Ment Dis 1993;181:522.

31. Pedersen D, Kienzler H, Gamarra J. Llaki and nakary: idioms of distress and suffering among the highland Quechua in the Peruvian Andes. Cult Med Psychiatry 2010;34:279–300.

32. Hinton DE, Good B. Culture and panic disorder. Stanford (CA): Stanford University Press; 2009.

33. Groleau D, Young A, Kirmayer LJ. The McGill Illness Narrative Interview (MINI): an interview schedule to elicit meanings and modes of reasoning related to illness experience. Transcult Psychiatry 2006;43:671–91.

34. American Psychiatric Association. DSM-5 task force. Diagnostic and statistical manual of mental disorders: DSM-5. 5th edition. Washington, DC: American Psychiatric Association; 2013.

35. de Jong JT, Reis R. Kiyang-yang, a West-African postwar idiom of distress. Cult Med Psychiatry 2010;34:301–21.

36. Hinton DE, Lewis-Fernandez R. Idioms of distress among trauma survivors: subtypes and clinical utility. Cult Med Psychiatry 2010;34:209–18.

37. Kleinman A, Kleinman J. Suffering and its professional transformation: toward an ethnography of interpersonal experience. Cult Med Psychiatry 1991;15: 275–301.

38. Coker EM. "Traveling pains": embodied metaphors of suffering among Southern Sudanese refugees in Cairo. Cult Med Psychiatry 2004;28:15–39.

39. Zarowsky C. Writing trauma: emotion, ethnography, and the politics of suffering among Somali returnees in Ethiopia. Cult Med Psychiatry 2004;28:189–209 [discussion: 211–20].

40. Worthington E Jr, Aten J. Forgiveness and reconciliation in social reconstruction after trauma. In: Martz E, editor. Trauma rehabilitation after war and conflict. New York: Springer; 2010. p. 55–71.

41. Volkan VD. Individual and large-group identity: parallels in development and characteristics in stability and crisis. Croat Med J 1999;40:458–65.

42. Thomas NK. There's always a villain to punish: group processes contributing to violence and its remediation. Int J Group Psychother 2015;65:89–107.

43. United Nations, Office of the High Commissioner for Human Rights. Istanbul protocol: manual on the effective investigation and documentation of torture and

other cruel, inhuman, or degrading treatment or punishment. 1 edition. New York: United Nations; 2004 [review].

44. Perera C, Verghese A. Implementation of Istanbul Protocol for effective documentation of torture—review of Sri Lankan perspectives. J Forensic Leg Med 2011;18: 1–5.

45. Robinson R. Reflections on the debriefing debate. Int J Emerg Ment Health 2008; 10:253–9.

46. Tol WA, Barbui C, Bisson J, et al. World Health Organization guidelines for management of acute stress, PTSD, and bereavement: key challenges on the road ahead. PLoS Med 2014;11:e1001769.

47. Agger I, Igreja V, Kiehle R, et al. Testimony ceremonies in Asia: integrating spirituality in testimonial therapy for torture survivors in India, Sri Lanka, Cambodia, and the Philippines. Transcult Psychiatry 2012;49:568–89.

48. Cook CT, Kalu K. The political economy of health policy in Sub-Saharan Africa. Med Law 2008;27:29–51.

49. Hobfoll SE, Watson P, Bell CC, et al. Five essential elements of immediate and mid-term mass trauma intervention: empirical evidence. Psychiatry 2007;70: 283–315 [discussion: 316–69].

50. Salcioglu E, Basoglu M. Control-focused behavioral treatment of earthquake survivors using live exposure to conditioned and simulated unconditioned stimuli. Cyberpsychol Behav Soc Netw 2010;13:13–9.

51. Basoglu M, Salcioglu E, Livanou M. Single-case experimental studies of a self-help manual for traumatic stress in earthquake survivors. J Behav Ther Exp Psychiatry 2009;40:50–8.

52. McMullen J, O'Callaghan P, Shannon C, et al. Group trauma-focused cognitive-behavioural therapy with former child soldiers and other war-affected boys in the DR Congo: a randomised controlled trial. J Child Psychol Psychiatry 2013; 54:1231–41.

53. Murray LK, Dorsey S, Haroz E, et al. A common elements treatment approach for adult mental health problems in low- and middle-income countries. Cogn Behav Pract 2014;21:111–23.

54. van Dijk JA, Schoutrop MJ, Spinhoven P. Testimony therapy: treatment method for traumatized victims of organized violence. Am J Psychother 2003;57:361–73.

55. Agger I, Raghuvanshi L, Shabana S, et al. Testimonial therapy. A pilot project to improve psychological wellbeing among survivors of torture in India. Torture 2009;19:204–17.

56. Neuner F, Schauer M, Klaschik C, et al. A comparison of narrative exposure therapy, supportive counseling, and psychoeducation for treating posttraumatic stress disorder in an African refugee settlement. J Consult Clin Psychol 2004; 72:579–87.

57. Ter Heide FJ, Mooren TM, Kleijn W, et al. EMDR versus stabilisation in traumatised asylum seekers and refugees: results of a pilot study. Eur J Psychotraumatol 2011. [Epub ahead of print].

58. Mello PG, Silva GR, Donat JC, et al. An update on the efficacy of cognitive-behavioral therapy, cognitive therapy, and exposure therapy for posttraumatic stress disorder. Int J Psychiatry Med 2013;46:339–57.

59. Patel N, Kellezi B, Williams AC. Psychological, social and welfare interventions for psychological health and well-being of torture survivors. Cochrane Database Syst Rev 2014;(11):CD009317.

60. Martz E. Trauma rehabilitation after war and conflict community and individual perspectives. New York: Springer; 2010. 1 online resource (xviii, 436 p.).

61. Agger I. Calming the mind: healing after mass atrocity in Cambodia. Transcult Psychiatry 2015. [Epub ahead of print].
62. Patel V, Boyce N, Collins PY, et al. A renewed agenda for global mental health. Lancet 2011;378:1441–2.
63. Keough ME, Samuels MF. The Kosovo family support project: offering psychosocial support for families with missing persons. Soc Work 2004;49:587–94.
64. Chapman AR, Spong B. Religion & reconciliation in South Africa: voices of religious leaders. Philadelphia: Templeton Foundation Press; 2003.
65. UNHCR. War's human cost. Geneva (Switzerland): UNHCR; 2013.
66. Buhmann CB. Traumatized refugees: morbidity, treatment and predictors of outcome. Not Found In Database 2014;61:B4871.
67. Wilson JP, Droždek B. Broken spirits: the treatment of traumatized asylum seekers, refugees, war, and torture victims. New York: Brunner-Routledge; 2004.
68. Steinhausen HC, Bearth-Carrari C, Winkler Metzke C. Psychosocial adaptation of adolescent migrants in a Swiss community survey. Soc Psychiatry Psychiatr Epidemiol 2009;44:308–16.
69. Neto F. Loneliness and adaptation among second-generation Portuguese migrants to France: roles of perceived responsibility and control. Percept Mot Skills 2000;91:115–9.
70. Rew KT, Clarke SL, Gossa W, et al. Immigrant and refugee health: cross-cultural communication. FP Essent 2014;423:30–9.
71. Jang JS, Cho KI, Jin HY, et al. Meta-analysis of cytochrome P450 2C19 polymorphism and risk of adverse clinical outcomes among coronary artery disease patients of different ethnic groups treated with clopidogrel. Am J Cardiol 2012;110: 502–8.
72. Martis S, Peter I, Hulot JS, et al. Multi-ethnic distribution of clinically relevant CYP2C genotypes and haplotypes. Pharmacogenomics J 2013;13:369–77.
73. Oppedal B, Idsoe T. The role of social support in the acculturation and mental health of unaccompanied minor asylum seekers. Scand J Psychol 2015;56: 203–11.
74. Shannon PJ, Vinson GA, Cook TL, et al. Characteristics of successful and unsuccessful mental health referrals of refugees. Adm Policy Ment Health 2015. [Epub ahead of print].
75. Eisenman DP, Keller AS, Kim G. Survivors of torture in a general medical setting: how often have patients been tortured, and how often is it missed? West J Med 2000;172:301–4.
76. Mohlen H, Parzer P, Resch F, et al. Psychosocial support for war-traumatized child and adolescent refugees: evaluation of a short-term treatment program. Aust N Z J Psychiatry 2005;39:81–7.
77. Olsen DR, Montgomery E, Bojholm S, et al. Prevalent musculoskeletal pain as a correlate of previous exposure to torture. Scand J Public Health 2006;34: 496–503.
78. Olsen DR, Montgomery E, Carlsson J, et al. Prevalent pain and pain level among torture survivors: a follow-up study. Dan Med Bull 2006;53:210–4.
79. Palic S, Elklit A. Psychosocial treatment of posttraumatic stress disorder in adult refugees: a systematic review of prospective treatment outcome studies and a critique. J Affect Disord 2011;131:8–23.
80. Drozdek B, Kamperman AM, Bolwerk N, et al. Group therapy with male asylum seekers and refugees with posttraumatic stress disorder: a controlled comparison cohort study of three day-treatment programs. J Nerv Ment Dis 2012;200: 758–65.

81. Bolton P, Lee C, Haroz EE, et al. A transdiagnostic community-based mental health treatment for comorbid disorders: development and outcomes of a randomized controlled trial among Burmese refugees in Thailand. PLoS Med 2014;11:e1001757.
82. Palic S, Carlsson J, Armour C, et al. Assessment of dissociation in Bosnian treatment-seeking refugees in Denmark. Nord J Psychiatry 2015;69:307–14.
83. Kohrt BA, Jordans MJ, Koirala S, et al. Designing mental health interventions informed by child development and human biology theory: a social ecology intervention for child soldiers in Nepal. Am J Hum Biol 2015;27:27–40.
84. Amone-P'Olak K, Lekhutlile TM, Meiser-Stedman R, et al. Mediators of the relation between war experiences and suicidal ideation among former child soldiers in Northern Uganda: the WAYS study. BMC Psychiatry 2014;14:271.
85. Klasen F, Reissmann S, Voss C, et al. The guiltless guilty: trauma-related guilt and psychopathology in former Ugandan child soldiers. Child Psychiatry Hum Dev 2015;46:180–93.
86. Betancourt TS, Newnham EA, McBain R, et al. Post-traumatic stress symptoms among former child soldiers in Sierra Leone: follow-up study. Br J Psychiatry 2013;203:196–202.
87. Jones L, Rrustemi A, Shahini M, et al. Mental health services for war-affected children: report of a survey in Kosovo. Br J Psychiatry 2003;183:540–6.
88. Dalgaard NT, Montgomery E. Disclosure and silencing: a systematic review of the literature on patterns of trauma communication in refugee families. Transcult Psychiatry 2015. [Epub ahead of print].
89. UNICEF. Silent harm. Geneva (Switzerland): UNICEF; 2012.
90. Tezer H, Ozkaya-Parlakay A, Kanik-Yuksek S, et al. Syrian patient diagnosed with meningococcal meningitis serogroup B. Hum Vaccin Immunother 2014;10:2482.
91. Pacione L, Measham T, Rousseau C. Refugee children: mental health and effective interventions. Curr Psychiatry Rep 2013;15:341.
92. Rousseau C, Measham T, Nadeau L. Addressing trauma in collaborative mental health care for refugee children. Clin Child Psychol Psychiatry 2013;18:121–36.
93. Onyut LP, Neuner F, Schauer E, et al. Narrative Exposure Therapy as a treatment for child war survivors with posttraumatic stress disorder: two case reports and a pilot study in an African refugee settlement. BMC Psychiatry 2005;5:7.

How Health Reform is Recasting Public Psychiatry

Roderick Shaner, MD[a],*, Kenneth S. Thompson, MD[b], Joel Braslow, MD, PhD[c,d], Mark Ragins, MD[e], Joseph John Parks III, MD[f], Jerome V. Vaccaro, MD[g]

KEYWORDS

- Community mental health • Public psychiatry • Health care reform
- Integrated behavioral health care • Managed behavioral health care
- Involuntary treatment • Telepsychiatry

KEY POINTS

- Milestones in the history of public psychiatry explain how health care reform is transforming the field through changes in financing, clinical integration, and care management.
- New features of community mental health include changing patient populations, increased importance of psychiatric consultation to primary care, telepsychiatry, practice in health homes, and greater participation in managed care.
- The future of public psychiatry encompasses new funding streams, collaboration in integrated health systems, evolving roles for recovery principles and involuntary treatment, and further academic partnerships.
- Public psychiatry leadership must help guide health care reform, emphasizing access to quality care, promotion of recovery and social engagement, and active participation in policy development.

INTRODUCTION

This article reviews ways that the fiscal, programmatic, clinical, and cultural forces of health care reform are transforming the work of public psychiatrists. Reform was

---

Disclosures: The authors have nothing to disclose.

[a] Los Angeles County Department of Mental Health, Keck School of Medicine, University of Southern California, 550 South Vermont Avenue, 12th Floor, Los Angeles, CA 90020, USA; [b] Pennsylvania Psychiatric Leadership Council, 6108 Kentucky Avenue, Pittsburgh, PA 15206, USA; [c] Department of Psychiatry and Biobehavioral Sciences, University of California, Los Angeles, Box 951759, CHS 33-251, Los Angeles, CA 90095-1759, USA; [d] Department of History, UCLA Wilshire Center, University of California, Los Angeles, Suite 300, 10920 Wilshire Boulevard, Los Angeles, CA 90024, USA; [e] MHA Village Integrated Service Agency, 456 Elm Avenue, Long Beach, CA 90802, USA; [f] Missouri Institute of Mental Health, University of Missouri–St. Louis, Dome Building, 5400 Arsenal, St Louis, MO 63139, USA; [g] Right Path HC, Ingenuity Health, 10 Fox Den Road, Mounts Kisco, NY 10549, USA
* Corresponding author.
E-mail addresses: rshaner@dmh.lacounty.gov; rshaner@aol.com

Psychiatr Clin N Am 38 (2015) 543–557
http://dx.doi.org/10.1016/j.psc.2015.05.007
0193-953X/15/$ – see front matter © 2015 Elsevier Inc. All rights reserved.

spurred by the fact that health care consumes some 17% of the national gross domestic product of the United States, yet provided relatively poor outcomes and left 40 million people uninsured. In addition to expanding access to care, the intent of health care reform is to achieve the triple aim of better health outcomes, improved quality and experience of care, and reduced costs.[1]

Tenets of health care reform, namely, increased access, parity, primary care–focused service integration, accountability with risk-bearing payment arrangements, and outcomes-driven treatment, arguably transform psychiatric practice more than other medical specialties, given psychiatry's enormous dependence on government funding.[2] Public psychiatry, long embedded in mental health systems essentially untethered from physical health care structures, has been especially upended as health care reform has occurred during an era of fiscal austerity in the face of increased service demands, corroding the midcentury foundations of community mental health. Public psychiatrists are challenged to create new practice models that respond to novel demands and preserve cherished values.

While recognizing variations of public psychiatric practice, this article focuses on public psychiatric activities practiced in community mental health systems by physicians supported directly or indirectly by governmental funding. Given the large funding roles of Medicare and Medicaid, this focus encompasses a sizable fraction of working psychiatrists.

Exciting new applications of public psychiatric practice in integrated primary health care environments and population health management are emerging.[3] Simultaneously, there is an opportunity, perhaps fleeting, to imbue a freshly minted health care system with therapeutic ethics that public psychiatry has long nurtured in sometimes unhelpful isolation. Effectively seizing this moment requires an understanding of key history, emerging psychiatric practices in safety-net systems, and some major issues for the future of public psychiatry.

A RECENT HISTORY OF PUBLIC PSYCHIATRY IN THE UNITED STATES

Public psychiatrists developed their identity as "community psychiatrists" in the clinical environments codified by the federal Community Mental Health Centers Act of 1963.[4] Freed from the confines of state hospitals, they now worked closely with community social agencies, local public hospitals, and associated academic institutions. Their clinical skills broadened to include more psychotherapies, and consultation and liaison psychiatry. Their contributions to the academic literature enhanced the scientific rigor of the subdiscipline.

Unfortunately, the transition from state hospital to community clinics was hampered by underplanning and underfunding.[5] The most severely mentally ill had more difficulty accessing treatment than did less severely affected patients seeking psychotherapy. Alliances with local general health systems often led to unfairly low budgets for mental health treatment, fueled by stigmatization of mental illness. Advocates successfully campaigned to separate administrative, programmatic, and fiscal supports for public mental health from those for the general health system.

This separation sometimes led to remarkable gains in community mental health services in general, but the effects on public psychiatry were profound. Public psychiatrists lost some previous connections with academia, general medical systems, and general psychiatry, and the decreased medical focus of the carve-out led to loss of many of their administrative functions.[6] Clinical practice narrowed, with prescribing eclipsing psychotherapy. The growing importance of empowerment and social support as mainstays of community treatment were occasionally contrasted with a negatively described "medical model" that included psychiatric interventions. The popularity of careers in public psychiatry, and especially community psychiatry, reached a low point in the 1970s.

Public psychiatry was reenergized in the 1980s when the roles of psychiatrist in community mental health systems were strengthened by renewed funding to treat severe and persistent mental illness, the rise of informed psychopharmacology, the proclamation of the "decade of the brain,"[7] and the Olmstead Decision in 1999.[8] With the leadership of the American Association of Community Psychiatry (AACP), founded in 1985, public psychiatrists reestablished ties with mainstream psychiatry and academia and forged strong new alliances with other community mental health disciplines, patients, and families. The "recovery model" of mental illness was deepened and embraced by many public psychiatrists, and a robust model of psychiatric service delivery in community mental health settings flourished by the turn of the century.

This relatively sunny model of community psychiatry is now challenged. New attention to population health and more sophisticated cost management are fundamental tenets of national health care reform, yet are still unfamiliar to many public psychiatrists. The relationship between health care funding and recovery model values of independence and self-reliance raises serious questions concerning proper funding priorities for psychiatric services. Reintegration of community mental health with primary care is almost universally embraced, but fully successful integrated programs are still exceptions. This unprecedented combination of forces challenges public psychiatrists to develop new clinical roles and theoretical models that will be effective and relevant in the emerging health care system.[9,10]

TOWARD A NEW PUBLIC PSYCHIATRY

The essence of public psychiatry is evolving, and this section examines 4 areas of rapid changes:

1. New patient populations
2. Renewed emphasis on consultation and primary care collaboration
3. Worksite transformation
4. Evolution of care management practices

Changes in Patient Population

Patients with disabling mental illness have always been a central responsibility of public mental health systems, sometimes to the exclusion of patients with other problems, including substance abuse.

Health care reform has expanded the population of Medicaid beneficiaries to childless individuals between the ages of 18 and 65 who may not be disabled.[11] Public psychiatrists are expected to care for individuals with new and sometimes complex medical needs, such as those with eating disorders and neurologically mediated behavioral syndromes stemming from traumatic brain injuries and neurodegenerative diseases. These new groups often require specific psychotherapeutic and care coordination skills.[12]

The population of individuals with severe mental illness (SMI) has also changed. A substantial number of people in this group always avoided mental health treatment, preferring to seek primary care services or avoid care altogether. Public health public insurance plans are now required to screen new beneficiaries for significant behavioral disorders and make community mental health center (CMHC) referrals for individuals with SMI who are often more ambivalent about seeking mental health services and may have other general medical health conditions. These individuals are often challenging to engage in treatment and less likely to collaborate with care planning.[13]

Increasingly, public psychiatrists must address more unstable patients who have been urgently referred. Newly mandated requirements for quicker access to mental health care are eliminating weeks-long wait lists that often caused unstable patients to end up in emergency care settings before CMHC intakes were available.[14] Abbreviated assessments and quick decisions about involuntary detention and transport to psychiatric emergency facilities are more necessary. The potential for self-destructive and assaultive behavior at first visit has increased. CMHC staff in some "restraint-free" outpatient settings has become uneasy about personal safety.

New Community Mental Health Center Psychiatric Consultation and Collaboration

CMHC consultation to primary care had become vestigial by the 1980s, but the integrative demands of health care reform are necessitating redevelopment of robust consultation services. The success of Medicaid health plans is predicated on efficient provision of primary care, and efficiency is greatly enhanced when primary care clinicians deliver a modicum of basic psychiatric services, supported by effective psychiatric consultation and collaborative care for individuals with comorbid physical and behavioral health conditions.

Academic/public partnerships have developed innovative psychiatric consultation models for newly integrated public systems,[15] but significant barriers to wholesale adoption must be surmounted.[16] To begin with, there are simply not enough public psychiatrists to provide for the consultation needs of the new beneficiary populations in publicly funded primary care who have a high prevalence of behavioral health conditions. Furthermore, primary care sites and CMHCs are only uncommonly colocated, inconveniencing patients and interfering with collaboration between consultants and primary care staff who are separated by both geography and organizational culture.

Separate record systems, and more stringent confidentiality requirements for mental health and substance abuse treatment information, present additional obstacles to consultation and integration between primary care and behavioral health specialists.[17] One unfortunate result is that community psychiatrists may seem unresponsive to other medical care providers, and the success of behavioral treatments is obscured.

Finally, the benefits of efficiency that are reaped from access to public psychiatric consultation currently accrue mostly to primary care while consulting CMHCs are rewarded with increased referrals and displacement of public psychiatrists from providing in-clinic care. This situation may be mitigated by carefully constructed arrangements with health plans and other payers (eg, at-risk medical groups), in which consultative services are reimbursed commensurate with the value they create through care efficiencies and improved medical and behavioral health outcomes.

To overcome long-standing barriers, reinvented public psychiatric consultation maximizes efficiency, supports appropriate primary care provision of mental health treatment, and identifies cases that should be transferred to specialty mental health.[18] Public psychiatrists increasingly practice indirect consultation to primary care. In traditional direct consultation, the consultant provides face-to-face assessment of the patient, either in person or through tele-technology. A summary of findings and interventions is available to the referring clinician, and a physician/patient relationship is established between consultant and patient.

By contrast, the indirect consultant does not participate in face-to-face assessment of a patient or initiation of care, and no physician/patient relationship is established.

The consultant discusses cases presented by primary care treatment teams, develops treatment strategies, provides in-service education, and facilitates selected referrals to specialty mental health services. This approach has been used successfully in other medical specialty areas with great success. One such program, SynerMed e-Consult, has demonstrated its efficacy in decreasing wait times, improving satisfaction, and decreasing costs for patients in areas as diverse as dermatology, radiology, and now psychiatry (Mason, 2014, personal communication).

Digital technologies increasingly support public psychiatric consultation, including secure video assessment and Web-based reviews of clinical records, recently coined "eConsultation."[19,20] The development of secure, Web-based registries mitigates difficulties of separate electronic health records (EHRs) by integrating data from different EHRs into a secure Web site.[21] While these technologies are powerful, experience thus far indicates that some physical presence of public psychiatrists in primary care sites is extremely helpful in building relationships that can be subsequently support eConsultation (Ricardo Mendoza, MD, Chief Psychiatrist, Telepsychiatry, Los Angeles County Department of Mental Health, Los Angeles CA, 2014, personal communication).

Beyond consultation, ongoing collaboration between public psychiatrists and primary care for treatment of shared patients is increasingly provided through on-site psychiatric services in primary care medical homes.[22,23] Significant mental health input into individual care plans is required of public health insurance plans. CMHC-based psychiatrists must collaborate with primary care when treating patients with general medical conditions likely to be influenced by behavioral abnormality or psychopharmacologic intervention. University-based collaborative care models focusing on patient-centered and population-based care have spread to some public systems.

Worksite Transformation

At least 3 novel public psychiatry worksites are sprouting in response to health care integration. Each has unique advantages and drawbacks: (1) colocation of public psychiatric services within primary care clinics; (2) behavioral health homes; and (3) tele-mental health hubs.[24]

Colocating mental health specialty services within the primary care home centralizes services, minimizes patient travel, promotes provider collaboration, and simplifies administrative overlay. Successful efforts to mesh the separate cultures of primary care and psychiatry under a single roof have demonstrated efficiencies and improved outcomes through joint setting of shared treatment targets, a unified medical record, and continuous formal and informal interaction. This model most easily lends itself to a future in which public psychiatry is no longer embedded in a separate mental health system.[25,26]

Despite its attractiveness, there are challenges inherent in this model. A relative lack of psychiatric expertise in primary care can lead practitioners either to overlook psychiatric problems or to address them through efforts to refer rather than collaborate. Current primary care sites often have an insufficient range of staff competencies on which public psychiatrists rely to fully address the psychotherapeutic and social services and community integration needs of individuals with significant psychiatric morbidity. Primary care clinics may have difficulties managing some forms of psychopathology that require more nuanced behavioral approaches.[27,28]

Behavioral health homes, essentially CMHCs augmented by on-site provision of primary care services, capitalize on preexisting resources that allow public psychiatrists and other behavioral health staff to function with maximum effectiveness while adding primary care presence. SMI populations, often with high rates of physical illness and challenges to navigate primary care service sites, can receive basic physical treatment.[29] The disadvantages include limited infrastructure for quality primary care, physical separation from medical specialty consultation, and perpetuation of challenges to administrative integration of health care. Nurse practitioners and related disciplines, however, can help bridge these gaps. The relatively few prototypic models are in the earliest developmental stages, but many advocates consider behavioral health homes as the health care delivery site of choice for many SMI consumers.

Dedicated tele-mental health service hubs, staffed by public psychiatrists, a nurse practitioner, and a small administrative team, can provide both tele-psychiatric and in-person services at distant sites.[30] These hubs house tele-technologies for diagnostic assessment, consultation, and psychotherapy to patients in primary care settings and many nonmedical settings, including group residential facilities and patient homes.[31] Indirect tele-consultation, often called eConsultation in its Web-based form, is augmented through specially designed software that focuses consultation questions arising in primary care settings, transmits medical record elements to psychiatrists, delivers responses, and modulates subsequent cross-talks between the consultant and the referring party.[20] Hubs address the need for both technology and efficient case discussion among psychiatric colleagues that makes "work at home" a less ideal option for public psychiatrists, and addresses the common desire for a set of responsibilities more varied than computer correspondence or video interactions.

Technology-based models for health care integration can improve collaborative efficiency and overcome some of the problems of physical and administrative separation. However, technology is an insufficient platform for some valuable types of interaction,[32] and requires substantial investment in hardware and software. It further requires participating patient sites to develop unfamiliar end-user procedures, including patient and equipment monitoring, staff training in use of the technology,[33] and on-site behavioral health-related emergency procedures. These drawbacks are becoming less significant as the technologies evolve and spread.

New Forms of Care Management

Managed care now increasingly affects public psychiatric practice.[34,35] Some public systems have turned over management of their behavioral health services to Managed Behavioral Health Organizations (MBHOs); others have adopted managed care techniques themselves. "Carved-out" management by MBHOs is giving way to reintegrated management of behavioral health and general health funding. This development presages a future in which managed care principles and lessons learned on both sides of the "carve-out" become intertwined and continue to iterate. Public psychiatrists, often responsible for decisions about costly resources such as psychiatric hospitalization and newer medications, are especially affected by these emerging approaches.[36,37]

Health care reform efforts to reduce the per-capita cost of health care have reenergized the fields of care management and population health management.[38] There is some compatibility between these approaches and community mental health. Both take a population-based view that recognizes distinctions among need levels of populations; managed care dedicates attention to high-risk/high-cost (HRHC) patients, while mental health care similarly views SMI group needs. Both recognize that outcomes are powerfully influenced by complex interplay among traditional medical/psychiatric interventions and those involving social, psychological, and economic matters.

Managed care places new practice requirements on public psychiatrists. First, new elements may be introduced into patient assessments and documentation.

Protocol-driven assessments increasingly determine the array of services that are available to public patients without additional procedures to authorize reimbursement. Often, assessments are used to assign patients to "levels of care,"[39] such as LOCUS[40] and MORS,[41] and to monitor measurable outcomes. Most MBHOs still rely on external care review to prospectively authorize reimbursement, especially for high-cost cases common in public specialty mental health. Public psychiatrists are often unused to scheduling and documentation requirements associated with such processes, and the CMHC infrastructure is ill-adapted to provide support.

Fortuitously, earlier versions of managed care with heavy administrative burdens have been supplanted by newer data-driven processes and novel approaches to payment, broadly characterized as value-based purchasing (VBP).[42] So-called fourth-generation systems foster efficient care through selection of provider networks that most effectively use resources to achieve given outcomes, whether or not the providers are bound by fee-for-service or risk-sharing arrangements.[43] As nontraditional providers pursue opportunities to deliver care to CMHC populations, VBP will change practices in community mental health care that have heretofore been sheltered from selection for efficiency. An emerging pattern harnesses the same forces that led the Centers for Medicare and Medicaid Services to initiate the accountable care organization (ACO) effort whereby groups of providers assume clinical and financial responsibility for entire populations of patients. Most health plans, and many state payers, have adopted these principles in their public sector health care delivery, and some states have placed provider groups at financial and clinical risk. A few states even have integrated medical and behavioral health funding streams for SMI patients, potentially facilitating the development of fully integrated SMI health homes.

SPECIAL ISSUES
The Impact of Funding Sources and Methodology in the Growth and Development of Community Psychiatry

The CMHC Act of 1963 and the appearance of Medicare/Medicaid in 1966 provided the funding and payment methodologies that allowed psychiatrists to treat seriously mentally ill persons in the community. From 1964 to 1981, the CMHC Act provided federal grants directly to local communities to provide a full range of mental health services within that community. The grant-funding structure did not require billing individual services for specific individual patients (fee-for-service). This method allowed psychiatrists in the CMHCs to provide innovative services and devote time for administrative work, staff training, planning, advocacy, and community leadership. Meanwhile, Medicaid and Medicare provided reliable funding for specific treatment to individual patients covered under those programs, allowing the CMHC block grant to be used for the uninsured and for services that traditional insurance payments would not cover.

Rapid rises in Medicaid spending engendered by this environment led to new funding limitations. The CMHC Act was replaced in 1981 by Mental Health Block Grants to states, which forced CMHCs to focus on care for persons with serious mental illness to reduce state hospital census, progressively restricted services for the uninsured, and limited the use of relatively expensive psychiatrists to only those services that could not be provided by less costly disciplines.[44] Lobbying by the pharmaceutical industry and focused mental health advocacy maintained fairly open access to psychiatric medications, despite much higher costs for newly developed agents. This reinforced the role of public psychiatrists as medication managers and limited the availability of funding to support the role of psychiatrists in providing other therapies, administrative work, teaching, and community leadership.

Thus, economic forces opened up community to psychiatry and then, 15 years later, substantially restricted the scope of what they could do in the community. The effect was mitigated in part by an increased use of 1115 demonstration waivers in the 1990s under which states were allowed to use Medicaid funding for innovative services not usually covered in the standard Medicaid budget, such as assertive community treatment (ACT) teams in support of employment.[45]

After the turn of the century, 2 major new developments began to reverse the fiscal policies that limited community psychiatry roles. First, epidemiological research demonstrated that persons with serious mental illness had a high burden of chronic medical illnesses.[46] Furthermore, economic analyses of several treatment outcome studies repeatedly found that high-cost, high-utilizing patients had an extremely high prevalence of behavioral health disorders. Increasing evidence that persons with serious mental illness were commonly both the medically sickest and most expensive led health care delivery system leaders to explore new funding mechanisms for community mental health systems.

Second, the Affordable Care Act passed in 2008 offered multiple opportunities for providers to receive lump-sum payments for all care provided to a population as capitation payments to ACOs, per-member per-month payments to health homes in person-centered medical homes, or global payments for episodes of care. These payment methodologies restore funded support for psychiatric involvement that goes beyond direct patient care[47]; recognize that relying on CMHC psychiatrists to directly provide the great bulk of medication management and associated psychotherapy is not fiscally sustainable; and suggest that psychiatric expertise is more effectively used through a consultative and collaborative supervision delivery model.

Taking advantage of these new opportunities will require that community psychiatrists reeducate themselves to work as physicians in medical settings, to act as consultants and supervisors rather than simply direct care providers in mental health settings, and to work as administrators and leaders in organizations. In addition, they will need to enhance their skills at negotiation, budgeting, and leadership, and become passionate about achieving measurable improvement in outcomes and keeping within budget without losing their passion for recovery and social justice.

The Recovery Movement in Integrated Health Care Settings

Recovery practices, with their emphasis on core values of recovery, namely independence, self-reliance, and individual responsibility, have fundamentally transformed both mental health practices and the fundamental goals of community mental health. Furthermore, community mental health systems are developing new recovery-oriented services that are a bulwark against misusing the model as a therapeutic rationale for linking service reduction to the best interests of patients.[48] According to New York's strategic plan for 1997 to 2001, "As the public mental health system moves into a managed care environment, the development of recovery-oriented services becomes increasingly important…Recovery is the ultimate positive outcome, and services that enhance the likelihood of recovery are the most cost-effective."[49]

A pressing concern is that the advances in both practice and program culture made by Recovery Movement will be lost as a result of integrating with medical model primary care settings and their funding systems.[50] There is, however, an opportunity for the recovery model and behavioral health to influence primary care despite our relatively small size and resources.[51] Primary care is struggling to move from a system that treats and triages acute illnesses to become a system that successfully manages complex, chronic illnesses, many of which depend on changing the behavior of persons. Many of the elements of "chronic care models" are versions of recovery-based practices (ie, self-coordinated care, activated patients, social supports, team based care, and so forth).[52] It may be that the relationship-based elements of the recovery model could address serious issues within primary care (such as the increasing rates of opiate overdose, low chronic medication compliance rates, repetitive emergency room usage patterns, and poor self-care behavioral change rates) more effectively than technology and managed care.[53,54]

Key recovery model practices that could transform primary care clinics into health homes include: (1) outreach, welcoming, and engagement; (2) commitment to improving lives beyond ameliorating illness, including building protective factors and resilience; and (3) collaboration with patients to reduce rates of treatment dropout.[55]

Health Reform and the Future of Involuntary Treatment

Nothing has been more divisive in public mental health than the issue of involuntary treatment. The controversy is exacerbated by a lack of definitive evidence for its effectiveness.[56,57] On the one side consumer, civil rights, antipsychiatry, and recovery groups (eg, the Bazelon Center for Mental Health Law, the National Empowerment Center, Substance Abuse and Mental Health Services Administration) have the elimination of involuntary treatment and all its attendant trauma and abuse as a fundamental goal. These groups cite constitutional issues and the dehumanizing, destructive impact of involuntary hospitalizations on trust and treatment engagement; they propose good, engaging, community-based services where there would be no need for involuntary treatment. Consistent with the Olmstead Decision, they reject involuntary detention as an alternative for persons that avoid using underfunded programs.

On the other side, many families, mental health professionals, and communities at large (eg, the National Alliance on Mental Illness Treatment Advocacy Center) think that expecting someone severely impaired by mental illness to make good choices on their own behalf is illogical. Instead of leaving them untreated (confused, suffering, disabled, destructive, and even dangerously violent) until they further deteriorate or seek treatment, caring, responsible people should assist them, forcibly if necessary, to get the treatment they need and deserve to get well, restore their capabilities, and regain control of their lives and the ability to make their own choices. Although they agree that community-based services should be better, they cite anosognosia, the biologically caused inability to recognize that one is ill, as the primary, and sometimes treatable, cause of treatment refusal. These proponents believe that leaving someone to "rot with their rights on" is inexcusable.[58–60]

In fact, funding changes have drastically decreased the use of involuntary hospitalization and treatment. Reimbursement limitations based on increasingly restrictive definitions of "medical necessity" have shortened acute hospital stays dramatically and have driven many hospitals out of business. Many people who at least initially might meet the legal requirements for involuntary treatment holds (usually being a danger to self or others, or gravely disabled) are released rather than admitted. Budgets of state-funded, long-term locked institutions have been slashed, and some of the remaining beds have been diverted from civil commitments to mentally ill criminals. Getting a long-term bed in many communities is more difficult than obtaining a conservatorship. Transfer of large numbers of inmates with mental illnesses to mental institutions is similarly obstructed by long waiting lists.

Driven by decreased funding for involuntary inpatient treatment, the battle over involuntary treatment has increasingly shifted to the community, with many states following New York's lead with the 1999 Kendra's Law providing for court-ordered Assisted Outpatient Treatment (AOT). Whether outcomes are improved is controversial, and study results vary according to the predispositions of those evaluating the data. Overall it does seem that involuntary, expensive (although cheaper than incarceration or hospitalization), targeted ACT services improve lives (whether the coercive component is always needed is in doubt) and that coercive treatment in the community decreases coercive institutionalization in hospitals and jails. On this basis, individuals thus treated may be freer overall. It seems likely that AOT programs will continue to spread and that increased funding will be allocated to them, although diverted from what remains to be seen. There is some risk that, like our inpatient mental health system, our public community mental health system will become predominantly involuntary over time as resources are reallocated to AOT.[61]

A few aspects of this trend deserve further consideration. First, there are a great number of frustrating, uncooperative persons in our communities who fall under the ever broadening definitions of mental illness. Who will decide who gets access to AOT, and on what basis? Mental health professionals may not agree with families about who should be "forced to take their meds." Many current programs, created through political compromise, exclude the very people for whom their frustrated family members had been advocating. Others advocate for including alcoholics and drug addicts, perpetrators of domestic violence, child abusers, sex offenders, and people with brain damage, all of whom are frustratingly treatment-rejecting, but usually not the target of mental health funding, expertise, or ACT services.

Second, involuntary community-based treatment requires collaboration between mental health and criminal justice staff and systems. Such collaborations have historically been challenging. However, partnerships between police in the community and mental health workers have been remarkably successful nationwide, generating active mental health training programs for police, integrated teams of one police and one social worker who respond to mental health crisis calls, and community policing teams focusing on mentally ill and homeless people (eg, the Quality of Life police in Long Beach, California). In the absence of such collaboration, unilateral law enforcement attempts to simply transport people to mental health programs usually proceed poorly. Given that mental health and drug courts are expensive propositions, it remains uncertain whether sufficient criminal justice resources will be diverted to community police, probation and parole, and dedicated courtrooms.[62,63]

Third, the past deinstitutionalization movement and the current decriminalization movement both occurred without the agreement of most communities. Communities do not easily tolerate and support people with either mental illnesses or drug addictions (and definitely not sex offenders). Many mental health and criminal laws are designed to limit participation in the community rather than facilitate it. For AOT to truly succeed, for it to be a tool for recovery and community integration, our communities have to be engaged in substantive ways to welcome and include the persons enrolled in such programs: the very same people who, for whatever reasons, have frustrated voluntary treatment efforts.

Academia and Public Psychiatry

Public psychiatry drifted away from mainstream academia since early pioneering work. Psychiatric residents were often exposed to public clinics and hospitals only in the context of convenient training sites in which to learn certain skills necessary for later private or academic work. Renewed focus on treatment of SMI in the early 1980s reawakened interest in specialized academic training for public psychiatrists. Starting in 1981 with the New York State Office of Mental Health's funding of a public psychiatric fellowship at New York State Psychiatric Institute at Columbia University Medical Center, public mental health systems used economic incentives for academic programs to select and train early career psychiatrists with talent, passion, and dedication to public service.[64] At present, there are some 15 public psychiatric fellowships in the United States.

The effects of new public/academic psychiatry partnerships are likely to grow. Although salaries and advancement in public mental health systems are not yet closely linked to fellowship training, applicants with this background are now sought. The funding provided by public mental health systems to academia increasingly influences faculty selection and general psychiatry curricula. Affiliation agreements between academic institutions and public systems lead to joint curriculum planning, exchange of theoretical and clinical perspectives, and a narrowing of the gaps between psychiatric training, research, and public practice. There has been rapid expansion of direct funding of general residency positions by public systems in exchange for curriculum changes and residency participation in patient care. Grant incentives contained in the Affordable Care Act may continue to spur this growth.

An Agenda for Public Psychiatric Leadership in Health Care Reform

The authors believe that the first task on the public psychiatry agenda is to ensure that community mental health and access to associated psychiatric services is properly placed within a system centered on primary care, with a focus on accountable, high-quality, whole-person health care. Obviously this requires psychiatric engagement, but how and to what extent? Fortunately, public psychiatrists are familiar with the tools of organizational change, and leaders in the field have the skills to engage in ongoing development of policy and initiatives with other architects of health care reform.

A second task is to continue the momentum to reform clinical practice. American public psychiatry has been the leading edge in incorporating recovery techniques into psychiatric practice. Although public psychiatrists are concerned that integration with primary care may impede this progress, the authors are heartened that terms such as the "activated patient," "engagement," "the social determinants of health," and "whole person health care" are entering primary care parlance. From this perspective recovery, and psychiatry along with it, actually stand to gain by having its methods become the core of all American health care.

A third agenda item emerges from the efforts to promulgate the recovery-oriented approach to care. Public psychiatry must complete the struggle to become the soul of general psychiatry's work and the core of our profession's social contract. With this shift in perspective, the psychiatric profession will better recognize how critical our primary population and payers are to the profession, and will seek more successful partnerships with government and private systems to train, recruit, and retain excellent psychiatrists dedicated to public service.

A fourth agenda item for public psychiatric leadership is to more actively engage in national policy formulation and implementation to promote and protect the well-being of both people with psychiatric challenges and the community as a whole. In part this requires a form of "inside baseball" that focuses on how public mental health care services are managed as a domain unto itself. However, public psychiatry leadership must also think "outside of the ball park" and consider the larger frame of mental health stewardship. This approach requires us to help ensure that policies and social resources are in place to help people avoid mental illness in the first place in addition to protecting them and helping them recover. The promotion of public service and social welfare by public psychiatrists is a critical element of our role as key stewards of the nation's mental health. In the end, public service psychiatry is a public health profession that should exercise expertise in national, state, and local policy development and implementation. Leaders and followers must enter into the debates shaping the broad range of government policies, taking a "health and mental health in all policies" approach.

There is a final agenda that is necessary for accomplishing the aforementioned. We must reliably create public psychiatry leaders capable of advancing public service and the public psychiatry agenda. For many years promotion of psychiatric leadership has been focused on research, academic health centers, commerce, or private practice. Meanwhile, the numbers of psychiatrists leading mental health services in federal, state, or local government agencies had become negligible, excepting the valiant work of the remaining Medical Directors in the National Association of State Mental Health Program Directors. But there are some bright spots. Although the academic presence of community psychiatrists is a mere shadow of its former self, there is resurgence in fellowship training in community psychiatry. The American Association of Community Psychiatrists, in large part responsible for this phenomenon, continues to develop as an influential platform for public psychiatry leadership. The tasks facing public psychiatry leaders, including the job of better connecting public psychiatrists and focusing their voice, will require adaptation, flexibility, and focus on key issues and effective solutions.[65] Perhaps this review of the state of public psychiatry and proposed agenda, or something like it, will further the unique activities and goals of public psychiatrists and, most importantly, contribute to the success of health care reform for our patients and the well-being of our communities.

REFERENCES

1. Berwick DM, Nolan TW, Whittington J. The triple aim: care, health, and cost. Health Aff 2008;27:759–69.
2. Alakeson V, Frank R. Health care reform and mental health care delivery. Psychiatr Serv 2010;61:1063.
3. Maust DT, Oslin DW, Marcus SC. Mental health care in the accountable care organization. Psychiatr Serv 2013;64:908–10.
4. Rochefort DA. Origins of the third psychiatric revolution: the community mental health centers act of 1963. J Health Polit Policy Law 1984;9:1–30.
5. Feldman JM. History of community psychiatry. In: McQuistion HL, Sowers WE, Ranz JM, et al, editors. Handbook of community psychiatry. New York: Springer; 2012. p. 669–76.
6. Feldman JM. Chronic mentally ill populations. In: Ruiz P, Primm A, editors. Disparities in psychiatric care clinical and cross-cultural perspectives. Baltimore (MD): Lippincott Williams & Wilkins; 2010. p. 189–97.
7. Bush G. Decade of the brain, 1990–1999. Presidential proclamation 6158. Federal Register 55, no. 140 (1990): 29553.
8. Olmstead V.L.C. (98–536) 527 U.S. 581. 1999.
9. Thornicroft G, Tansella M. Community mental health care in the future: Nine proposals. J Nerv Ment Dis 2014;202:507–12.
10. Kennedy PJ, Greden JF, Riba M. The next 50 years: a new vision of community of mental health. Am J Psychiatry 2013;170:1097–8.
11. Crowley RA, Golden W. Health policy basics: Medicaid expansion. Ann Intern Med 2014;160:423–5.
12. Decker SL, Kostova D, Kenney GM, et al. Health status, risk factors, and medical conditions among persons enrolled in Medicaid vs uninsured low-income adults potentially eligible for Medicaid under the Affordable Care Act. JAMA 2013;309:2579–86.

13. Salsberry PJ, Chipps E, Kennedy C. Use of general medical services among Medicaid patients with severe and persistent mental illness. Psychiatr Serv 2005;56:458–62.
14. State of California Department of Health Care Services. Coordinated care initiative. Executive summary fact sheet updated March 2013. Available at: http://www.calduals.org/wp-content/uploads/2013/03/1-CCI-Overview.pdf. Accessed January 28, 2015.
15. Ratzliff A, Unutzer J, AIMS Center. Primary Care Consultation Psychiatry. 2012. Available at: http://aims.uw.edu/sites/default/files/IntroductiontoPrimaryCarePsychiatricConsultation.pdf. Accessed January 28, 2015.
16. Grazier KL, Hegedus AM, Carli T, et al. Integration of care: integration of behavioral and physical health care for a Medicaid population through a public-public partnership. Psychiatr Serv 2003;54:1508–12.
17. Jost TS. Appendix B. Constraints on sharing mental health and substance-use treatment information imposed by federal state and medical records privacy laws. In: Institute of Medicine (US) Committee, editor. Crossing the quality chasm: adaptation to mental health and addictive disorders. Improving the quality of health care for mental and substance-use conditions. Washington, DC: National Academies Press; 2006. p. 405–22.
18. Yellowlees P, Odor A, Parish MB, et al. A feasibility study of the use of asynchronous telepsychiatry for psychiatric consultations. Psychiatr Serv 2010;61:838–40.
19. Shore JH. Telepsychiatry: videoconferencing in the delivery of psychiatric care. Am J Psychiatry 2013;170:256–62.
20. eConsult Overview updated 05/14/13 [Internet]. L.A. care health plan. Available at: http://econsultla.com/sites/all/files/econsult/2014%200328%20Flyer%20-%20What%20is%20eConsult.pdf. Accessed January 28, 2015.
21. Gliklich RE, Dreyer NA, Leavy MB. Registries for evaluating patient outcomes: a user's guide. U.S. Agency for Health Care Research and Quality/AHRQ. Washington, DC: Government Printing Office; 2014.
22. Katon WJ, Lin EH, Von Korff M, et al. Collaborative care for patients with depression and chronic illnesses. N Engl J Med 2010;363:2611–20.
23. Kilbourne AM, Nord KM, Bauer MS, et al. Mental health collaborative care and its role in primary care settings. Curr Psychiatry Rep 2013;15(8):383.
24. Bao Y, Casalino LP, Pincus HA. Behavioral health and health care reform models: patient-centered medical home, health home, and accountable care organization. J Behav Health Serv Res 2013;40:121–32.
25. Grant R, Greene D. The health care home model: Primary health care meeting public health goals. Am J Public Health 2012;102:1096–103.
26. Fogarty CT, Mauksch L. The development of joint principles: integrating behavioral health care into the patient-centered medical home. Families, Systems & Health 2012;32(2):153.
27. Smith T, Sederer L. A new kind of homelessness for individuals with serious mental illness? The need for a mental health home. Psychiatr Serv 2009;60:528–33.
28. Massa I, Miller BF, Kessler R. Collaboration between NCQA patient-centered medical homes and specialty behavioral health and medical services. Transl Behav Med 2012;2:332–6.
29. Behavioral health homes for people with mental health and substance abuse conditions. The core clinical features SAMHSA-HRSA Center for Integrated Health Solutions. 2012. Available at: http://www.integration.samhsa.gov/clinical-practice/cihs_health_homes_core_clinical_features.pdf. Accessed January 28, 2015.

30. Mendoza R. Telehealth–leveraging technology to foster awareness and integration. Presented at the 10th Annual Statewide Conference: Integrating Substance Use, Mental Health, and Primary Care Services. Los Angeles, October 23–24, 2013.

31. Grady B, Myers KM, Nelson E-L, et al. Evidence-based practice for telemental health. Telemed J E Health 2011;17:131–48.

32. Hilty DM, Nesbitt TS, Marks SL, et al. Effects of telepsychiatry on the doctor-patient relationship: communication, satisfaction, and relevant issues. Primary Care Psychiatry 2002;9:29–34.

33. Kim Y, Chen AH, Keith E, et al. Not perfect, but better: primary care providers experiences with electronic referrals in a safety net health system. J Gen Intern Med 2009;24:614–9.

34. Isett KR, Ellis AR, Topping S, et al. Managed care and provider satisfaction in mental health settings. Community Ment Health J 2009;45:209–21.

35. Cuffel BJ, Snowden L, Masland M, et al. Managed care in the public mental health system. Community Ment Health J 1996;32:109–24.

36. Busch AB, Frank RG, Lehman AF. The effect of a managed behavioral health carve-out on quality of care for Medicaid patients diagnosed as having schizophrenia. Arch Gen Psychiatry 2004;61:442–8.

37. Dickey B, Normand SLT, Hermann RC, et al. Guideline recommendations for treatment of schizophrenia: the impact of managed care. Arch Gen Psychiatry 2003;60:340–8.

38. Rust G, Strothers H, Miller WJ, et al. Economic impact of a Medicaid population health management program. Popul Health Manag 2011;14:215–22.

39. Jarvis D, Rosenberg L. The money woes in Medicaid managed care states. Behav Healthc 2006;26:28–9.

40. Sowers W, Pumariega A, Huffine C, et al. Best practices: level-of-care decision making in behavioral health services: the LOCUS and the CALOCUS. Psychiatr Serv 2003;54:1461–3.

41. Fisher DG, Pilon D, Hershberger SL, et al. Psychometric properties of an assessment for mental health recovery programs. Community Ment Health J 2009;45:246–50.

42. Eldridge GN, Korda H. Value-based purchasing: the evidence. Am J Manag Care 2011;17:e310.

43. Kushner JN, Moss S. Purchasing managed care services for alcohol and other drug treatment. Bethesda (MD): Center for Substance Abuse Treatment; 1995.

44. Frank RG, Glied S. Better but not well mental health policy in the United States since 1950. Baltimore (MD): Johns Hopkins University Press; 2006.

45. Mechanic D. Mental health services then and now. Health Aff 2007;26:1548–50.

46. Parks J, Svendsen D, Singer P, et al. Morbidity and mortality in people with serious mental illness. Alexandria (VA): National Association of State Mental Health Program Directors (NASMHPD) Medical Directors Council; 2006.

47. Raney LE. Integrated care: working at the interface of primary care and behavioral health. Arlington (VA): American Psychiatric Pub; 2014.

48. Shern D, Jones K, Chen H, et al. Medicaid managed care and the distribution of societal costs for persons with severe mental illness. Am J Psychiatry 2008;165:254–60.

49. Strategic Plan Framework. Albany (NY): New York Office of Mental Health; 2007. p. 3. Available at: http://www.omh.ny.gov/omhweb/budget/2007-2008/strategic_framework.pdf.

50. Davidson L, O'Connell M, Tondora J, et al. The top ten concerns about recovery encountered in mental health system transformation. Psychiatr Serv 2006;57:640–5.

51. CalMEND, Integration of Mental Health, Substance Abuse, and Primary Care Services Vol. 1 Embracing our Values from a Client and Family Member Perspective 2011. Available at: http://www.integration.samhsa.gov/sliders/slider_10.3.pdf. Accessed January 30, 2015.
52. Wagner EH, Austin BT, Davis C, et al. Improving chronic illness care: translating evidence into action. Health Aff 2001;20:64–78.
53. Druss BG, Zhao L, von Esenwein SA, et al. The health and recovery peer (HARP) program: a peer-led intervention to improve medical self-management for persons with serious mental illness. Schizophr Res 2010;118:264–70.
54. Ragins M. Top 10 strategies from the world of recovery and serious mental illness that should be used in medical and behavioral health homes. Los Angeles (CA): Mental Health America of Los Angeles; 2013. Available at: http://static1.1. sqspcdn.com/static/f/1084149/23741355/1382467980850/article_Top_10_Strategies_ for_Health_Homes.pdf?token=q4frrTqwtVLqOUNDT7MZCw%2BrbiU%3D. Accessed January 28, 2015.
55. Pollack D, Ragins M. Recovery and community mental health. In: Yeager K, Cutler DL, Svendsen D, et al, editors. Modern community mental health: an interdisciplinary approach. Oxford (United Kingdom): Oxford University Press; 2013. p. 385–404.
56. Phelan J, Sinkewicz M, Castille D, et al. Effectiveness and outcomes of assisted outpatient treatment in New York State. Psychiatr Serv 2010;61:137–43.
57. Munetz MR, Ritter C, Teller JL, et al. Mental health court and assisted outpatient treatment: perceived coercion, procedural justice, and program impact. Psychiatr Serv 2014;65(3):352–8.
58. Appelbaum PS, Gutheil TG. Rotting with their rights on: constitutional theory and clinical reality in drug refusal by psychiatric patients. Bull Am Acad Psychiatry Law 1979;7:306–15.
59. Swartz M, Wilder C, Swanson J, et al. Assessing outcomes for consumers in New York's assisted outpatient treatment program. Psychiatr Serv 2010;61:976–81.
60. Treatment Advocacy Center, Assisted Outpatient Treatment Laws 2011. Available at: http://www.treatmentadvocacycenter.org/solution/assisted-outpatient-treatment-laws. Accessed January 28, 2015.
61. Ragins M. Important considerations for implementing assisted outpatient treatment: a collaborative advocacy agenda 2014. Los Angeles (CA): Mental Health America of Los Angeles; 2014. Available at: http://static1.1.sqspcdn.com/static/ f/1084149/25167959/1408663597870/111ImportantConsiderationsforImplementing AssistedOutpatientTreatment.pdf?token=DNKoMGIKhYKp1cJ%2FSu93S%2FGW ugw%3D. Accessed January 28, 2015.
62. Lamb HR, Weinberger LE, DeCuir WJ. The police and mental health. Psychiatr Serv 2002;53:1266–71.
63. Almquist L, Dodd E, Center J, et al. Mental health courts: a guide to research-informed policy and practice. Washington, DC: Council of State Governments, Justice Center; 2009.
64. Ranz JM, Deakins SM, LeMelle SM, et al. Public-academic partnerships: core elements of a public psychiatry fellowship. Psychiatr Serv 2008;59:718–20.
65. Heifetz R. "Build the stomach for the journey". In: Levy B, Gaufin J, editors. Mastering public health: essential skills for effective practice. Oxford (United Kingdom): Oxford University Press; 2012. p. 311–2.

Telepsychiatry

Effective, Evidence-Based, and at a Tipping Point in Health Care Delivery?

Donald Hilty, MD[a],*, Peter M. Yellowlees, MBBS, MD[b],
Michelle B. Parrish, MA[c], Steven Chan, MD, MBA[d]

KEYWORDS

- Telepsychiatry • Telemedicine • Models • Integrated and stepped care
- Effectiveness

KEY POINTS

- Telepsychiatry is effective compared with in-person care for adults and many populations, disorders, and settings.
- Telepsychiatry adds versatility to clinical practice and new models of care, if applied judiciously and incrementally.
- Good telepsychiatric care depends on time-tested principles of good patient-doctor engagement, the therapeutic relationship, communication, bio-psycho-socio-cultural treatment, and integrated care.
- Participants in care, particularly patients, feel empowered through technology and inform us of virtual care options for the future.

INTRODUCTION

Telepsychiatry is at a "tipping point" and, after more than 50 years of slow clinical implementation around the world, is finally being widely introduced. This article helps the reader to (1) learn and be able to apply the evidence base on telepsychiatry to

Disclosures: The authors have no financial conflict of interest.
[a] Psychiatry & Behavioral Sciences, Telehealth, USC Care Health System, Keck School of Medicine, University of Southern California, 2250 Alcazar Street, CSC Suite 2200, Los Angeles, CA 90033, USA; [b] Psychiatry & Behavioral Sciences, Health Informatics Graduate Program, University of California, Davis School of Medicine and Health System, 2450 48th Street, Suite 2800, Sacramento, CA 95817, USA; [c] Telepsychiatry and Health Informatics, University of California, Davis School of Medicine & Health System, 2450 48th Street Suite 2800, Sacramento, CA 95817, USA; [d] Department of Psychiatry & Behavioral Sciences, University of California, Davis School of Medicine & Health System, 2150 Stockton Boulevard, Sacramento, CA 95817, USA
* Corresponding author.
E-mail address: hilty@usc.edu

Psychiatr Clin N Am 38 (2015) 559–592
http://dx.doi.org/10.1016/j.psc.2015.05.006
0193-953X/15/$ – see front matter © 2015 Elsevier Inc. All rights reserved.

psych.theclinics.com

clinical practice; (2) adjust or change current systems of care as they implement telepsychiatry (eg, how to use technology, get paid, and adhere to legal issues), and (3) compare telepsychiatric models of care to in-person care for different ages, disorders, and bio-psycho-socio-cultural treatment modalities. The article uses a clinical vignette to illustrate the objectives.

HOW CAN THE EVIDENCE BASE FOR TELEPSYCHIATRY TO CLINICAL PRACTICE BE APPLIED?

Patient-centered health care confronts us with a question about how to deliver quality, affordable, and timely care in a variety of settings,[1] without stigma and with sensitivity to culture and diversity.[2,3] Technology and empowerment have been linked for some time,[4] and patients have been very satisfied with telemental health (TMH) care. Systems are trying to increase clinical operating efficiency by integrating care and providing care at multiple points of service[5] and use it to leverage interdisciplinary team members' clinical, administrative, and other care coordination expertise.[6] The World Health Organization, too, is surveying telemedicine opportunities and developments in member states.[7]

Evaluation of telepsychiatry TMH has gone through 3 phases.[3] First, TMH was found to be effective in terms of increasing access to care, acceptance, and good educational outcomes.[3] Second, it was noted to be valid and reliable compared with in-person services.[8] In addition to comparison (or as good as) studies, telepsychiatric outcomes are not inferior to in-person care (ie, noninferiority studies).[9] Third, frameworks are being used to approach complex themes like costs and models.[8,10,11]

Most clinicians, administrators, and other leaders want to ensure good care, do it ethically, and be remunerated. Time-tested quality care in psychiatry is mostly attributed to the patient-doctor engagement, the therapeutic relationship, shared decision-making, the role of stories and narratives, and biopsychosocial treatment.[12] As for technology as an innovation, folks accept "innovation represents a potential efficacy in solving a perceived need or problem."[13] Systems of care and their leaders are moving fast now with traditional video/synchronous telepsychiatry (STP), novel (eg, asynchronous or asynchronous telepsychiatry [ATP], social media), and emerging (eg, Web- and mobile/wireless-based) models.

CLINICAL VIGNETTE

Identification Info

A 14-year-old Latino American boy was struggling in school, in social situations, and at home. Parents attributed this to "ADD." He had a 9-year-old sister, a 7-year-old brother, and a 3-year-old brother. They lived in small rural community of 12,000 with a small K-12 school, one private and one public health clinic juxtaposed, and one adult mental health (MH) therapist (social worker for adults).

History of Present Illness and Referral

The boy was born in Mexico, and his father and mother immigrated 10 and 6 years earlier, respectively. A public health nurse with 25 years of experience supported the physician ordering the consultation, because the pediatrician was not sure how to proceed. "It seems like attention deficit hyperactivity disorder (ADHD), but I am not sure as there may be some depression, too," according to the brief consultation request faxed to the academic center 100 miles away. The concerning events had been focused in these 2 areas: (1) inattention, poor follow-up on homework, being seen as "hyperactive" in class, and (2) "moody," "angry," and making comments like "I might as well be dead."

Consultation and Technology

The telemedicine consultation used a unit with transmission speeds at 384 kilobits per second (KBPS) and far-end camera control for the provider of an academic health center. Payment for the visit was only through Medicaid/Medicare, which did not cover the true costs.

Evaluation

A 90-minute telepsychiatric consultation was completed by a general telepsychiatrist; child psychiatrists were not available. The interview was in stages: the child, mother, and 2 older siblings; the child; the mother; and all parties. Findings included some mood change (probably depression), no imminent suicidal ideation, disruptive behavior linked to teen-father issues (discipline, absence of the father for truck-driving work), and some decent relationships with peers; no clear use of substances or conduct disordered behavior.

TELEPSYCHIATRY IS EFFECTIVE

For specifics of evaluating outcomes, there are 3 main resources in the literature. The first resource is the American Telemedicine Association (ATA) TMH expert consensus that produced a lexicon for outcomes in the following areas: patient satisfaction (ie, access, distance to service, use of), provider satisfaction, process of care (eg, no-shows, coordination, completion of treatment), communication (eg, rapport), reliability/validity (eg, assessment, treatment vs in-person), specific disorder measures (eg, symptoms), cost (ie, length of service, travel, hardware and software), and other administrative factors (eg, facility management, team staffing).[10] Second, another resource looks in-depth at clinical, cost, program evaluation, and other areas of TMH care—the focus is on how to prioritize, make decisions, and implement program change based on iterative feedback.[11] Finally, a review on effectiveness systematically describes patient outcomes, models of care, and how to adjust TMH to different populations and settings.[3]

Clinical Outcome Evidence

More information is available over the last decade to compare TMH services with in-person care (**Table 1**). Telemedicine simulates real-time experiences in terms of audio and video quality at 384+ KBPS. Comparison and noninferiority studies show TMH is as good as in-person care in terms of diagnosis and treatment.[9] Reports include less length of hospitalization,[14,15] more medication use,[14,16] symptom reduction of disorders,[14,16] and therapy judged as evidence-based for posttraumatic stress disorder (PTSD).[17,18]

Child telepsychiatry research is now beyond feasibility, acceptability, and good initial outcomes.[19] For some populations (eg, autism spectrum patients), it might be better than in-person care (**Table 2**).[20] ADHD is being treated as synchronous and asynchronous collaborative care partly using Web-based data systems.[21]

Geriatric data are emerging, but more studies are needed in medicine and TMH.[22] Obstacles include access to service, functional challenges, primary care provider (PCP) attitudes, and lack of psychiatrists,[23] and perhaps what could be called a lack of nursing home "ownership" by any one provider to formalize a clinical approach. Nursing home TMH studies have been effective in terms of informal measures, mainly focusing on depression or dementia, with evaluation more facile and more efficient use of consultant time; some would have gotten no service otherwise.[24] Assessment, cognitive intervention, and outcomes have been similar to in-person and a new

Table 1
Summary of clinical/outcome studies by population age, disorder, or culture

Study	N	Patients	KBPS/Frames	Location	Comments
Geriatric					
Lyketsos et al, 2001	NAP	Geriatric outpatients	NS	USA	Video reduced "unneeded" hospitalizations
Poon et al, 2005	22	Geriatric dementia patients	1.5 Mb	China	Significant, comparable cognitive improvement in video and in-person; high satisfaction; feasible assessment, intervention, and outcomes
Rabinowitz et al, 2010	106	Nursing home residents	384	USA	Reduced travel time, fuel costs, physician travel time, personnel costs
Weiner et al, 2011	85	Adult and geriatric dementia patients	NS	USA	Feasible alternative to face-to-face care in patients with cognitive disorders who live in remote areas
Adult					
Graham et al, 1996	39	Adult outpatients	768	USA	Video reduced "unneeded" hospitalizations
Zaylor et al, 1999	49	Adult depressed or schizoaffective outpatients	128	USA	Video equals in-person in GAF scores at 6-mo follow-up
Hunkeler et al, 2000	302	Adult primary care outpatients	NS	USA	Video by nurses improved depressive symptoms, functioning, and had high satisfaction vs in-person
Ruskin et al, 2004	119	Adult veterans	384	USA	Depression outcomes video and in-person equal as were adherence, satisfaction, cost
Manfredi et al, 2005	15	Adult inmates	384	USA	Feasibility from an urban university to rural jail; less need for inmate transport
Sorvaniemi et al, 2005	60	Adult emergency patients	384	Finland	Minor technical problems occurred Assessment and satisfaction fine
Modai et al, 2006	24/15	Adult outpatients	NS	Israel	Video > in-person cost per service and more hospitalization cost (less available per usual care)

Study	N	Population	Bandwidth	Country	Findings
Urness et al, 2006	39	Adult outpatients	384	Canada	Video < in-person for encouragement; improved outcomes for both
O'Reilly et al, 2007	495	Adult outpatients	384	Canada	Video equal to in-person in outcomes. Satisfaction: 10% less expensive per video
Yellowlees et al, 2011	60	Nonemergency adult patients	NAP	USA	First ATP to demonstrate feasibility
All ages					
De Las Cuevas et al, 2006	130	All ages: outpatients	384–768	Spain	Video equals in-person, including those in remote areas with limited resources
Depression					
Ruskin et al, 2004	119	Adult veterans	384	USA	Video equals in-person for adherence, patient satisfaction, and cost
Fortney et al, 2007	177	Adult outpatients	NS	USA	Video can help adapt collaborative care model in small primary care clinics and symptoms improved more rapidly in intervention group vs usual care group
Moreno et al, 2012	167	Adult patients	NS	USA	Video may close gap in access to culturally and linguistically congruent specialists; improves depression severity, functional ability, and quality of life
Fortney et al, 2013	364	Adult patients	NS	USA	Video collaborative care group > reductions in severity than usual care
Titov et al, 2011	37	Adult patients	384+/Internet	USA	Depression reduction at 3-mo follow-up after 8 weekly CBT sessions
Johnston et al, 2013	129	Adult patients	384+/Internet	USA	Both sole diagnosis and those with comorbid disorders had significant symptom reduction by CBT
Posttraumatic stress disorder or panic disorder					
Bouchard et al, 2004	21	Adults, panic disorder	384/NS	Canada	Video 81% of patients panic-free posttreatment and 91% at 6-mo follow-up via CBT

(continued on next page)

Table 1 (continued)					
Study	N	Patients	KBPS/Frames	Location	Comments
Frueh et al, 2007	38	Adult male veterans, PTSD	384/NS	USA	Video equals in-person in clinical outcomes and satisfaction at 3 mo follow-up. Video < comfort vs in-person in talking with therapist posttreatment and had worse treatment adherence
Morland et al, 2010	125	Adult male veterans, PTSD	384/NS	USA	Video CBGT for PTSD-related anger is feasible for rural/remote veterans, with reduced anger
Germain et al, 2009	48	Adult patients, PTSD	NS	Canada	Video equals in-person in reducing PTSD over 16–25 wk
Hedman et al, 2014	570	Adult patients	384+	Sweden	Video CBT over 6 wk significantly improved symptoms
Fortney et al, 2015	296	Adult patients in VA community clinics, PTSD	384+	USA	Cognitive processing therapy for the treatment group > usual care group over 12-mo follow-up
Substance abuse					
Frueh et al, 2005	14	Adult male outpatients	384/NS	USA	Video had good attendance, comparable attrition, and high satisfaction
Developmental disability					
Szeftel et al, 2012	45	Adolescents	NS	USA	Video led to changed Axis I psychiatric diagnosis (excluding developmental disorders) 70%, and changed medication 82% of patients initially, 41% at 1 y and 46% at 3 y. Video helped PCPs with recommendations for developmental disabilities

Study	N	Population	Connection	Country	Findings
Hispanic					
Moreno et al, 2012	167	Adult patients	NS	USA	Video lessens depression severity and raises functional ability and quality of life; improves access to culturally and linguistically congruent specialists
Chong et al, 2012	167	Adult patients	NS	USA	Video acceptable to low-income depressed Hispanic patients, but its feasibility is questionable
Yellowlees et al, 2013	127	English- and Spanish-speaking patients	NS	USA	ATP equal for English- and Spanish-speaking patients
American Indian					
Shore et al, 2008	53	Male adult patients	NS	USA	Video equals in-person assessment, interaction, and satisfaction; comfort level high and culturally accepted
European					
Mucic, 2010	61	Adult outpatients	2 Mbit (Denmark) 10 Mbit (Sweden)	Denmark	Video improved access, reduced waiting time, and reduced travel to see bilingual psychiatrists; high satisfaction Video preferred via "mother tongue" rather than interpreter-assisted care
Asian					
Ye et al, 2012	19	Adult outpatients	NS	USA	Primary language facilitates expression of feelings, emotional discomfort, or social stressors
Sign language					
Lopez et al, 2004	1	Adult woman, deaf since birth	NS	USA	Video communication fine with American Sign Language interpreter and psychiatric symptoms improved

Abbreviations: GAF, global assessment of function; NAP, not applicable.
Data from Refs.[2,14–18,21,24,65,118–142]

Table 2
Summary of clinical outcome studies for child and adolescent telemental health (not inclusive of satisfaction-only studies)

Citation	Design	Sample	Assessment	Findings
Blackmon et al, 1997	Descriptive	43 children, parents	Routine clinical	All children and 98% of parents report satisfaction equal to in-person care
Elford et al, 2000	RCT	25 children, various diagnoses	Diagnostic interviews	96% concordance between video and in-person evaluations; no difference in satisfaction
Elford et al, 2001	Descriptive	23 children	Routine clinical	Diagnosis and treatment recommendation: equal to usual, in-person care
Glueckauf et al, 2002	Modified RCT Pre vs post	22 adolescents 36 parents	Issue-specific measures of family problems Teen functioning (Social Skills Rating System) Working Alliance Inventory Adherence to appointments	Improvement for problem severity and frequency in all conditions. Therapeutic alliance high; teens rated alliance lower for video
Nelson et al, 2003	RCT	28 children depression	Diagnostic interview and scale	Video = in-person for improvement of depressive symptoms in response to therapy
Myers et al, 2004	Comparative	159 youth (age 3–18)	Comparison of patients evaluated through TMH vs in-person in clinic	Video basically similar to in-person outpatients demographically, clinically, and by reimbursement Video > "adverse case mix"
Greenberg, 2006	Descriptive	NS children 35 PCPs and 12 caregivers	Not specified Focus groups with PCPs, interviews with caregivers	PCP and caregiver satisfied with video; frustrated with limitations of local supports Family caretakers and service providers frustrated with limitations of the video
Myers et al, 2006	Descriptive	115 incarcerated youth (age 14–18)	11-item satisfaction survey	80% successfully prescribed medications and expressed confidence in the psychiatrist by video Youth expressed concerns about privacy

Myers et al, 2007	Descriptive	172 patients (age 2–21) and 387 visits	11-item provider/PCP satisfaction survey	Video to patients at 4 PCP sites: high satisfaction with services; pediatricians > family physicians
Bensink et al, 2008	Descriptive	8 youth Pediatric cancer	Feasibility and satisfaction ratings	Video (by phone) used to families with a child diagnosed with cancer: technically feasible and high parental satisfaction
Clawson et al, 2008	Descriptive	15 youth (age 8 mo to 10 y)	VC feasibility with pediatric feeding disorders	Video feasible and resulted in cost-savings
Fox, 2008	Pre-/post	190 youth in juvenile detention	Goal Attainment Scale	Improvement in the rate of attainment of goals associated with family relations and personality/behavior
Morgan et al, 2008	RCT	27 parents, child age ≤25 mo	Video vs telephone for children with congenital heart disease, anxiety ratings	Video > phone for reducing parent anxiety enabling significantly greater clinical information than phone
Myers et al, 2008	Descriptive	172 patients, parental satisfaction	12-item Parent Satisfaction Survey	Parents with school-aged children endorsed higher satisfaction than those with adolescents. Adherence high for return appointments
Shaikh et al, 2008	Pre-/post	99 youth (age: 1–17)	Diagnostic assessment, weight measurement	Video consultations resulted in substantial changes/additions to diagnoses; subset with repeated consultations led to improved health behaviors (eg, weight maintenance or loss)
Wilkinson et al, 2008	RCT	16 youth (age not reported)	Children with cystic fibrosis, assessment of quality of life, anxiety, depression, service utilization	Video = in-person for quality of life, anxiety levels, depression levels, admissions to hospital or clinic attendances, general practitioner calls, or intravenous antibiotic use between the 2 groups

(continued on next page)

Table 2
(continued)

Citation	Design	Sample	Assessment	Findings
Witmans et al, 2008	Descriptive	89 children sleep disorders	Sleep diary; Childhood Sleep Habits Questionnaire; Pediatric QOL Questionnaire; Client Satisfaction Quest	Patients were very satisfied with the delivery of multidisciplinary pediatric sleep medicine services over video
Yellowlees, 2008	Pre-/post	41 children in rural primary care	CBCL	At 3-mo, improvements in the Affect and Oppositional Domains of the CBCL
Pakyurek et al, 2010	Descriptive	12 children, autism spectrum in primary care	Routine clinical	Video might actually be superior to in-person for consultation
Myers et al, 2010	Descriptive	701 patients, 190 PCPs	Collection of patient demographics, diagnoses, and utilization of services	Video feasible; psychiatrists adjust practice from in-person well
Lau et al, 2011	Descriptive and advanced assessment	45 children/adolescent	Patient characteristics, reason for consultation, and treatment recommendations	Video reaches a variety of children, with consultants providing diagnostic clarification and modifying treatment
Mulgrew et al, 2011	Descriptive	25 children pediatric obesity	Consulting providers' listening skills and ease of instruction to patients; Comfort level of parents in discussing health concerns	Video = in-person for parent satisfaction between consultations for weight management
Stain, 2011	Descriptive and RCT	11 adolescents/young adults	Diagnostic Interview for Psychosis–Diagnostic Module	Strong correlation of assessments done in-person vs video
Storch et al, 2011	RCT	31 children and teenagers	Routine clinical and measures 1. ADIS-IV-C/P 2. Clinician-admin. CY-BOCS 3. Clinical Global Impressions Scales (CGI) 4. Others: obsessive, anxiety, depression inventory	Video was superior to in-person on all primary outcome measures, higher % meeting remission. Consultants providing diagnostic clarification and modifying treatment
Himle et al, 2012	RCT	20 children, Tourette disorder or chronic motor tic disorder	Routine clinical assessment with Yale Global Tic Severity Scale; Parent Tic Questionnaire (Clinician Global Severity & Improvement Scales; CGI-S and CGI-I)	Both treatment delivery modalities resulted in significant tic reduction with no between group differences

Author, year	Study type	Sample	Measures	Results
Jacob et al, 2012	Descriptive	15 children (age 4–18; mean 9.73)	Routine clinical; 12-item Parent Satisfaction Survey	Patient satisfaction high and PCPs found recommendations helpful; outcomes pending on follow-up
Nelson et al, 2012	Service utilization chart review	22 children	Routine clinical	No factor inherent to the video delivery mechanism impeded adherence to national ADHD guidelines
Reese et al, 2012	Pre-/post	8 children; Asian	Routine clinical ADHD	Families reported improved child behavior and decreased parent distress via video format of Group Triple P Positive Parenting Program
Szeftel et al, 2012	Descriptive Chart review	45 patients; 31 ≤ 18 y old	Routine clinical-medication changes, frequency of patient appointments, diagnostic changes, symptom severity and improvement	Video led to changed Axis I psychiatric diagnosis (excluding developmental disorders) 70%, and changed medication 82% of patients initially, 41% at 1 y and 46% at 3 y; Video helped PCPs with recommendations for developmental disabilities
Heitzman-Powell et al, 2013	Pre-/post	NS youth 7 parents	OASIS training program Problem Behavior Recording Incidental Teaching Checklist	Parents increased their knowledge and self-reported implementation of behavioral strategies
Xie et al, 2013	RCT	22 children behavioral disorder	Routine clinical Parent Child Relationship Questionnaire, Vanderbilt Assessment Scales, CGAS, CGIS	Parent training through video was as effective as in-person training and was well accepted by parents
Reese et al, 2013	Descriptive and RCT	21 children; 90% Caucasian	Autism Diagnostic Observation Schedule (ADOS), Module 1 Autism Diagnostic Interview–Revised (ADI-R) Parent satisfaction	No difference in reliability of diagnostic accuracy, ADOS observations, ratings for ADI-R parent report of symptoms, and parent satisfaction

(continued on next page)

Table 2
(continued)

Citation	Design	Sample	Assessment	Findings
Davis et al, 2013	Descriptive	58 youth pediatric obesity	Body mass index 24-h dietary recall ActiGraph - physical activity duration and intensity CBCL Behavioral Pediatrics Feeding Assessment Scale	Both groups showed improvements in body mass index, nutrition, and physical activity, and the groups did not differ significantly on primary outcomes
Freeman et al, 2013	Descriptive	71 youth, diabetes adherence	Baseline metabolic control Conflict Behavior Questionnaire Diabetes Responsibility and Family Conflict Scale–Parent and Youth Working Alliance Inventory	No differences were found in therapeutic alliance between the groups
Hommel et al, 2013	Descriptive	9 youth, irritable bowel disease, adherence	Pill count Pediatric Ulcerative Colitis Activity Index Partial Harvey-Bradshaw Index Feasibility Acceptability Questionnaire	Video improved adherence and cost-savings across patients
Lipana et al, 2013	Descriptive	243 youth, pediatric obesity	Review of medical records	Video > in-person in enhancing nutrition, increasing activity, and decreasing screen time
Rockhill et al, 2013	RCT	223 children with ADHD ± ODD ± Anxiety	Caregiver distress assessed with Patient Health Questionnaire-9, Parenting Stress Index, Caregiver Strain Questionnaire, Family Empowerment Scale	Parents of children with ADHD and a comorbid disorder had significantly more distress than those with ADHD alone

Comer et al, 2014	Pre-/post	5 children (age 4–8)	Behavioral intervention with child, facilitated by parent; OCD rating scale by parent	Child OCD symptoms and diagnoses declined; child global functioning improved
Myers et al, 2015	RCT	223 children with ADHD ± ODD ± anxiety	CBCL screening, DISC-IV diagnostic assessment, ADHD rating scales (inattention, hyperactivity, combined, ODD, role performance) and Columbia Impairment Scale	Caregivers reported significantly greater improvement for inattention, hyperactivity, combined ADHD, ODD, role performance for video vs those treated in primary care. Teachers reported significantly greater improvement in ODD and role performance for video group, too
Tse et al, 2015	RCT subsample	37 caregivers of children with ADHD ± ODD ± anxiety	CaBT delivered via CBCL screening, DISC-IV diagnostic assessment, ADHD rating scales (inattention, hyperactivity, combined, ODD, role performance) and Columbia Impairment Scale	Caregivers reported comparable improvements for children's outcomes whether CaBT video = in person; no improvement in caregivers' distress when CaBT provided through video
Rockhill et al, in press	Descriptive; telepsychiatrists in RCT	223 children with ADHD ± ODD ± anxiety, the telepsychiatrists, and PCPs	Telepsychiatrists' adherence to guidelines-based care, ADHD outcomes by prescriber based on comorbidity status	Telepsychiatrists adhered to guideline-based care, used higher medication doses than PCPs, and their patients reached target of 50% reduction in ADHD symptoms more often than with PCPs

Note: CaBT acronym is not standard, but created to avoid first glance confusion with cognitive behavioral therapy.
Abbreviations: ADIS-IV-C/P, Anxiety Disorders Interview Schedule-IV-Child/Parent Version; CaBT, caregiver behavioral training; CY-BOCS, Children's Yale-Brown Obsessive-Compulsive Scale; DISC, diagnostic interview schedule for children; NS, not specified; OCD, obsessive compulsive disorder; ODD, oppositional defiant disorder; QOL, quality of life; VC, videoconferencing.
Data from Refs.[20,21,62,114,137,143–179]

development is telemonitoring of depression in the home, which facilitates connectedness.[25]

Telepsychiatry has been studied in culturally diverse populations.[3,8,11] The culturally diverse populations include Hispanics/Latinos, Asians, Native American, Eastern Europeans, and other populations (eg, sign language). Language is a key factor, and a common practice is to use interpreters on-site, but sometimes relatives or untrained interpreters miscommunicate medical complaints[26] or de-emphasize information.[27] Ironically, telephone translation may be best when the perceived ethnicity of an interpreter (eg, Asian American) does not match the language spoken (eg, Spanish). Nurses, too, do a little better with concrete medical complaints than capturing the narrative or cultural metaphors.[28]

Special settings and populations also include involuntary, inpatient, and incarcerated—and those in emergency rooms—and adjustments may be needed to ensure quality of care, informed consent, and privacy. Preliminary guidelines for emergency telepsychiatry need to be evaluated[3,29] and a survey describing services of different programs.[30]

Cost and economic outcomes depend on the program and the measures used per a framework,[3] sites/settings (eg, rural),[31] service (eg, ATP as cost-effective),[32] or all of the above.[10] There are different types of cost analyses: cost-offset; cost-minimization; cost-effectiveness; and cost-benefit analysis. Cost studies have differences in data sought, its collection, and how it is analyzed. Savings may be shown versus in-person with high consultation rates, break-even, or other thresholds used (eg, number of consultations per year), or when patient's travel, time, and food are included.

Application to the Clinical Vignette

1. Starting with the correct diagnosis enables specific treatment (first, a selection of psychotherapy instead of medications; second, if medication is needed, an antidepressant rather than a stimulant). In one study, specialists changed the diagnosis and medications in 91% and 57% of cases, respectively, which led to clinical improvements in 56% of cases.[33]
2. Furthermore, provider knowledge and skills improve over time,[34] particularly in rural PCPs,[35] so the impact is directly to the patient seen and indirectly to the population that the PCP serves.
3. Culturally sensitive treatment helps with patient engagement and outcomes, presumably.
4. Finally, a child and adolescent–trained therapist aligns better with teenage patients.

Psychotherapy Evidence Base

The evidence base for therapy by TMH is growing. Initial studies focused on satisfaction, working alliance between the patient-provider, and communication changes,[3,36] and it seemed that no significant problems were arising once the technology bandwidth had increased.[3] Studies in adults generally involve patients with depression and anxiety—often military populations with PTSD—and these studies show comparative efficacy of TMH to in-person services (**Table 3**). Incidentally, a preliminary study on therapeutic alliance and attrition among participants receiving anger management group therapy showed that no significant differences, except a lower alliance with the telegroup leader than those in the in-person condition.[37] The core issues are the impact of technology, patient education, exploring the virtual connection,[38] and adjusting some behaviors (eg, handing a tissue box, sighing, pat on the shoulder, handshake) to verbal statements conveying the same thing (eg, empathy).[36]

Table 3
Summary of clinical outcome studies for telemental health versus in-person psychotherapy (not including satisfaction-only studies)

Study	N	Sample	Intervention	Findings
Bastien et al, 2004	21	Adults, panic disorder	CBT for PD delivered via TMH compared with in-person	Significant reduction in PD symptoms and increase in the number of PD-free patients at follow-up; equivalent to in-person
Grady & Melcer, 2005	81	Active duty/retired personnel and adult family members	Retrospective review of TMH care compared with in-person	Improved patient adherence for both, but better follow-up adherence with TMH
Cluver et al, 2005	9	Adults, terminally ill cancer, adjustment disorder or depression	Psychotherapy alternated between in-person and TMH	Therapy delivery mode made no difference in patient reports; TMH feasible
Frueh et al, 2007	38	Adults, combat related PTSD	CBT for PTSD delivered via TMH compared with in-person	No significant differences in clinical outcomes for TMH vs in-person
Morgan et al, 2008	186	Adult male inmates	Therapy for mood disorder and psychosis via TMH compared with in-person	No significant differences in inmates' satisfaction, postsession mood, or work alliance with the MH professional
Ertelt et al, 2008	128	Adults, DSM-IV criteria for BN or eating disorder	CBT delivered for BN via TMH compared with in-person	Acceptable to participants and equivalent in outcome to therapy delivered in-person
Germain et al, 2009	48	Adults, PTSD	CBT delivered via TMH compared with in-person	Significant decline in symptoms in both groups; effectiveness same
Germain et al, 2010	46	Adults, PTSD	Therapeutic alliance via TMH compared with in-person	Equivalent in both groups on Working Alliance Inventory, Videoconference Telepresence Scale, and other measures
King et al, 2009	37	Adults, opioid-agonist treatment	Addiction counseling delivered via TMH compared with in-person	No significant difference between assistance in both groups

(*continued on next page*)

Table 3
(continued)

Study	N	Sample	Intervention	Findings
Marrone et al, 2009	116	adults, BN	CBT delivered for BN via TMH compared with in-person	Reduction in binge eating at week 6 TMH and week 8 for in-person
Tuerk et al, 2010	47	Adult veterans, PTSD	Prolonged exposure therapy via TMH compared with in-person comparison group	Statistically significant decreases in self-reported pathology for veterans TMH > in-person
Morland et al, 2010	125	Adult male veterans, PTSD	CBT for anger management via TMH compared with in-person	TMH viable; does not compromise a therapist's ability to effectively structure & manage patient care
Gros et al, 2011	89	Veterans, PTSD	Exposure therapy for trauma via telemedicine compared with in-person	Findings support the utility of TMH services to provide effective, evidence-based psychotherapies
Yuen et al, 2013	24	Adults, social anxiety disorder	12 sessions of weekly CBT for generalized social anxiety via TMH	Significant improvements in social anxiety, depression, disability, quality of life, and experiential avoidance
King et al, 2014	85	Adults, substance use	Addiction counseling delivered via TMH compared with in-person	Similar rates of counseling attendance and drug-positive urinalysis results
Khatri et al, 2014	18	Adults, depression and anxiety	CBT for depression anxiety via TMH compared with in-person	Pre-/postintervention scores for depression comparable in-person vs TMH
Fortney et al, 2015	133	Veterans, PTSD	Collaborative care, therapy, psychiatry via TMH compared with in-person	Significant decrease in PTSD symptoms TMH > in-person at 6 and 12 mo. Participation in cognitive processing therapy predicted improvement

Abbreviations: BN, bulimia nervosa; CBT, cognitive behavioral therapy; PD, panic disorder.
Data from Refs.[17,18,39–41,70,134,180–189]

Indeed, TMH sometimes is better,[39–41] which is similar to one child pilot study.[20] Guidelines for therapy by videoconferencing have been explored,[42] as have systematic reviews[43] and broadly defined e-therapy.[44]

HOW CAN CURRENT SYSTEMS OF CARE BE CHANGED AND TELEPSYCHIATRY (EG, USE TECHNOLOGY, GET PAID, AND ADHERE TO REGULATORY ISSUES) BE SUCCESSFULLY IMPLEMENTED?

Overview

The ATA adult guidelines[8] review scope, clinical applications, and clinical/administrative/technical procedures for practice. Assessments (ie, obtaining a history, mental status examination), treatments (eg, psychotherapy), and other factors such as cultural competency are described. Specific groups of patients, difficult settings (eg, emergency department TMH), and ethical considerations are reviewed. The American Association of Child and Adolescent Psychiatry has distributed a "Practice Parameter for Telepsychiatry with Children and Adolescents"[45] and Minimal Standards that focus on specific dimensions (eg, patient appropriateness, sites, therapeutic space, technology, how to select a model of care, and risk management).

Organizational Leadership and Program Evaluation

Organizational leadership and program evaluation have become increasingly important to meet program, patient, provider, and externally driven (eg, Joint Commission)[46] needs; it is key to preserve the standard of care and use best practices. Assessment typically includes satisfaction, technology, cost, clinical measures, and process of care with an iterative feedback loop for quality improvement. Financial feasibility is assessed based on technical cost, patient volume, appointment adherence, payment model (eg, pay for time whether show or not), patient mix in terms of complexity, payer or payers mix, and other issues. Studies are now being conducted using economic modeling,[47,48] clinical encounter costing and data sets,[49] health care reform,[50] health care costs with changes in health risks among employers of all sizes,[51] and prototypes of existing health systems (eg, Veterans Affairs).[52]

Technology

The key issue for many providers is determining whether to pick a telemedicine group or technology-only support system. Full commercial models hire clinicians and provide patient contracts, hardware, software, technical support, and business support (more costly). Business support provides the secure Web site with software and the clinician/group does the rest; security of the system is the central factor in this arrangement (less costly). The terms of service and level of equipment vary widely. A reasonable analogy for this is the difference between an in-person private, solo practice versus a group practice with organizational infrastructure. Generally, the more aspects of the TMH that providers feel comfortable managing, the less support they will need. Unanticipated events are now very infrequent, but planning ahead for disruption in connection is advisable (range from reboot, to phone alternative, to other).

The ATA Videoconferencing Guidelines[8] review organizations' technical responsibilities to ensure the equipment readiness, safety, effectiveness, security of data, connectivity, and compliance with legal/regulatory guidelines. Policies and procedures are recommended for a wide range of functions, including informed consent, privacy, clinical care, staff roles, evaluation/quality improvement, and education/training.

Credentialing, Licensing, and Malpractice

Centers for Medicare & Medicaid Services (CMS) regulatory requirements include a mechanism for hospitals and critical access hospitals to use proxy credentialing, whose responsibility it is (eg, distance site), and written agreement requirements (eg, code series 42 CFR. (Code of Federal Regulations) 48X). Sometimes, privileging is required at the distant-site hospital providing the telemedicine services, and that has its own requirements. Finally, an organization must attend to telehealth standards, clinical guidelines, and other Joint Commission specifications on credentialing and privileging, environment of care, patient rights, confidentiality and privacy, training, and preparation. Other issues vary per location and population, like licensing (usually in the state where the patient is), definition of "in-person," informed consent, and scope of practice. Risk management issues related to telepsychiatry have been explored.[53]

Reimbursement

A review of reimbursement in the United States notes that private payers have administrative rules regarding telehealth reimbursement that are barriers to services and reimbursement, and that some providers would benefit from being better informed about billing and coding for telehealth services and how to advocate for telehealth services reimbursement.[54] Key factors are the sites involved (eg, critical access hospital; federally qualified health center; rural health clinic), current procedural terminology (CPT) coding (usually same as in-person unless a rural site designation specifier is used), and ensuring an eligible practitioner (ie, medical doctor, nurse practitioner, social worker; registered nurse).

Application to the Clinical Vignette

1. Technology support for care is from technology-only support to "wrap-around" support (including hiring, business, and other dimensions).
2. Clinicians must fully understand the legal and regulatory aspects of in-person care, learn the new specification for emerging technologies, and apply knowledge to unforeseen situations that may arise in clinical care (eg, patient's use of text or e-mail to signal life-threatening behavior).
3. Federal, state, private company, and other specifications are crucial to review to provide care and bill legally.
4. For clinic populations with indigent, high proportions of patients with minimal reimbursement by the payers, accommodations for remuneration are critical to enlist providers (eg, balancing a payer mix, contracts with rural hospital networks to reimburse providers whether time is used or not).

MODELS OF CARE: THE E-CONTINUUM TOWARD INTEGRATED AND STEPPED CARE FOR DIFFERENT POPULATIONS, DISORDERS, AND TREATMENTS
Models of Care: How to Select Them and Impact on Evaluation

A summary of TMH models of care reviewed the pros and cons of each model.[3,7,55]

Low intensity

- Case review of diagnosis and follow-up after a discussion[56]
- Telepsychiatric consultation to primary care help to align PCPs' diagnosis or diagnoses and medication treatments,[33] with an indirect benefit over time of improving PCPs' knowledge and skills[34,35]
- In-person, telephone, or e-mail doctor-to-doctor "curbside" consultations may arise during patient care in day-to-day practice[57] and meet approximately 33%

of informational PCPs' needs "in-time."[58] Both telephone and face-to-face contacts occur; the former are purposeful and timely, and the latter are random and prone to delays. More recently, e-mail consultations that do not include patient evaluations are valuable, inexpensive, brief, and more readily available,[59] including a multispecialty phone and e-mail consultation system to PCPs for the care of adults and children with developmental disabilities.[60]

- Cultural consultation to rural primary care using telemedicine[61]

Moderate intensity

- An integrated program of mental health screening, therapy on site, telepsychiatric consultation (phone, e-mail, or video), continuing medical education, and staff training on screening questionnaires has improved patient outcomes and site-based staff skills.[62]
- A randomized controlled trial (RCT) for depression in adults using disease management and telepsychiatric consultation versus usual care over a period of 12 months improved the care of both groups; the latter group benefited from the Hawthorne effect and providers' application of skills from the intervention group.[63]
- ATP is feasible, valid, reliable, and cost-effective in English- and Spanish-speaking patients in primary care.[2,32,61] (Similar methods are used in radiology, dermatology, ophthalmology, cardiology, and pathology.) One ATP model uses a basic questionnaire for screening by the provider of the patient, video capture of that interview, and uploading of patient histories for a remote psychiatrist to review in a HIPAA-adherent manner.[64]

High intensity

- Collaborative care, which has now been more formally applied to telemedicine,[9,16,65] has encouraging results. The virtual collaborative care team was able to produce better outcomes than the traditional gold-standard methodology of primary care psychiatry.[65]
- Child collaborative care for children with ADHD at a distance used STP and ATP (ie, Web-based approaches for further training, data collection, and monitoring, which showed positive clinical outcomes).[21]

Integrated Care

Integrated care and stepped care models provide efficient expertise to the point of service; TMH further enhances that. The core characteristics of integrated care are (1) responsibility, decision-making, and oversight of patient care; (2) colocation of services, both literally and virtually, that applies to both inpatient and outpatient sector care; (3–5) integrated funding, evaluation, and outcome measurement; (6) an e-platform; and (7) reimbursement, preferably aligned (eg, a capitated or sole Medicare population) rather than unaligned (ie, mixed populations). Stepped care models may be the most cost-effective models in the health system, where the effectiveness of the intervention is maximized by making the best use of resources adequately available at the right time.[66,67]

Patient-Centered Medical Home

These services are in development and need to be better studied, although costs are dramatically decreasing. The patient-centered medical home (PCMH) is a concept founded on the presence of inadequate treatment in primary care and an inability to access needed services.[68] Under oversight of the PCP, PCMH allows telepsychiatric input at home and has been shown to improve patient care and health,[69,70] including desk-mounted video systems convenient for patients with cancer to get therapy.

Internet or Web-Based Care

Patients benefit from tools for self-directed habit, lifestyle or illness changes, prompts for appointments, and evidence-based treatments via the Internet (eg, anxiety disorders). "Fear Fighter," a computer-guided self-exposure approach to treat phobia/panic, fills a hole when qualified and trained therapists are scarce.[71] "PTSD Coach" is designed to help veterans learn about, manage symptoms, and augment MH interventions after trauma.[72] Recent patient-centered strategies that increase patient compliance are simple e-mail, telephone, or short messaging service (SMS) reminders that have been shown to be an effective way to support patient attendance to follow-up appointments.[73,74] Internet-based cognitive behavioral therapy (ICBT) interventions are as effective as traditional in-person care and a 30-month follow-up study for treatment of social phobia and panic disorder.[75,76] ICBT combined with monitoring by text messages (mobile CBT) and minimal therapist support by e-mail and telephone help prevent depression relapse.[77] Interestingly, a review of virtual reality reports it has been used in the treatment of many MH conditions, including eating disorders, autism spectrum disorders, pain management, and stroke.[78] Finally, a schizophrenic can create a virtual representation of the scary voices using an avatar, then work with a therapist in real time to manage the avatar speaking the voices.[79]

Caregivers, too, may benefit by the use of telecommunication technology. A review of Internet-based interventions for medical and MH disorders showed that approximately two-thirds of open or RCTs reduced stress and improved quality of life—at least significantly in terms of specific measured outcomes.[80] Family caregivers located in rural areas found e-health support to be beneficial in comparison with conventional caregiver support, by using interactive communities, bulletin board chatting, and therapy groups.[81] Patient populations included MH (dementia, schizophrenia, anorexia) and medical (older adults/aging, heart transplant, traumatic brain injury, hip fracture, cancer, stroke).[81] Caregivers' outcomes improved, and they are satisfied and comfortable with support services delivered by cell phones.[82]

WHAT CAN BE LEARNED AND WHAT MUST BE CONTENDED WITH, IN TERMS OF EMERGING MODELS OF E-CARE AND COMMUNICATION?

The traditional models of care have been in-person, STP, and more recently, ATP; that is really only the beginning, and emerging models are sprouting quickly. In general, that is how technology affects basic clinical practice. Its impact on clinical boundaries, communication, and engagement has been under review.[83] The American Psychiatric Association has a guideline on e-prescribing.[84] The effect on professionalism and education and training of the next generations has been explored.[85]

Telepsychiatry can extend beyond videoconferencing modalities to other mechanisms, including the following:

- New digital communication from one user to another user using standard protocols: e-mail, SMS text messaging, multiple messaging service (MMS) messaging, instant messaging
- New digital communication from one user to another user using proprietary networks: Twitter direct messages, Facebook Messenger, Epic MyChart electronic medical record messaging, My HealtheVet electronic medical record messaging
- New social media communication platforms that transmit from one to many users: Internet forums, Facebook pages and profiles, Twitter streams

Digital Communication—e-Mail, Messaging Services, Web Sites, and Online Profiles

Online digital information is an important source of information for today's online user. As of January 2014, 90% of adults have a cell phone and 58% have a smartphone.[86] In the public health space, 35% of US adults have gone online to research health information and learn from other patients' experiences.[87] Aside from entertainment purposes, those aged 13 to 54 years in the United States use most of their smartphone time to socialize and interact with others manage themselves, including their health, and research information.[88]

This finding has implications for psychiatrists. First, online messaging is required for providers caring for Medicare and Medicaid patients under federal electronic medical record guidelines as required by meaningful use stage 2 by 2014.[89] In fact, the government's financial incentives and penalties program requires more than 5% of unique patients to be sending secure messages to clinicians, thus incentivizing the use of messaging. Although the general public may use e-mail, SMS, and MMS, these do not, by default, provide HIPAA-compliant encryption.

There are also implications for patient-centered Googling and other Internet searches in which clinicians search for publicly available information about their patient. There are literature reports on how checking Facebook has helped resolve emergencies and aid in forensic psychiatric evaluations.[90] Psychiatrists, in general, should consider their intentions in searching for such information, whether it is for patient care purposes, what the effect may be, and the value or risk for treatment.[91] Indeed, the patient's best interests must be kept in mind.

Social Media Communication

Advantages of social media

The modern psychiatrist can take advantage of, but also be cautious with, the use of social media by patients. All ages are using social media for a variety of applications, sense of being heard, consumer health social networking (CHSN), and other health complaints (eg, suicidal ideation).[92] Child and adolescent populations, also known as digital natives, are more adept at using social media, and multiple social media channels can assist in destigmatizing the conversation over mental health. Analogous to sexual health and high-risk behaviors, users may want a credible source of reliable information that is personalized and maintains their anonymity and confidentiality.[93] More treatments are being done by mobile phones.[94]

Social networks also enhance social connectedness. These modalities help boost social support for cancer survivors,[95] new mothers' well-being,[96] and older adult users and the elderly with family and friends.[97,98] Social networks also provide an access point for those reluctant to seek help in-person. For instance, 33% of soldiers unwilling to speak to an in-person counselor were willing to use technology-based social networks for mental health care.[99] Of young college students, 68% indicated they would use the Internet for mental health support, and 94% of participants with mental illnesses used social networking sites.[100] Finally, social networks also provide a modality for those who cannot access traditional mental health, such as those with mental illness in rural areas.[101]

Cautions about, and guidelines for, social media use

Preliminary guidelines discuss concerns about patient privacy, professional image, confidentiality, and defined expectations for use in general[102,103] and for social media.[104] Providers should consider the professional and ethical responsibilities for routes of communication, absences, or any other changes in accessibility in advance.

Guidelines for social media use generally include discussions with the patient in advance, as part of the informed consent process:

- Using e-mail, text, instant messaging, only for patients who maintain in-person follow-up
- Consider the pros and cons of gathering information about patients: intent, use, and implications
- Psychoeducation with online educational resources with patients: accuracy and reputable?
- Physician-produced blogs, microblogs, and comments: "pause before posting" and "step back" to consider what is conveyed to the public about the physician and the profession
- Digital venues for communicating with colleagues about patient care: ensure security/privacy and follow policies of institution

Many organizations have specifically made recommendations about professionalism and social media (eg, The American College of Physicians, Canadian Medical Association, and British Medical Association),[105,106] focusing on communication with patients, gathering information, online education, and other topics. Separation of personal and professional life is suggested,[107,108] if it can be done.[109] In fact, physicians should assume that one's private profile can be found. The *Journal of Medical Internet Research* provided guidelines based on a review of over 100 articles, Web sites, policies, and reports[110]:

- Maintain professionalism at all times—follow institutional policies, "assume that all information exchanged is public and posted in a medium no different than a newspaper," and maintain a disclaimer.
- Be authentic, have fun, and do not be afraid—"the only way to create meaningful relationships over social media is to be genuine."
- Ask for help—pay attention to "how people interact (eg, etiquette)" and "mimic the social media service and community's practices (so long as they are professional)."
- Focus, grab attention, engage, and take action—based on the Dragonfly model, social media users must "identify a single, concrete, and measurable goal for using social media"; "make others look at content by saying or posting something interesting"; "foster personal connections by discussing…interests with like-minded people"; and "enable and empower others."

"Friend" requests on sites like Facebook have resulted in decidedly mixed views: shall we engage or exercise caution?[111–113] If a provider engages patients with social media, the provider may consider having both a private and a professional account[112] for privacy and maintaining therapeutic boundaries. The provider may also consider how parties will interpret the "friend" connection and compare it to a true friendship, where a more equal exchange of private information and confidences would normally exist.[112] Even with private accounts, privacy settings may be insufficient to prevent certain elements from being visible publicly.

Requests for contact between visits (eg, texts, Facebook visits) are increasing because of the time spent online.[83] Asynchronous written or e-mail language does not have nuances with pitch modulations, changing volume, meaningful pauses, and accompanying body language; this may lead to misinterpretations and have unexpected consequences. E-mails should be sent during regular working hours to attend to expectation and boundary issues.[83]

Additional guidelines are available for addressing youth patients[114] and addressing privacy issues.[115] Additional ethics codes from the American Psychological

Association, American Counseling Association, and the American Psychiatric Association are available for mental health professionals on managing ethical concerns and avoid ethical violations.

The future virtual presence for doctors

Leading physicians in the digital health space advocate for the profession and individual physicians to own their virtual presence. They recommend maintaining profiles for LinkedIn professional networking platform, Facebook social networking platform, Doximity physician communication platform, and Healthgrades physician rating network. In fact, maintaining an online presence is so important that leading institutions are implementing medical school curriculum in social media communication, patient engagement, and Wikipedia article management. Avoiding online media puts the health care practitioner at risk in allowing others to spread misinformation[85,86] and jeopardizing public health and safety.[87]

Application to the Clinical Vignette

1. Models allow versatile care approaches.
2. TMH disseminates expertise "in-time" and in context to the patient and provider's needs.
3. Patient empowerment is enhanced by applying user-friendly, everyday technologies to health care: better access, more options, and a sense of confidence or self-efficacy (akin to what "good education" does for novice learners like medical students).

DISCUSSION, CLINICAL VIGNETTE PART II, AND SUMMARY

Today, TMH services are unquestionably effective in most regards, although more analysis is needed. They are effective for diagnosis and assessment, across many populations (adult, child, geriatric, and ethnic), and in disorders in many settings (emergency, home health) are comparable to in-person care, and complement other services in primary care. Additional evaluation (ie, randomized trials, lack of inferiority designs) would be helpful for some treatments (eg, psychotherapy), populations (eg, child and adolescent, geriatric), disorders (eg, anxiety, substance use, psychotic), and settings (eg, emergency room, schools, home MH).

Several findings from the evidence base of studies are quite interesting. First, it is clear that TMH is a versatile way to increase access and empower patients, similarly when applied to systems of care it helps providers and administrators integrate care. Second, TMH can be done in a variety of e-models (e-mail, telephone, video, and other asynchronous options), and it can facilitate clinical care models (eg, collaborative care into services in primary care settings). Care more thoughtfully conducted, with attention to culture, diversity, and language "better" care at a distance nationally and internationally—this is now within reach.

It has been seen for some populations that it is easier or more conducive for some patients (eg, autism spectrum, home-based patients with anxiety),[20] and it may have distinct advantages to in-person care as evidenced by the therapy results.[39–41] The authors suggest 3 factors have a hand in this: (1) the extra preparation of TMH service (consent, discussions) may result in readiness for treatment; (2) the hands-on approach by the interdisciplinary team (eg, telemedicine coordinator, nurse, others) may enhance the therapeutic alliance; and (3) access to treatment, in general, and in-time may empower the patient.

Finally, although inconceivable to everyone in the 1990s, when systematic application and evaluation of TMH began, it may be a tipping point in which all the little things that

TMH makes possible start adding up, and changing the framework and approach to health care: as one moves from a new way to practice and a new standard of practice.[115] The major results of the Children's ADHD Telemental Health Treatment Study[19] show better dissemination of evidence-based treatments and new modalities of treatment of many psychiatric disorders delivered at a distance can be better disseminated—this would apply *even if* the patient is not particularly geographically isolated. A new way to practice is "hybrid models care," which uses in-person and technology-delivered care,[115,116] and by implication, multiple levels of technological complexity (ie, from low-intensity e-mail and phone to high intensity videoconferencing).

CLINICAL VIGNETTE

Treatment Plan

1. *Evaluation for ADHD with Conner's scales by parents and teacher were done 3 weeks later; the scores were at 68 (parent version; borderline) and 50 (teacher version; below diagnostic threshold). This was consistent with the clinician impression that ADHD was not the primary problem, which seemed localized to home.*

2. *Short-term therapy by a child psychiatry fellow, with supervision from faculty, was obtained (eg, 6 sessions over 12 weeks when father was in town); it was fortuitous that the fellow was Latino American, and she eagerly sought the opportunity for a brief therapy case in Spanish. The goals were to provide supportive therapy for depression, to engage father with the son's life (time together, more communication), and work on codiscipline by mother and father on key issues (ie, so father is not the "bad" person).*

3. *Culture and language integration: the telemedicine-based psychotherapy allowed the patient to speak in the primary language, which along with supervision on cultural themes per DSM-5[117] eliminated a communication issue as a reason for errant diagnosis. The use of the primary language also increases rapport, adds meaning, and allows full range of expression on sentimental themes.[27,28]*

Follow-up: An immediate medication prescription may have been misfired on cases like this by a PCP. At 2-month follow-up, the patient's behavior and mood at home were better. There was an issue, though, with the patient's interest in texting the provider and bringing up her Facebook page. The main issues here are

4. *The clinician should evaluate the impact of technology on clinical issues including, but not limited to, safety, boundaries, and professionalism—and spell out expectations and limitations during informed consent discussions and in accompanying documents.*

5. *The clinician should evaluate the need/preference for synchronous versus asynchronous modes of communication for the care participants—and should educate others before and as opportunities arise on such issues.*

ACKNOWLEDGMENTS

American Telemedicine Association, the Mental Health Interest Group, the Department of Psychiatry and Behavioral Sciences at the University of Southern California, and the Department of Psychiatry and Behavioral Sciences at UC Davis are gratefully acknowledged.

REFERENCES

1. Akinci F, Patel PM. Quality improvement in healthcare delivery utilizing the patient-centered medical home model. Hosp Top 2014;92(4):96–104.
2. Yellowlees PM, Odor A, Iosif A, et al. Transcultural psychiatry made simple: asynchronous telepsychiatry as an approach to providing culturally relevant care. Telemed J E Health 2013;19(4):1–6.

3. Hilty DM, Ferrer D, Callahan EJ, et al. The effectiveness of telemental health: a 2013 review. Telemed J E Health 2013;19(6):444–54.
4. Davis MH, Everett A, Kathol R, et al. American Psychiatric Association ad hoc work group report on the integration of psychiatry and primary care, 2011. Available at: http://naapimha.org/wordpress/media/Integration-of-Psychiatry-and-Primary-Care.pdf. Accessed April 1, 2015.
5. Yellowlees P. Your guide to E-Health: third millennium medicine on the internet. Queensland, Australia: University of Queensland PR; 2001.
6. Hilty DM, Green J, Nasatir-Hilty SE, et al. Mental healthcare to rural and other underserved primary care settings: benefits of telepsychiatry, integrated care, stepped care and interdisciplinary team models. J Nursing Care, in press.
7. World Health Organization. Telemedicine opportunities and developments in member states. Results of the second global survey on eHealth. Geneva (Switzerland): WHO Press; 2011.
8. Yellowlees PM, Shore JH, Roberts L, et al. Practice guidelines for videoconferencing-based telemental health. Telemed J E Health 2010;16(10): 1074–89.
9. Richardson L, McCauley E, Katon W. Collaborative care for adolescent depression: a pilot study. Gen Hosp Psychiatry 2009;31:36–45.
10. Shore JH, Mishkind MC, Bernard J, et al. A lexicon of assessment and outcome measures for telemental health. Telemed J E Health 2013;3:282–92.
11. Hilty DM, Yellowlees PM, Nasatir SE, et al. Program evaluation and practical, step-by-step program modification in telemental health. Behavioral telehealth series volume 1—clinical video conferencing: program development and practice. New York: Springer Press; 2014. p. 105–34.
12. Hilty DM, Srinivasan M, Xiong G, et al. Lessons from psychiatry and psychiatric education for medical learners and teachers. Int Rev Psychiatry 2013;25: 329–37.
13. Rogers EM. Diffusion of innovations. 4th edition. New York: Free Press; 1995.
14. O'Reilly R, Bishop J, Maddox K, et al. Is telepsychiatry equivalent to face to face psychiatry: results from a randomized controlled equivalence trial. Psychiatr Serv 2007;258:836–43.
15. De Las Cuevas C, Arrendondo MT, Cabrera MF, et al. Randomized controlled trial of telepsychiatry through videoconference versus face-to-face conventional psychiatric treatment. Telemed J E Health 2006;12:341–50.
16. Fortney JC, Pyne JM, Edlund MJ, et al. A randomized trial of telemedicine-based collaborative care for depression. J Gen Intern Med 2007;22(8):1086–93.
17. Morland LA, Greene CJ, Rosen CS, et al. Telemedicine for anger management therapy in a a rural population of combat veterans with posttraumatic stress disorder: a randomized noninferiority trial. J Clin Psychiatry 2010;71:855–63.
18. Frueh BC, Monnier J, Yim E, et al. Randomized trial for post-traumatic stress disorder. J Telemed Telecare 2007;13:142–7.
19. Myers KM, Palmer NB, Geyer JR. Research in child and adolescent telemental health. Child Adolesc Psychiatr Clin N Am 2011;20(1):155–71.
20. Pakyurek M, Yellowlees PM, Hilty DM. The child and adolescent telepsychiatry consultation: can it be a more effective clinical process for certain patients than conventional practice? Telemed J E Health 2010;16(3):289–92.
21. Myers KM, Vander Stoep A, Zhou C, et al. Effectiveness of a telehealth service delivery model for treating attention-deficit hyperactivity disorder: results of a community-based randomized controlled trial. J Am Acad Child Adolesc Psychiatry 2015;54(4):263–74.

22. Botsis T, Demiris G, Peterson S, et al. Home Telecare technologies for the elderly. J Telemed Telecare 2008;14:333–7.
23. Sheeran T, Dealy J, Rabinowitz T. Geriatric telemental health. In: Myers K, Turvey CL, editors. Telemental health. New York: Elsevier; 2013. p. 171–95.
24. Rabinowitz T, Murphy KM, Amour JL, et al. Benefits of a telepsychiatry consultation service for rural nursing home residents. Telemed J E Health 2010;16(1): 34–40.
25. Sheeran T, Rabinowitz T, Lotterman J, et al. Feasibility and impact of telemonitor-based depression care management for geriatric homecare patients. Telemed J E Health 2011;17:620–6.
26. Brooks TR. Pitfalls in communication with Hispanic and African-American patients: do translators help or harm? J Natl Med Assoc 1992;84(11):941.
27. Brua C. Role-blurring and ethical grey zones associated with lay interpreters: three case studies. Community Med 2008;5(1):73.
28. Elderkin-Thompson V, Silver RC, Waitzkin H. When nurses double as interpreters: a study of Spanish-speaking patients in a US primary care setting. Soc Sci Med 2001;52:1343–58.
29. Yellowlees PM, Burke MM, Marks SL, et al. Emergency telepsychiatry. J Telemed Telecare 2008;14:277–81.
30. Williams M, Pfeffee M, Boyle, et al. Telepsychiatry in the emergency department: Overview and case studies. California HealthCare Foundation, 2010. Available at: http://www.chcf.org/publications/2009/12/telepsychiatry-in-the-emergency-department-overview-and-case-studies. Accessed April 1, 2015.
31. Shore JH, Brooks E, Savin DM, et al. An economic evaluation of telehealth data collection with rural populations. Psychiatr Serv 2007;58(6):830–5.
32. Butler TN, Yellowlees P. Cost analysis of store-and-forward telepsychiatry as a consultation model for primary care. Telemed J E Health 2012;18(1):74–7.
33. Hilty DM, Marks SL, Urness D, et al. Clinical and educational applications of telepsychiatry: a review. Can J Psychiatry 2004;49(1):12–23.
34. Hilty DM, Yellowlees PM, Nesbitt TS. Evolution of telepsychiatry to rural sites: change over time in types of referral and PCP knowledge, skill, and satisfaction. Gen Hosp Psychiatry 2006;28(5):367–73.
35. Hilty DM, Nesbitt TS, Kuenneth TA, et al. Telepsychiatric consultation to primary care: rural vs. suburban needs, utilization and provider satisfaction. J Rural Health 2007;23(2):163–5.
36. Hilty DM, Nesbitt TS, Marks SL, et al. How telepsychiatry affects the doctor-patient relationship: communication, satisfaction, and additional clinically relevant issues. Prim Psychiatr 2002;9(9):29–34.
37. Greene CJ, Morland LA, Macdonald A, et al. How does tele-mental health affect group therapy process? Secondary analysis of a noninferiority trial. J Consult Clin Psychol 2010;78(5):746–50.
38. Glueck D. Establishing therapeutic rapport in telemental health. In: Myers K, Turvey CL, editors. Telemental health. New York: Elsevier; 2013. p. 29–46.
39. Grady BJ, Melcer T. A retrospective evaluation of TeleMental Healthcare services for remote military populations. Telemed J E Health 2005;11(5):551–8.
40. Tuerk PW, Yoder M, Ruggiero KJ, et al. A pilot study of prolonged exposure therapy for posttraumatic stress disorder delivered via telehealth technology. J Trauma Stress 2010;23(1):116–23.
41. Fortney JC, Pyne JM, Kimbrell TA, et al. Telemedicine-based collaborative care for posttraumatic stress disorder: a randomized clinical trial. JAMA Psychiatry 2015;72(1):58–67.

42. Nelson EL, Duncan AB, Lillis T. Special considerations for conducting psycho-therapy via videoconferencing. In: Myers K, Turvey CL, editors. Telemental health: clinical, technical and administrative foundations for evidenced-based practice. San Francisco (CA): Elsevier; 2013. p. 295–314.

43. Backhaus A, Agha Z, Maglione ML, et al. Videoconferencing psychotherapy: a systematic review. Psychol Serv 2012;9(2):111–31.

44. Postel MG, de Haan HA, de Jong CA. E-Therapy for mental health problems: a systematic review. Telemed J E Health 2008;14(7):707–14.

45. Myers K, Cain S, Work Group on Quality Issues, American Academy of Child and Adolescent Psychiatry Staff. Practice Parameter for Telepsychiatry with Children and Adolescents. J Am Acad Child Adolesc Psychiatry 2008;47(12): 1468–83.

46. Joint Commission and Joint Commission International. Available at: http://www.jcrinc.com/. Accessed April 1, 2015.

47. Crane M. Exploring telehealth models. Med Econ 2014;91(14):17–20.

48. Mazzolini C. Telemedicine's next big leap. Med Econ 2013;90(20):64–6.

49. Barker G, McNeill KM, Krupinski EA, et al. Clinical encounters costing for tele-medicine services. Telemed J E Health 2004;10(3):381–8.

50. Thompson S, Kohli R, Jones C, et al. Evaluating health care delivery reform ini-tiatives in the face of "cost disease". Popul Health Manag 2015;18(1):6–14.

51. Musich S, White J, Hartley SK, et al. A more generalizable method to evaluate changes in health care costs with changes in health risks among employers of all sizes. Telemed J E Health 2014;17(5):297–305.

52. Grady B. A comparative cost analysis of an integrated military telemental health-care service. Telemed J E Health 2002;8(3):293–300.

53. Cash C. Telepsychiatry and risk management. Innov Clin Neurosci 2011;8: 26–30.

54. Antoniotti NM, Drude KP, Rowe N. Private payer telehealth reimbursement in the United States. Telemed J E Health 2014;20(6):539–43.

55. Hilty DM, Yellowlees PM, Cobb HC, et al. Models of telepsychiatric consultation-liaison service to rural primary care. Psychosomatics 2006;47(2):152–7.

56. Dobbins ML, Roberts N, Vicari SK, et al. The consulting conference: a new model of collaboration for child psychiatry and primary care. Acad Psychiatry 2011;35:260–2.

57. Manian FA, Janssen DA. Curbside consultations. JAMA 1996;275:145–6.

58. Dee C, Blazek R. Information needs of the rural physician. A descriptive study. Bull Med Libr Assoc 1993;81:259–64.

59. Bergus GR, Sinift D, Randall CS, et al. Use of an e-mail curbside consultation service by family physicians. J Fam Pract 1998;47(5):357–60.

60. Hilty DM, Ingraham RL, Yang RP, et al. Multispecialty phone and email consul-tation to primary care providers for patients with developmental disabilities in ru-ral California. Telemed J E Health 2004;10:413–21.

61. Yellowlees PM, Marks SL, Hilty DM, et al. Using e-health to enable culturally appropriate mental health care in rural areas. Telemed J E Health 2008;14(5): 486–92.

62. Yellowlees PM, Hilty DM, Marks SL, et al. A retrospective analysis of child and adolescent e-mental health. J Am Acad Child Adolesc Psychiatry 2008;47(1):1–5.

63. Hilty DM, Marks SL, Wegeland JE, et al. A randomized controlled trial of disease management modules, including telepsychiatric care, for depression in rural pri-mary care. Psychiatry 2007;4(2):58–65.

64. Yellowlees PM, Odor A, Patrice K, et al. PsychVACS: a system for asynchronous telepsychiatry. Telemed J E Health 2011;17(4):299–303.

65. Fortney JC, Pyne JM, Mouden SP, et al. Practice-based versus telemedicine-based collaborative care for depression in rural federally qualified health centers: a pragmatic randomized comparative effectiveness trial. Am J Psychiatry 2013;170(4):414–25.

66. Haaga DA. Introduction to the special section on stepped care models in psychotherapy. J Consult Clin Psychol 2000;68:547–8.

67. van't Veer-Tazelaar N, van Marwijk H, van Oppen P, et al. Prevention of anxiety and depression in the age group of 75 years and over: a randomized controlled trial testing the feasibility and effectiveness of a generic stepped care program among elderly community residents at high risk of developing anxiety and depression versus usual care. BMC Public Health 2006;1:186.

68. Rosenthal TC. The medical home: growing evidence to support a new approach to primary care. J Am Board Fam Med 2008;21(5):427–40.

69. Hollingsworth JM, Saint S, Hayward RA, et al. Specialty care and the patient-centered medical home. Med Care 2011;49(1):4–9.

70. Cluver JS, Schuyler D, Frueh BC, et al. Remote psychotherapy for terminally ill cancer patients. J Telemed Telecare 2005;11:157–9.

71. Kenwright M, Liness S, Marks I, et al. Reducing demands on clinicians by offering computer-aided self-help for phobia/panic. Feasibility study. Br J Psychiatry 2001;179(5):456–9.

72. National Center for Telehealth and Technology. PTSD Coach [Internet]. PTSD Coach | t2health, 2013. Available at: http://www.t2.health.mil/apps/ptsd-coach. Accessed April 1, 2015.

73. Luxton DD, McCann RA, Bush NE, et al. mHealth for mental health: integrating smartphone technology in behavioral healthcare. Prof Psychol Res Pract 2011; 42(6):505–12.

74. Kunigiri G, Gajebasia N, Sallah D. Improving attendance in psychiatric outpatient clinics by using reminders. J Telemed Telecare 2014;20(8):464–7.

75. Carlbring P, Nordgren LB, Furmark T, et al. Long-term outcome of Internet-delivered cognitive-behavioural therapy for social phobia: a 30-month follow-up. Behav Res Ther 2009;47(10):848–50.

76. Kiropoulos LA, Klein B, Austin DW, et al. Is internet-based CBT for panic disorder and agoraphobia as effective as face-to-face CBT? J Anxiety Disord 2008;22(8):1273–84.

77. Kok G, Bockting C, Berger H, et al. Mobile cognitive therapy: adherence and acceptability of an online intervention in remitted recurrently depressed patients. Internet Interv 2014;1(2):65–73.

78. Yellowlees PM, Holloway KM, Parish MB. Therapy in virtual environments—clinical and ethical issues. Telemed J E Health 2012;18(7):558–64.

79. Leff J, Williams G, Huckvale M, et al. Avatar therapy for persecutory auditory hallucinations: what is and how does it work? Psychosis 2014;6(2):166–76.

80. Hu C, Kung S, Rummans TA, et al. Reducing caregiver stress with internet-based interventions: a systematic review of open-label and randomized controlled trials. J Am Med Inform Assoc 2015;22:e194–209.

81. Blusi M, Dalin R, Jong M, et al. The benefits of e-health support for older family caregivers in rural areas. J Telemed Telecare 2014;20(2):63–9.

82. Chi NC, Demiris G. A systematic review of telehealth tools and interventions to support family caregivers. J Telemed Telecare 2015;21(1):37–44.

83. Hilty DM, Belitsky R, Cohen MB, et al. Impact of the information age residency training: the impact of the generation gap. Acad Psychiatry 2015;39:104–7.

84. APA Electronic Prescribing Guideline. Available at: http://www.psych.org/practice/managing-a-practice/electronic-prescribing. Accessed April 1, 2015.

85. DeJong SM, Benjamin S, Anzia JA, et al. Professionalism and the internet in psychiatry: what to teach and how to teach it. Acad Psychiatry 2012;36(5):356–62.

86. Pew Research Center; 2013. Internet survey. Available at: http://www.pewinternet.org/~/media//Files/Reports/PIP_HealthOnline.pdf or smart phone information http://www.pewinternet.org/data-trend/mobile/cell-phone-and-smart phone-ownership-demographics/. Accessed April 1, 2015.

87. Fox S, Maeve D. Health Online 2013. Available at: https://www.evernote.com/shard/s277/nl/36107944/281a93a5-fc31-4de9-a1df-76cfc7d2d33f/. Accessed April 1, 2015.

88. How people really use mobile. Harv Bus Rev 2013;91(1):30–1.

89. HealthIT.gov. Meaningful Use Definition & Objectives. EHR Incentives & Certification. 2014. Available at: http://www.healthit.gov/providers-professionals/meaningful-use-definition-objectives. Accessed April 1, 2015.

90. Mossman D, Farrell HM. Facebook: social networking meets professional duty. Current Psychiatry 2012;11(3). Available at: http://www.currentpsychiatry.com/index.php?id=22661&tx_ttnews[tt_news]=176674. Accessed April 1, 2015.

91. Clinton BK, Silverman BC, Brendel DH. Patient-targeted Googling: the ethics of searching online for patient information. Harv Rev Psychiatry 2010;18(2):103–12.

92. Hidy B, Porch E, Reed S, et al. Social networking and mental health. In: Myers K, Turvey CL, editors. Telemental health. New York: Elsevier; 2013. p. 367–95.

93. Yonker LM, Zan S, Scirica CV, et al. Friending teens: systematic review of social media in adolescent and young adult health care. J Med Internet Res 2015;17(1):e4.

94. Seko Y, Kidd S, Wiljer D, et al. Youth mental health interventions via mobile phones: a scoping review. Cyberpsychol Behav Soc Netw 2014;17(9):591–602.

95. McLaughlin M, Nam Y, Gould J, et al. A videosharing social networking intervention for young adult cancer survivors. Comput Human Behav 2012;28(2):631–41.

96. McDaniel BT, Coyne SM, Holmes EK. New mothers and media use: associations between blogging, social networking, and maternal well-being. Matern Child Health J 2012;16(7):1509–17.

97. Sundar SS, Oeldorf-Hirsch A, Nussbaum J, et al. Retirees on Facebook: can online social networking enhance their health and wellness?. In: CHI'11 extended abstracts on human factors in computing systems. Scottsdale, AZ: ACM; 2011. p. 2287–92.

98. Hogeboom DL, McDermott RJ, Perrin KM, et al. Internet use and social networking among middle aged and older adults. Educ Gerontol 2010;36(2):93–111.

99. Wilson JA, Onorati K, Mishkind M, et al. Soldier attitudes about technology-based approaches to mental health care. Cyberpsychol Behav 2008;11(6):767–9.

100. Horgan A, Sweeney J. Young students' use of the Internet for mental health information and support. J Psychiatr Ment Health Nurs 2010;17(2):117–23.

101. O'Dea B, Campbell A. Healthy connections: online social networks and their potential for peer support. Stud Health Technol Inform 2011;168:133–40.

102. Recupero P. E-mail and the psychiatrist-patient relationship. J Am Acad Psychiatry Law 2005;33:465–75.

103. Frankish K, Ryan C, Harris A. Psychiatry and online social media: potential, pitfalls and ethical guidelines for psychiatrists and trainees. Australas Psychiatry 2012;20:181–7.

104. Koh S, Cattell GM, Cochran DM, et al. Psychiatrists' use of electronic communication and social media and a proposed framework for future guidelines. J Psychiatr Pract 2013;19(3):254–63.

105. Farnan JM, Snyder Sulmasy L, Worster BK, et al. Online medical professionalism: patient and public relationships: policy statement from the American College of Physicians and the Federation of State Medical Boards. Ann Intern Med 2013;158(8):620–7.

106. American Medical Association. Opinion 9.124-Professionalism in the Use of Social Media. AMA Code of Medical Ethics 2011. Available at: http://www.ama-assn.org/ama/pub/physician-resources/medical-ethics/code-medical-ethics/opinion9124.page?. Accessed April 1, 2015.

107. Behnke S. Ethics in the age of the Internet. Mon Psychol 2008;39(7):74.

108. Canadian Medical Association. Social media and Canadian physicians - issues and rules of engagement. Available at: http://www.cma.ca.libproxy.usc.edu/socialmedia. Accessed March 15, 2015.

109. British Medical Association. Using social media: practical and ethical guidance for doctors and medical students. [2013-10-27]. Available at: http://www.medschools.ac.uk/SiteCollectionDocuments/social_media_guidance_may2011.pdf. Accessed March 15, 2015.

110. Grajales FJ, Sheps S, Ho K, et al. Social media: a review and tutorial of applications in medicine and health care. J Med Internet Res 2014;16(2):e13.

111. Mitchell KJ, Ybarra M. Social networking sites: finding a balance between their risks and benefits. Arch Pediatr Adolesc Med 2009;163(1):87–9.

112. Bishop M, Yellowlees P, Gates C, et al. Facebook goes to the doctor. New York: ACM Press; 2011. p. 13–20.

113. Camargo K, Grant R. Public health, science, and policy debate: being right is not enough. Am J Public Health 2015;105(2):232–5.

114. Regan H. The Disneyland measles outbreak likely came from overseas. Time 2015. Available at: http://time.com/3688914/disneyland-measles-outbreak-overseas/. Accessed 1 April 1, 2015.

115. Hilty DM, Yellowlees PM. Collaborative mental health services using multiple technologies – the new way to practice and a new standard of practice? J Am Acad Child Adolesc Psychiatry 2015;54(4):245–6.

116. Yellowlees PM, Nafiz N. The psychiatrist-patient relationship of the future: anytime, anywhere? Harv Rev Psychiatry 2010;18(2):96–102.

117. American Psychiatric Association. Diagnostic criteria from DSM-5. Via Table 1. Washington, DC: American Psychiatric Publishing; 2013.

118. Lyketsos C, Roques C, Hovanec L. Telemedicine use and reduction of psychiatric admissions from a long-term care facility. J Geriatr Psychiatry Neurol 2001;14:76–9.

119. Poon P, Hui E, Dai D, et al. Cognitive intervention for community-dwelling older persons with memory problems: telemedicine versus face-to-face treatment. Int J Geriatr Psychiatry 2005;20:285–6.

120. Weiner M, Rossetti H, Harrah K. Videoconference diagnosis and management of Choctaw Indian dementia patients. Alzheimers Dement 2011;7:562–6.

121. Graham MA. Telepsychiatry in Appalachia. Am Behav Sci 1996;39:602–15.

122. Zaylor C. Clinical outcomes in telepsychiatry. J Telemed Telecare 1999;5:59–60.

123. Hunkeler EM, Meresman JF, Hargreaves WA, et al. Efficacy of nurse telehealth care and peer support in augmenting treatment of depression in primary care. Arch Fam Med 2000;9:700–8.

124. Ruskin PE, Silver-Aylaian M, Kling MA, et al. Treatment outcomes in depression: comparison of remote treatment through telepsychiatry to in in-person treatment. Am J Psychiatry 2004;161:1471–6.
125. Manfredi L, Shupe J, Batki S. Rural jail telepsychiatry: a pilot feasibility study. Telemed J E Health 2005;11(5):574–7.
126. Sorvaniemi M, Ojanen E, Santamäki O. Telepsychiatry in emergency consultations: a follow-up study of sixty patients. Telemed J E Health 2005;11(4):439–41.
127. Modai I, Jabarin M, Kurs R, et al. Cost effectiveness, safety, and satisfaction with video telepsychiatry versus face-to-face care in ambulatory settings. Telemed J E Health 2006;12:515–20.
128. Urness D, Wass M, Gordon A, et al. Client acceptability and quality of life – telepsychiatry compared to in-person consultation. J Telemed Telecare 2006;12(5): 251–4.
129. Yellowlees PM, Odor A, Burke MM, et al. A feasibility study of asynchronous telepsychiatry for psychiatric consultations. Psychiatr Serv 2010;61(8):838–40.
130. Moreno FA, Chong J, Dumbauld J, et al. Use of standard Webcam and Internet equipment for telepsychiatry treatment of depression among underserved Hispanics. Psychiatr Serv 2012;63(12):1213–7.
131. Titov N, Dear BF, Schwencke G, et al. Transdiagnostic internet treatment for anxiety and depression: a randomised controlled trial. Behav Res Ther 2011;49(8): 441–52.
132. Johnston L, Titov N, Andrews G, et al. Comorbidity and internet-delivered transdiagnostic cognitive behavioural therapy for anxiety disorders. Cogn Behav Ther 2013;42(3):180–92.
133. Bouchard S, Paquin B, Payeur R, et al. Delivering cognitive-behavior therapy for panic disorder with agoraphobia in videoconference. Telemed J E Health 2004; 10(1):13–25.
134. Germain V, Marchand A, Bouchard S, et al. Effectiveness of cognitive behavioural therapy administered by videoconference for posttraumatic stress disorder. Cogn Behav Ther 2009;38(1):42–53.
135. Hedman E, Ljótsson B, Rück C, et al. Effectiveness of internet-based cognitive behaviour therapy for panic disorder in routine psychiatric care. Acta Psychiatr Scand 2013;128(6):457–67.
136. Frueh BC, Henderson S, Myrick H. Telehealth service delivery for persons with alcoholism. J Telemed Telecare 2005;11(7):372–5.
137. Szeftel R, Federico C, Hakak R, et al. Improved access to mental health evaluation for patients with developmental disabilities using telepsychiatry. J Telemed Telecare 2012;18(6):317–21.
138. Chong J, Moreno FA. Feasibility and acceptability of clinic-based telepsychiatry for low-income Hispanic primary care patients. Telemed J E Health 2012;18(4): 297–304.
139. Shore JH, Brooks E, Savin D, et al. Acceptability of telepsychiatry in American Indians. Telemed J E Health 2008;14(5):461–6.
140. Mucic D. Transcultural telepsychiatry and its impact on patient satisfaction. J Telemed Telecare 2010;16(5):237–42.
141. Ye J, Shim R, Lukaszewski T, et al. Telepsychiatry services for Korean immigrants. Telemed J E Health 2012;18(10):797–802.
142. Lopez AM, Cruz M, Lazarus S, et al. Use of American sign language in telepsychiatry consultation. Via Table 2. Telemed J E Health 2004;10(3):389–91.
143. Blackmon LA, Kaak HO, Ranseen J. Consumer satisfaction with telemedicine child psychiatry consultation in rural Kentucky. Psychiatr Serv 1997;48:1464–6.

144. Elford R, White H, Bowering R, et al. A randomized, controlled trial of child psychiatric assessments conducted using videoconferencing. J Telemed Telecare 2000;6:73–82.

145. Elford DR, White H, St John K, et al. A prospective satisfaction study and cost analysis of a pilot child telepsychiatry service in Newfoundland. J Telemed Telecare 2001;7:73–81.

146. Glueckauf RL, Fritz SP, Ecklund-Johnson EP, et al. Videoconferencing-based family counseling for rural teenagers with epilepsy: phase 1 findings. Rehabil Psychol 2002;47(1):49–72.

147. Nelson EL, Barnard M, Cain S. Treating childhood depression over videoconferencing. Telemed J E Health 2003;9:49–55.

148. Myers KM, Sulzbacher S, Melzer SM. Telepsychiatry with children and adolescents: are patients comparable to those evaluated in usual outpatient care? Telemed J E Health 2004;10(3):278–85.

149. Greenberg N, Boydell K, Volpe T. Pediatric telepsychiatry in Ontario: caregiver and service provider perspectives. J Behav Health Serv Res 2006;33(1):105–11.

150. Myers K, Valentine J, Morganthaler R, et al. Telepsychiatry with incarcerated youth. J Adolesc Health 2006;38(6):643–8.

151. Myers KM, Valentine JM, Melzer SM. Feasibility, acceptability, and sustainability of telepsychiatry for children and adolescents. Psychiatr Serv 2007;58:1493–6.

152. Bensink M, Armfield N, Irving H, et al. A pilot study of videotelephone-based support for newly diagnosed paediatric oncology patients and their families. J Telemed Telecare 2008;14(6):315–21.

153. Clawson B, Selden M, Lacks M, et al. Complex pediatric feeding disorders: using teleconferencing technology to improve access to a treatment program. Pediatr Nurs 2008;34(3):213–6.

154. Fox KC, Conner P, McCullers E, et al. Effect of a behavioural health and specialty care telemedicine programme on goal attainment for youths in juvenile detention. J Telemed Telecare 2008;14(5):227–30.

155. Morgan GJ, Craig B, Grant B, et al. Home videoconferencing for patients with severe congential heart disease following discharge. Congenit Heart Dis 2008;3(5):317–24.

156. Myers KM, Valentine JM, Melzer SM. Child and adolescent telepsychiatry: utilization and satisfaction. Telemed J E Health 2008;14(2):131–7.

157. Shaikh U, Cole SL, Marcin JP, et al. Clinical management and patient outcomes among children and adolescents receiving telemedicine consultations for obesity. Telemed J E Health 2008;14(5):434–40.

158. Wilkinson OM, Duncan-Skingle F, Pryor JA, et al. A feasibility study of home telemedicine for patients with cystic fibrosis awaiting transplantation. J Telemed Telecare 2008;14(4):182–5.

159. Witmans MB, Dick B, Good J, et al. Delivery of pediatric sleep services via telehealth: the Alberta experience and lessons learned. Behav Sleep Med 2008; 6(4):207–19.

160. Myers KM, Vander Stoep A, McCarty CA, et al. Child and adolescent telepsychiatry: variations in utilization, referral patterns and practice trends. J Telemed Telecare 2010;16:128–33.

161. Lau ME, Way BB, Fremont WP. Assessment of SUNY Upstate Medical University's child telepsychiatry consultation program. Int J Psychiatry Med 2011;42(1):93–104.

162. Mulgrew KW, Shaikh U, Nettiksimmons J, et al. Comparison of parent satisfaction with care for childhood obesity delivered face-to-face and by telemedicine. Telemed J E Health 2011;17(5):383–7.

163. Stain HJ, Payne K, Thienel R, et al. The feasibility of videoconferencing for neu-ropsychological assessments of rural youth experiencing early psychosis. J Telemed Telecare 2011;17(6):328–31.

164. Storch EA, May JE, Wood JJ, et al. Multiple informant agreement on the anxiety disorders interview schedule in youth with autism spectrum disorders. J Child Adolesc Psychopharmacol 2012;22(4):292–9.

165. Himle MB, Freitag M, Walther M, et al. A randomized pilot trial comparing video-conference versus face-to-face delivery of behavior therapy for childhood tic disorders. Behav Res Ther 2012;50(9):565–70.

166. Jacob MK, Larson JC, Craighead WE. Establishing a telepsychiatry consultation practice in rural Georgia for primary care physicians: a feasibility report. Clin Pediatr (Phila) 2012;51(11):1041–7.

167. Nelson EL, Duncan AB, Peacock G, et al. Telemedicine and adherence to national guidelines for ADHD evaluation: a case study. Psychol Serv 2012;9(3):293–7.

168. Reese RJ, Slone NC, Soares N, et al. Telehealth for underserved families: an evidence-based parenting program. Psychol Serv 2012;9(3):320–2.

169. Heitzman-Powell LS, Buzhardt J, Rusinko LC, et al. Formative evaluation of an ABA outreach training program for parents of children with autism in remote areas. Focus Autism Developmental Disabilities 2013;29(1):23.

170. Xie Y, Dixon JF, Yee OM, et al. A study on the effectiveness of videoconferencing on teaching parent training skills to parents of children with ADHD. Telemed J E Health 2013;19(3):192–9.

171. Reese RM, Jamison R, Wendland M, et al. Evaluating interactive videoconfer-encing for assessing symptoms of autism. Telemed J E Health 2013;19(9):671–7.

172. Davis AM, Sampilo M, Gallagher KS, et al. Treating rural pediatric obesity through telemedicine: outcomes from a small randomized controlled trial. J Pediatr Psychol 2013;38(9):932–43.

173. Freeman KA, Duke DC, Harris MA. Behavioral health care for adolescents with poorly controlled diabetes via Skype: does working alliance remain intact? J Diabetes Sci Technol 2013;7(3):727–35.

174. Hommel KA, Greenley RN, Maddux MH, et al. Self-management in pediatric in-flammatory bowel disease: a clinical report of the North American Society for Pediatric Gastroenterology, Hepatology, and Nutrition. J Pediatr Gastroenterol Nutr 2013;57(2):250–7.

175. Lipana LS, Bindal D, Nettiksimmons J, et al. Telemedicine and face-to-face care for pediatric obesity. Telemed J E Health 2013;19(10):806–8.

176. Rockhill C, Violette H, Vander Stoep A, et al. Caregivers' distress: youth with attention-deficit/hyperactivity disorder and comorbid disorders assessed via tel-emental health. J Child Adolesc Psychopharmacol 2013;23(6):379–85.

177. Comer JS, Furr JM, Cooper-Vince CE, et al. Internet-delivered, family-based treatment for early-onset OCD: a preliminary case series. J Clin Child Adolesc Psychol 2014;43(1):74–87.

178. Tse YJ, McCarty CA, Vander Stoep A, et al. Teletherapy delivery of caregiver behavior training for children with attention-deficit hyperactivity disorder. Tel-emed J E Health 2015;21(6):451–8.

179. Rockhill C, Violette H, Vander Stoep A, et al. Telepsychiatrists' adherence to guidelines-based care, ADHD outcomes by prescriber based on comorbidity status. Telemed J E Health, in press.

180. Bastien CH, Morin CM, Ouellet MC, et al. Cognitive-behavioral therapy for insomnia: comparison of individual therapy, group therapy, and telephone con-sultations. J Consult Clin Psychol 2004;72(4):653–9.

181. Morgan RD, Patrick AR, Magaletta PR. Does the use of telemental health alter the treatment experience? Inmates' perceptions of telemental health versus face-to-face treatment modalities. J Consult Clin Psychol 2008;76(1):158–62.

182. Ertelt TW, Crosby RD, Marino JM, et al. Therapeutic factors affecting the cognitive behavioral treatment of bulimia nervosa via telemedicine versus face-to-face delivery. Int J Eat Disord 2011;44(8):687–91.

183. Germain V, Marchand A, Bouchard S, et al. Assessment of the therapeutic alliance in face-to-face or videoconference treatment for posttraumatic stress disorder. Cyberpsychol Behav Soc Netw 2010;13(1):29–35.

184. King VL, Stoller KB, Kidorf M. Assessing the effectiveness of an Internet-based videoconferencing platform for delivering intensified substance abuse counseling. J Subst Abuse Treat 2009;36:331–8.

185. Marrone S, Mitchell JE, Crosby R, et al. Predictors of response to cognitive behavioral treatment for bulimia nervosa delivered via telemedicine versus face-to-face. Int J Eat Disord 2009;42(3):222–7.

186. Gros DF, Price M, Strachan M, et al. Behavioral activation and therapeutic exposure: an investigation of relative symptom changes in PTSD and depression during the course of integrated behavioral activation, situational exposure, and imaginal exposure techniques. Behav Modif 2012;36(4):580–99.

187. Yuen EK, Herbert JD, Forman EM, et al. Acceptance based behavior therapy for social anxiety disorder through videoconferencing. J Anxiety Disord 2013;27(4):389–97.

188. King VL, Brooner RK, Peirce JM. A randomized trial of Web-based videoconferencing for substance abuse counseling. J Subst Abuse Treat 2014;46:36–42.

189. Khatri N, Marziali E, Tchernikov I, et al. Comparing telehealth-based and clinic-based group cognitive behavioral therapy for adults with depression and anxiety: a pilot study. Clin Interv Aging 2014;7(9):765–70.

Index

Note: Page numbers of article titles are in **boldface** type.

A

B

C

Psychiatr Clin N Am 38 (2015) 593–601
http://dx.doi.org/10.1016/S0193-953X(15)00067-2
0193-953X/15/$ – see front matter © 2015 Elsevier Inc. All rights reserved.

psych.theclinics.com

Moving?

Make sure your subscription moves with you!

To notify us of your new address, find your **Clinics Account Number** (located on your mailing label above your name), and contact customer service at:

Email: journalscustomerservice-usa@elsevier.com

800-654-2452 (subscribers in the U.S. & Canada)
314-447-8871 (subscribers outside of the U.S. & Canada)

Fax number: 314-447-8029

Elsevier Health Sciences Division
Subscription Customer Service
3251 Riverport Lane
Maryland Heights, MO 63043

*To ensure uninterrupted delivery of your subscription, please notify us at least 4 weeks in advance of move.

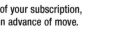

Printed and bound by CPI Group (UK) Ltd, Croydon, CR0 4YY

07/10/2024

01040499-0007